TREATING PAIN

with

Traditional Chinese Medicine

Dagmar Riley

Prescriptions by:

Liú Dé-Quán (刘德全) (Acupuncture)

Zhāng Chūn-Róng (张春荣) (Medicinal Formulas)

Paradigm Publications

Brookline Massachusetts and Taos New Mexico

2 0 0 3

Treating Pain with Traditional Chinese Medicine

Dagmar Riley

Copyright © 2001, 2003 Dagmar Riley

Edited by Michael Helme

International Standard Book Number (ISBN) 0-912111-71-2

Library of Congress Cataloging-in-Publication Data

Riley, Dagmar, 1969-
  Treating pain with traditional Chinese medicine / by Dagmar Riley.
    p. ; cm.
Includes bibliographical references and index.
  ISBN 0-912111-71-2 (pbk. : alk. paper)
  1. Pain--Treatment. 2. Medicine, Chinese.
  [DNLM: 1. Pain--therapy. 2. Medicine, Chinese Traditional. WL 704
R573t 2003] I. Title.
  RB127 .R55 2003
  616'.0472--dc21

                                        2003006773

Published by Paradigm Publications
www.paradigm-pubs.com
Brookline, Mass and Taos, New Mexico

Cover design by Herb Rich III
www.digidao.com

Council of Oriental Medical Publishers (C.O.M.P.) Designation: Compiled from primary Chinese sources. English terminology from Wiseman N., *A Practical Dictionary of Chinese Medicine,* Paradigm Publications, Brookline, MA and Taos, NM, 2000.

Table of Contents

Dedication

To Dr. Zhū Shēng-Ān (朱生安大夫), master of Chinese medicine and martial arts; and to my dear friend Zhāng Hóng (章虹).

Preface

"Chinese medicine is to be practiced remembering that life constitutes change. Once you have grasped the principles of Chinese medicine, you have to learn how to use them according to the nature of change. If you don't understand the nature of change, your knowledge is dead and useless. Remember that."

This is how my revered teacher, Dr. Wáng Hán-Wén (王寒雯), master of *Shāng Hán Lùn* [伤寒论], starts to teach every new disciple.

In this light, it becomes important to understand how to read any book that goes beyond the basic theories of Chinese medicine and interprets these basic theories according to a specific theme, as for example this book interprets the theories of Chinese medicine regarding the treatment of pain.

It is a grave misunderstanding to confuse the *interpretation* of the principles of Chinese medicine with yet a new set of principles. This misunderstanding leads to the accumulation of dead knowledge, which will prevent one from understanding change and which does not work in practice. It is therefore important to know that the prescriptions in this book have been written by two very different people:

The Chinese medicinal formulas in this book have been written by Professor Zhāng Chūn-Róng (张春荣), who divides his time between researching, writing, teaching, and treating patients at the Běijīng University of Chinese Medicine [北京中医药大学]. Professor Zhāng's academic achievements are outstanding. Thus, his choices of formulas and variations are based on an extremely well-founded academic standpoint. They can be apppreciated by anyone having completed studies of Chinese medicinals and formulas and are excellent for further developing the reader's ability to apply the principles of Chinese medicine to the treatment of pain.

The acupuncture prescriptions, on the other hand, were written by Dr. Liú Dé-Quán (刘德全), vice chief doctor of the Běijīng Xuānwǔ TCM Hospital [北京宣武中医医院], who has seen patients all day, six days a week, for over 40 years, averaging more than 80 patients on a normal day. His clinical mastery of acupuncture is outstanding and often puzzling; because of this wealth of experience, and because he comes from a family tradition of TCM practitioners, his treatments are perfectly adapted to the individual case of the patient yet are also often anything but "by the book." Nevertheless, he strictly applies the principles of Chinese medicine. Therefore, his examples of acupuncture prescriptions present a chance to step away from textbook knowledge and learn the "way of thought" [思路 *sī lù*] Dr. Liú has developed in using Chinese medicine principles according to the nature of change.

The Chinese herbal formulas and acupuncture prescriptions in the chapter on menstrual pain were written by Dr. Zhū Shēng- Ān [朱生安大夫], former director of the Confucius Temple Traditional Chinese Medicine Clinic in Beijing and 6th generation master of Qí Shì Tōngbèi Quán [祁氏通臂拳]. Dr. Zhū's medical education is founded on both a family tradition and a long and arduous education in Chinese martial arts, which he studied under the famous doctor and Qí Shì Tōngbèi Quán martial artist Wáng Xiá-Lín [王侠林]. Although Dr. Zhū later studied Chinese and Western medicine at university, he says that he would have no true understanding of Chinese Medicine if it was not for his traditional education with his master.

Dagmar Riley, Běijīng, July 2001

Note on the Acupuncture Prescriptions

For the most part, the acupuncture prescriptions in this book differ from textbook prescriptions. The reason for this is that I have used both prescriptions I have developed during my long years of clinical experience and prescriptions that have been handed down in my family.

Textbook theory cannot cover daily clinical practice and has to be combined with clinical experience to become alive. The prescriptions in this book only consist of points that are essential and have proven to be highly effective in a certain clinical context and a certain combination.

Liú Dé-Quán (刘德全), Beijing July 2001

CHAPTER 1

Causes of Pain

Understanding the different causes of pain is the basis for choosing the right treatment method. Several patients may display the same pain symptom, but that same pain symptom may be brought about by a different cause. Thus, different treatments may be needed to treat the same pain symptom, which is known as "unlike treatment of like disease" [同病异治 *tóng bìng yì zhì*]).

The different causes of pain are:

external contraction [外感 *wài gǎn*] of the six excesses [六淫 *liù yín*]

internal damage by the seven affects [内伤七情 *nèi shāng qī qíng*]

other causes:[1]

- excessive taxation [劳 *láo*] or leisure [逸 *yì*]
- blood stasis [瘀血 *yū xuè*]
- phlegm-rheum [痰饮 *tán yīn*]
- dietary irregularities [饮食失调 *yǐn shí shī tiáo*]

1.1 EXTERNAL CONTRACTION OF THE SIX EXCESSES

The climatic factors wind, cold, summerheat, dampness, dryness, and fire are called the six qì [六气 *liù qì*].

When the six qì cause disease by appearing in excess or out of season and invading the body from the exterior, they are called the "six excesses" [六淫 *liù yín*]. The six qì can also invade the body if body resistance is low.

---

[1] The three causes of disease are usually translated as external causes, internal causes, and neutral causes. In this instance, the author is not attributing all the traditionally described neutral causes of disease as a cause of pain, and therefore is citing "other causes" as the relevant subset of neutral causes. (Ed.)

The six excesses do not only appear in connection with the seasons but can also manifest in connection with a person's living conditions (e.g., a damp basement flat), work conditions (e.g., construction work, maritime work, working with certain materials), or personal habits (e.g., sleeping with an air conditioner running).

The six excesses often combine with each other. For example, wind, cold, and damp combine and give rise to impediment pattern [痹证 *bì zhèng*]. In such cases, it is important to establish whether there is a prevalence of any one of these excesses.

After entering the body, the six excesses can transform according to the patient's constitution. If, for example, the patient's body constitution tends towards exuberant yáng [阳盛 *yáng shèng*], external evils can transform into heat.

1.1.1   Wind

Wind is said to be the "chief of the 100 diseases" [风为百病之长 *fēng wéi bǎi bìng zhī zhǎng*]. It is one of the leading factors which cause pain and it often combines with other external excesses to form conditions such as wind-cold, wind-heat, and wind-damp.

Pain Characteristics – Wind

- Pain caused by wind mostly affects the upper part of the body, especially the head and face.
- Wind is a yáng evil and mostly invades the upper part (e.g., facial pain or headaches) and outer part of the body, the yáng channels, and the fleshy exterior. It causes pain by assailing the exterior, injuring construction [营 *yíng*] and defense [卫 *wèi*], and giving rise to disharmony of qì and blood.

- Wandering pain, or pain without a fixed location, is the result of wind.

- Wind is swift and changeable [风善行数变 *fēng shàn xíng shuò biàn*]; it is marked by a rapid onset of disease and swiftly changing manifestations. Thus, wind causes wandering pain that has no fixed location. An example is wind impediment [行痹 *xíng bì*]; impediment is caused by wind-cold-damp invading the sinews and joints and manifesting in joint pain, heaviness of the limbs, and so forth. When wind evil prevails over the other two evils, the impediment is characterized by wandering pain.

1.1.2   Cold

Cold is the most important cause of pain. Cold governs congealing [凝滞 *níng zhì*] and contracture and tautness [收引 *shōu yǐn*], which cause pain by inhibiting the normal flow of qì-blood, blocking the channels, and causing tension of the sinews.

Pain Characteristics – Cold

- Pain caused by cold is characterized by acuteness (intensity) and fixed location.
- Cold pain is relieved by the application of warmth and exacerbated by exposure to cold.
- It can appear anywhere in the body, including the torso, limbs, abdomen, back, sinews and bones, skin and flesh, channels, and internal organs.

1.1.3 Summerheat

This is an infrequent cause of pain. Hot summer weather can cause disease that is essentially either a heat pattern or a damp-heat pattern. The only exception is yīn summerheat [阴暑 *yīn shǔ*] that is caused by wind or by cold drinks and foods during summer.

Pain caused by summerheat, mostly headache or rib-side pain, will thus bear the characteristics of either heat or damp-heat (see below).

1.1.4 Dampness

Dampness, a yīn evil, easily causes pain by damaging yáng qì and obstructing the qì dynamic [气机 *qì jī*]. Dampness has a downward tendency and is heavy [重着 *zhòng zhuó*], viscous [黏滞 *nián zhì*], and lingering (i.e., dampness patterns are especially hard to cure).

Pain Characteristics – Dampness

- pain feels heavy
- pain remains in a fixed location
- often seen in the lower part of the body
- lingering, persistent, and recalcitrant

1.1.5 Dryness

Dryness is an infrequent cause of pain that is highly seasonal. In China, it is mostly seen during autumn and winter. Dryness easily damages the fluids [津液 *jīn yè*] and blood, which causes failure to nourish the network vessels [络脉 *luò mài*]. There is external dryness and internal dryness. The lung channel is most easily attacked by external dryness. Internal dryness is caused by a depletion of the body fluids or essence-blood, which may be brought about by excessive sweating. Commonly seen pain symptoms are sore throat, chest pain, and headache.

Pain Characteristics – Dryness

- mostly associated with the lung and the lung channel, such as the throat, nose, or chest
- often accompanied by a hard and rough feeling

1.1.6   Fire

Fire, a yáng evil, has an upward tendency and easily damages the fluids [津液 *jīn yè*] and blood. It frequently engenders wind [生风 *shēng fēng*] and stirs the blood [动血 *dòng xuè*].

Pain Characteristics – Fire

- pain accompanied by redness, swelling, and sensation of heat
- scorching pain that is relieved by the application of cold
- often severe pain
- Pain from fire appears anywhere in the body, but because of its yáng characteristics it appears more frequently in the upper body.

1.2   INTERNAL DAMAGE BY THE SEVEN AFFECTS [内伤七情 *nèi shāng qī qíng*]

The seven affects are joy, anger, anxiety, thought, sorrow, fear, and fright, and a balanced emotional life promotes the normal flow of the qì dynamic. However, when the seven affects are extreme or endure for too long, they damage the qì dynamic in the following ways:[2]

- Anger causes qì to rise [怒则气上 *nù zé qì shàng*].
- Joy causes qì to slacken [喜则气缓 *xǐ zé qì huǎn*].
- Sorrow causes qì to disperse [悲则气消 *bēi zé qì xiāo*].
- Fear causes qì to precipitate [恐则气下 *kǒng zé qì xià*].
- Fright causes derangement of qì [惊则气乱 *jīng zé qì luàn*].
- Thought causes qì to bind [思则气结 *sī zé qì jié*].

The organs primarily affected by the seven affects are the heart and the liver.

Heart

The heart stores the spirit [心藏神 *xīn cáng shén*], and any mental or emotional irritation or upset affects the heart. The heart also governs the blood and vessels [心主血脉 *xīn zhǔ xuè mài*]. Prolonged mental or emotional

---

[2] The following descriptions of how the individual affects influence qì come from *Elementary Questions* (素问 *Sù Wèn*), which does not provide such information for the 7th affect, anxiety. (Ed.)

disturbance negatively affects heart qì and impairs the heart's function of governing blood and vessels. This disturbs the normal flow of qì and blood and causes pain. Mental and emotional pain, if excessive or prolonged, can thus lead to physical pain.

Liver

The liver governs free coursing [肝主疏泄 *gān zhǔ shū xiè*], and binding depression of liver qì [肝气郁结 *gān qì yù jié*] denotes the liver not fulfilling its function of free coursing. This impairs the qì dynamic and leads to stagnation of the liver and the liver channel, which causes pain. Binding depression of liver qì is mainly caused by affect damage [内伤七情 *nèi shāng qī qíng*], especially anger and frustration. Other pain symptoms of the liver and the liver channel are distention and pain in the rib-side(s), lesser abdomen, and breasts, and oppression in the chest.

When affect damage by anger or frustration impairs free coursing, depressed liver qì easily transforms into fire, and fire damages yīn-blood. When damaged yīn-blood is not strong enough to restrain yáng, the result is ascendant hyperactivity of liver yáng [肝阳上亢 *gān yáng shàng kàng*]; a possible pain symptom is distending pain in the head.

Conclusion

The power of the seven affects should not be underestimated because they have a direct effect on the qì dynamic. On the one hand, when the seven affects are unbalanced, they can easily cause disharmony of qì and blood and of the internal organs, thus giving rise to pain. On the other hand, pain — especially chronic pain — can cause emotional distress. Emotional distress, a disharmony of one or several of the seven affects, will further damage the qì-dynamic according to the above principles, thus intensifying the pain and creating a vicious cycle.

Pain Characteristics – Seven Affects

- pain is related to emotional changes

- often located in the head, chest and rib-side, or abdomen

- often appears as distending pain [胀痛 *zhàng tòng*], which is mobile and penetrating[3]

---

[3] In Chinese the phrase "mobile and penetrating" usually describes the nature of medicinals; in this instance, tit is used as an accurate description of the nature of the pain. (Ed)

1.3   OTHER CAUSES

1.3.1   Excessive Taxation [劳 *láo*] or Leisure [逸 *yì*]

Excessive Taxation

Excessive taxation denotes continual taxation through mental [劳神 *láo shén*] or physical [劳力 *láo lì*] exhaustion or excessive sexual activity [房劳过度 *fáng láo guò dù*]. Mental taxation tends to damage the spleen and heart, physical taxation tends to damage the qì and blood, and sexual taxation tends to damage kidney essence. The resulting yīn-blood insufficiency, essential qì [精气 *jīng qì*] depletion, or failure to nourish the network vessels [络脉不养 *luò mài bù yǎng*] may cause pain.

Pain Characteristics – Vacuity Pattern [虚证 xū zhèng] Taxation

- dull pain [隐痛 *yǐn tòng*]
- empty pain [空痛 *kōng tòng*]
- continuous pain [绵痛 *mián tòng*]
- Pain from taxation is often located in the head, lumbus, chest, or abdomen.

Excessive Leisure

The term "excessive leisure" includes physical leisure while the mind is working. This makes excessive leisure an important disease-causing factor for anyone who has a desk job and does not exercise. Excessive leisure causes qì and blood to congest and stagnate [气血壅滞 *qì xuè yōng zhì*], thus causing pain.

Pain Characteristics – Leisure

- distending pain [胀痛 *zhàng tòng*]
- oppressive pain [闷痛 *mèn tòng*]
- numbness or tingling pain [麻木作痛 *má mù zuò tòng*]
- often manifests as a vacuity-repletion complex [虚实错杂 *xū shí cuò zá*]

Combination of Excessive Taxation and Excessive Leisure

A common scenario in our times is excessive mental taxation and excessive physical leisure, such as is caused by a stressful office job. This manifests as a vacuity-repletion complex [虚实错杂 *xū shí cuò zá*].

1.3.2   Blood stasis [瘀血 *yū xuè*]

External injury (trauma) [外伤 *wài shāng*] causes blood stasis. Moreover, qì vacuity, qì stagnation, cold congealing, blood heat, and phlegm obstruction may also bring about blood stasis.

As blood stasis is an evil that has a physical form and is thus considered yīn, the pain caused by blood stasis is lighter during daytime and worse during nighttime.

Pain Characteristics – Blood Stasis

- stabbing pain [刺痛 cì tòng]
- fixed pain location
- pain worse at night
- sometimes painful swelling, such as when caused by trauma
- pain refuses pressure [拒按 jù àn][4]

In many cases of pain due to blood stasis there is a history of trauma or medical operation.

1.3.3   Phlegm-Rheum [痰饮 *tán yǐn*]

Phlegm-rheum denotes fluids that accumulate in the body; "phlegm" denotes thick and "rheum" denotes thin pathological fluids. Phlegm-rheum arises when the movement and transformation of fluids within the body is impaired, which is mostly due to disturbed function of the lung, spleen, or kidney.

When phlegm-rheum accumulates in any part of the body it easily obstructs the qì-dynamic [气机 *qì jī*] and blocks the channels and network vessels, causing pain. Examples are phlegm-damp headache [痰湿头痛 *tán shī tóu tòng*] or phlegm lodged in the limbs [痰留肢体 *tán liú zhī tǐ*].

Pain Characteristics – Phlegm-Rheum

- oppressing-distending pain
- tends to be acute pain
- can occur in all parts of the body
- mostly fixed location

1.3.4   Dietary Irregularities [饮食失调 *yǐn shí shī tiáo*]

The term "dietary irregularities" means, among other things, the consumption of any food(s) in excess, particularly spicy-hot foods or alcohol. The modern diet found in northern Europe and the United States often includes large quantities of raw and cold foods, fatty foods, and sweet foods, which tend to harm the spleen and stomach and easily create dampness and phlegm.

---

[4] The characters 拒按 [*jù àn*] literally mean "refuses pressure," just as this term is translated herein. Its connotation is that if the painful spot were palpated, the pain would be exacerbated, particularly if the pain were due to blood stasis. (Ed.)

Dietary irregularities are an important cause of phlegm formation, as the spleen is the source of phlegm formation [脾为生痰之源 *pí wéi shēng tán zhī yuán*]. Because the spleen is in charge of moving and transforming fluids within the body, when this function is impaired dampness accumulates and transforms into phlegm, which may accumulate and cause pain (see the discussion of phlegm-rheum above).

Dietary irregularities can harm the qì dynamic of the spleen and stomach and cause spleen-stomach qì stagnation that results in abdominal pain.

CHAPTER 2
Pathomechanism of Pain

External contraction, internal damage by the seven affects, and the other causes of pain can give rise to all sorts of symptoms. They do not necessarily cause pain. For example, heat, one of the six excesses, can cause symptoms such as thirst, short voidings of reddish urine, and agitation, without actually generating pain. What process, then, has to happen within the body so that pain arises?

When There Is Stoppage, There Is Pain [不通则痛 *bù tōng zé tòng*].

"When there is stoppage, there is pain" is the common pathomechanism that is triggered by the different causes of pain. In this context, "stoppage" means the inhibition of the free flow of qì and/or blood, e.g., blood stasis or qì stagnation. Qì vacuity and blood vacuity are also considered forms of inhibited flow of qì and blood.

2.1 DIFFERENT CAUSES OF PAIN NEED DIFFERENT METHODS FOR RESTORING FLOW

From "when there is stoppage, there is pain" follows "when there is free flow, there is no pain" [通则不痛 *tōng zé bú tòng*]. However, depending on the mechanism that caused the stoppage, merely moving qì or quickening blood will not necessarily address the underlying cause of the stoppage.

Every cause of pain has its own characteristics and therefore brings about stoppage in a different way (see Chapter 1: Causes of Pain). Depending on the cause, one may have to indirectly move qì or quicken the blood by treating the root cause [治本 *zhì běn*]. For example, if the stoppage is due to cold contracting the channels and inhibiting the normal flow of qì and blood, then warming the channel and dissipating cold will restore a smooth flow of qì and blood.

It should be noted that when treating pain patients, one should always consider including treatment of the tip [治标 *zhì biāo*], i.e., the pain, especially if the pain is severe or chronic. This relieves unnecessary suffering and breaks through the vicious cycle of emotional distress (which is caused by pain) further damaging the qì dynamic and thus intensifying the pain and creating more emotional distress.

2.2   VISCERAL FUNCTIONS IN MAINTAINING THE FLOW OF QÌ AND BLOOD

The normal flow of qì and blood is dependent on specific functions of the viscera, which must be considered in the treatment process. The following viscera provide the driving force for the flow of qì and blood.

Heart: The heart governs the blood and vessels [心主血脉 *xīn zhǔ xuè mài*], and heart qì is the driving force that circulates the blood in the vessels. Heart qì vacuity may therefore lead to blood stagnation.

Lung: The lung governs qì [肺主气 *fèi zhǔ qì*] and plays an important role in the production of ancestral qì [宗气 *zōng qì*]. Ancestral qì is the most important driving force of the lung and the heart; thus it is also a major driving force for the flow of qì and blood. Ancestral qì gathers in the chest and respiratory tract and passes through the heart and vessels.

Kidney: The kidney is the root of yáng qì of the whole body and is most closely connected to the yáng qì of the heart, lung, and spleen. Thus it can be considered the root of the driving force of the flow of qì and blood. Furthermore, the warming function of yáng qì prevents the channels from contracting and constraining the flow of qì and blood.

Apart from the above visceral functions that provide the driving force for the flow of qì and blood, the following organs pave the way for smooth circulation.

Liver: The liver governs free coursing [肝主疏泄 *gān zhǔ shū xiè*] and thus ensures a smooth qì dynamic; when the qī dynamic functions smoothly, the channels are unobstructed and blood and qì are in harmony.

Spleen: The spleen governs movement and transformation [脾主运化 *pí zhǔ yùn huà*]. This function ensures the movement of water-damp that would otherwise obstruct the channels and the upbearing of the clear (essence of grain and water); by keeping the channels unobstructed, qì and blood naturally flow freely.

CHAPTER 3
Diagnosis of Pain Symptoms

3.1 TYPES OF PAIN

In general, the various types of pain give valuable clues toward the diagnosis and narrow the possible choice of patterns. As most types of pain indicate several possible patterns, they have to be evaluated together with the accompanying signs and symptoms (see below) to establish a definite pattern.

For example, aching pain [酸痛 *suān tòng*] can be a sign of vacuity, damp evil, or cold evil. In the case of scapulohumeral periarthritis, aching pain in the shoulder may be caused by invasion of wind-cold-damp or by qì-blood vacuity.

If the aching pain in the shoulder area feels cold, is exacerbated by wind and/or cold, relieved by warmth, and accompanied by aversion to wind and/or cold and a feeling of heaviness, tightness, or numbness and tingling in the shoulder, the aching pain is caused by cold-damp invasion.

If, however, the aching pain in the shoulder area is an enduring pain that is exacerbated by exertion and accompanied by signs such as aching lumbus and limp knees, dizziness and dizzy vision, lack of strength in the four limbs, torpid intake, and distention in the abdomen, the aching pain indicates qì-blood vacuity.

The following subsections introduce the various types of pain and associated patterns. They are followed by subsections that explain the accompanying signs and symptoms of the associated patterns.

3.1.1 Aching Pain [酸痛 *suān tòng*]

Aching pain [酸痛 *suān tòng*] is a sign of vacuity, damp evil, or cold evil. This type of pain is not severe and tends to be accompanied by a feeling of weakness in the affected body part. It mostly occurs in the limbs and trunk.

Examples: Aching pain in the lumbus and back that comes and goes and is relieved by rubbing and pressing may be due to liver and kidney depletion. Aching cold pain in the shoulder area may be due to invasion of wind-cold-damp.

3.1.2   Distending Pain [胀痛 *zhàng tòng*]

Distending pain [胀痛 *zhàng tòng*] is a sign of depressed qì dynamic. Depressed qì dynamic may be due to liver depression and qì stagnation, ascendant liver yáng, contraction of wind-heat, or phlegm and food collecting internally.

Examples: If in the case of painful menstruation there is distending pain that comes and goes, this is a sign of qì stagnation. Or if distending pain is experienced in the head, it may be due to ascendant liver yáng, liver fire flaming upward, or contraction of wind-heat. If distending pain occurs in the stomach duct, it may be due to liver qì invading the stomach or food collecting and stagnating.

3.1.3   Dull Pain [隐痛 *yǐn tòng*]

Dull pain is a sign of vacuity, especially if relieved by pressure and rubbing. It tends to be due to insufficiency of yáng-qì or yīn-blood depletion that causes failure to nourish the channels.

Examples: Dull pain in the stomach duct that is relieved by warmth and pressure indicates spleen-stomach vacuity cold. Dull pain in the head with dizziness and a bright white facial complexion indicates blood vacuity headache.

3.1.4   Empty Pain [空痛 *kōng tòng*]

Empty pain is often seen in vacuity patterns such as headaches due to kidney essence depletion.

Examples: Headache characterized by empty pain with dizziness and tinnitus points to kidney vacuity headache. Empty pain and dull pain [隐痛 *yǐn tòng*] in the area of one or more trigeminal nerve branches indicates trigeminal neuralgia due to qì and blood depletion.

3.1.5   Cold Pain [冷痛 *lěng tòng*]

Cold pain is a sign of cold evil obstructing the network vessels or of yáng qì vacuity. This type of pain is relieved by warmth.

Examples: Cold pain in the lumbus indicates cold-damp. Cold pain in the stomach duct indicates cold evil invading the stomach.

3.1.6   Gripping Pain [绞痛 *jiǎo tòng*]

Gripping pain is a sign of cold evil assailing the interior or of obstruction by tangible evils such as gallstones, blood stasis, or phlegm turbidity. Gripping pain is severe.

Examples: Gripping pain in the chest tends to be due to heart blood stasis in true heart pain [真心痛 *zhēn xīn tòng*]. Gripping pain in the smaller abdomen tends to be due to stones in stone strangury [石淋 *shí lín*].

3.1.7   Heavy Pain [重痛 *zhòng tòng*]

This refers to pain with a simultaneous feeling of heaviness. Heavy pain is a sign of dampness, which has a downward tendency and is heavy, viscous, and lingering.

Examples: Heavy pain in the head (bag-over-the-head sensation) indicates wind-damp. In the case of sciatica, heavy pain along the back and outer side of the leg (along the distribution area of the sciatic nerve) with disinclination to move and general heaviness of the legs indicates sciatica due to dampness evil obstructing the network vessels.

3.1.8   Pulling Pain [掣痛 *chè tòng*]

Pulling pain means either a painful pulling feeling or a pain that stretches from one point to another. Pulling pain is a sign of sinew vessels [筋脉 *jīn mài*] lacking nourishment. As the liver governs the sinews, the root of the disease tends to be the liver. Pulling pain may also be due to wind-cold-phlegm or blood stasis obstructing the sinew vessels.

Examples: If there is pulling pain in the face, it tends to be due to cold phlegm obstructing the network vessels. Alternatively, because the liver governs physical movement [肝主运动 *gān zhǔ yùn dòng*], pulling pain that regularly occurs during or after physical exertion (e.g., during sports) tends to be caused by the liver failing to nourish the sinew vessels.

3.1.9   Scorching Pain [灼痛 *zhuó tòng*]

Scorching pain is a sign of either repletion heat or vacuity heat.

Examples: In the case of trigeminal neuralgia, severe scorching pain in the area of one or more trigeminal nerve branches points to liver-gallbladder depression heat. Dull scorching pain in the stomach duct with dry mouth and throat is due to stomach yīn depletion.

3.1.10 Scurrying Pain [窜痛 *cuàn tòng*]

Scurrying pain moves about and has no fixed location. It is a sign of depressed qì dynamic or of moving impediment [行痹 *xíng bì*] (prevalence of wind, which is swift and changeable [风善行数变 *fēng shàn xíng shuò biàn*] and thus causes wandering pain that has no fixed location).

Examples: When wind, cold, and damp assail the knee, a prevalence of wind is characterized by wandering pain in the knee. Cholecystitis due to liver-gallbladder qì stagnation is characterized by scurrying and gripping [绞痛 *jiǎo tòng*] pain in the upper right abdomen with nausea, vomiting, dizziness, and bitter taste in the mouth.

3.1.11 Stabbing pain [刺痛 *cì tòng*]

Stabbing pain [刺痛 *cì tòng*] is a sign of blood stasis.

Examples: Stabbing pain in the heel is due to internal obstruction of static blood. If in the case of painful menstruation the pain is stabbing, constant, and relieved with the passing of blood clots and if there is more pain than distention in the lower abdomen, this is a sign of blood stasis.

3.2 ACCOMPANYING SIGNS AND SYMPTOMS FOR PATTERNS ASSOCIATED WITH PAIN

3.2.1 Qì Vacuity

Symptoms: Fatigue, lack of strength, shortage of qì [少气 *shǎo qì*], laziness to speak, faint voice, shortness of breath, poor appetite, white facial complexion, dizziness and dizzy vision, palpitations, spontaneous sweating. Pale tongue. Vacuous thin pulse.

3.2.2 Blood Vacuity

Symptoms: White or withered-yellow face and lusterless facial complexion, pale lips, dizziness, flowery vision, palpitations, sleeplessness, numbness of arms and legs, scant menstruation.. Pale tongue. Deep or thin pulse.

3.2.3 Yīn Vacuity

Symptoms: Emaciation, dry mouth and throat, sleeplessness, vexing heat in the five hearts [五心烦热 *wǔ xīn fán rè*], tidal heat effusion [潮热 *cháo rè*], night sweating, postmeridian heat effusion, short voidings of yellow or reddish urine, dry stool. Red tongue with scarce fur. Fine, rapid pulse.

3.2.4 Yáng Vacuity

Symptoms: Fear of cold and cold limbs, pale white complexion, fatigue and lack of strength, shortage of qì and laziness to speak, spontaneous sweating, bland taste in the mouth, no thirst, long voidings of clear urine, sloppy stool. Pale tender-soft tongue. Vacuous-slow or deep-weak pulse.

3.2.5 Qì Stagnation

Symptoms: Local feeling of distention, oppression, and fullness. Pain is scurrying (has no fixed location) and of varying severity. The distention, oppression, and fullness tend to be relieved by belching or passing of flatus. Qì stagnation is related to emotional factors (affects that cause binding depression). Frequent sighing. Thin tongue fur. Stringlike pulse.

3.2.6 Blood Stagnation

Symptoms: Rough, dry, and lusterless skin, soot-black complexion, speckles and macules under the skin, masses and swellings, menstrual irregularities. Dark purple tongue with stasis macules. Fine rough pulse.

3.2.7 Internal Phlegm Turbidity Obstruction

Symptoms: Cough and panting, expectoration of phlegm, oppression in the chest, glomus in the stomach duct, nausea, retching, torpid intake, dizziness and dizzy vision, numbness and tingling in the limbs, sound of phlegm in the throat. Slimy tongue fur. Slippery pulse.

3.2.8 Rheum Evil [饮邪 *yǐn xié*] Collecting Internally

Symptoms: Cough and expectoration of clear thin phlegm, oppression in the chest, panting, difficult breathing when lying down, no appetite, vomiting of clear water, swelling in the lower limbs. White slimy tongue fur. Sunken stringlike pulse.

3.2.9 Food Stagnation

Symptoms: Distention and fullness in the stomach duct and abdomen, acid regurgitation, belching of putrid qì, aversion to the smell of food, stool that smells of rotten eggs. Turbid slimy tongue fur. Slippery pulse.

3.2.10 Exterior Pattern

Symptoms: Aversion to cold and heat effusion, or aversion to wind, blocked runny nose.

(A) If aversion to cold is stronger than heat effusion, the nasal discharge is clear, and there is no sweating, the pain is due to exterior cold. Thin white tongue fur. Floating tight pulse.

(B) If heat effusion is stronger than aversion to cold, the nasal discharge is turbid, and there is sweating, the pain is due to exterior heat. Red tongue with dry fur. Floating rapid pulse.

3.2.11 Internal Cold Evil

Symptoms: Aversion to cold and liking for warmth, bland taste in the mouth, no thirst, cold limbs, sleeping curled up, long voidings of clear urine, sloppy stool. Moist white tongue fur. Slow pulse.

3.2.12 Internal Heat Evil

Symptoms: Red face and hot body, thirst and desire for cold drinks, vexation, short voidings of reddish urine, constipation. Red tongue. Rapid pulse.

3.2.13 Pain Responses to Pressure, Warmth, and Cold

- Pain exacerbated by the application of warmth is a sign of heat.

- Pain relieved by the application of warmth is a sign of cold.

- Acute, intense pain [疼痛剧烈 *téng tòng jù liè*] that refuses pressure [拒按 *jù àn*] is a sign of repletion.

- Pain relieved by rubbing and pressing is a sign of vacuity.

Examples: Cold pain in the smaller abdomen that is relieved by pressure and application of warmth indicates vacuity cold. Cold pain in the smaller abdomen that is relieved by application of warmth but refuses pressure is a sign of cold evil congealing and stagnating [寒邪凝滞 *hán xié níng zhì*], which is a repletion pattern.

3.3 LOCATION OF PAIN

The location of the pain can give clues as to which channels, bowels, and viscera are affected by pathological changes.

Be aware that the pathological changes of an affected organ may cause pain in locations other than the channel pathways (e.g., painful urination due to heart fire spreading heat to the small intestine, which settles in the bladder). Also, do not neglect the other accompanying signs and symptoms to establish a definite pattern.

3.3.1   Pathological Changes in the Liver and Gallbladder and in Their Respective Channels

According to the pathways of the foot reverting yīn liver channel [足厥阴肝经 *zú jué yīn gān jīng*] and foot lesser yáng gallbladder channel [足少阳胆经 *zú shào yáng dǎn jīng*], pain in the following areas typically indicates pathological changes in the liver/gallbladder and respective channels:

- vertex or the sides of the head
- ear
- rib-sides
- lesser abdomen
- yīn aspect (inside) of the thigh [股阴 *gǔ yīn*]
- yīn organs [阴器 *yīn qì*]

Moreover, according to the relations between the five phases, liver qì can invade the stomach and cause stomach pain. The liver opens at the eyes [肝开窍于目 *gān kāi qiào yú mù*] and can play a role in eye pain.

3.3.2   Pathological Changes in the Heart and Small Intestine and in Their Respective Channels

According to the pathways of the hand lesser yīn heart channel [手少阴心经 *shǒu shào yīn xīn jīng*] and hand greater yáng small intestine channel [手太阳小肠经 *shǒu tài yáng xiǎo cháng jīng*], pain in the following areas may indicate pathological changes in the heart/small intestine and respective channels:

- corners of the eyes
- face
- chest
- shoulder blade
- inside of the arms

Moreover, the heart opens at the tongue and heart fire flaming upwards may cause a painful tongue. Other pain may be caused by an inhibited function of the heart or small intestine, such as true heart pain [真心痛 *zhēn xīn tòng*] or painful urination (heart fire spreading heat to the small intestine [心火移热于小肠 *xīn huǒ yí rè yú xiǎo cháng*], which settles in the bladder).

3.3.3   Pathological Changes in the Spleen and Stomach and in Their Respective Channels

According to the pathways of the foot greater yīn spleen channel [足太阴脾经 *zú tài yīn pí jīng*] and foot yáng brightness stomach channel [足阳明胃经 *zú yáng míng wèi jīng*], pain in the following areas may indicate pathological changes in the spleen/stomach and respective channels:

- frontal vertex or forehead
- upper teeth
- tongue
- stomach duct
- greater abdomen [大腹 *dà fù*]
- outside of the legs

3.3.4 Pathological Changes in the Lung and Large Intestine and in Their Respective Channels

According to the pathways of the hand greater yīn lung channel [手太阴肺经 *shǒu tài yīn fèi jīng*] and hand yáng brightness large intestine channel [手阳明大肠经 *shǒu yáng míng dà cháng jīng*], pain in the following areas may indicate pathological changes in the lung/large intestine and respective channels:

- nose
- throat
- lower teeth
- shoulder and back
- chest
- anus
- elbow

3.3.5 Pathological Changes in the Kidney and Urinary Bladder and in Their Respective Channels

According to the pathways of the foot lesser yīn kidney channel [足少阴肾经 *zú shào yīn shèn jīng*] and foot greater yáng bladder channel [足太阳膀胱经 *zú tài yáng páng guāng jīng*], pain in the following areas may indicate pathological changes in the kidney/urinary bladder and respective channels:

- vertex
- spine
- back
- lumbus
- coccyx
- smaller abdomen
- feet

Other pain may be caused by an inhibited function of the kidney or urinary bladder, such as kidney vacuity fire flaming upwards causing discomforts such as toothache and ear pain.

CHAPTER 4
Headache

Pain in the whole head or in certain parts of the head, such as the forehead, occiput, sides, or vertex, is called headache.

Headache may be caused by six excesses external contraction [六淫外感 *liù yín wài gǎn*] or by bowel and visceral internal damage [脏腑内伤 *zàng fǔ nèi shāng*]. Pain is caused by impaired flow in the channels and network vessels, such as in cases of blocked yáng qì, turbid evils [浊邪 *zhuó xié*] that ascend and obstruct clear yáng, ascending liver yáng [肝阳上亢 *gān yáng shàng kàng*], essence marrow [精髓 *jīng suǐ*] depletion, or qì-blood depletion.

Headache can be classified according to the following nine forms:

1. Wind-cold headache [风寒型头痛 *fēng hán xíng tóu tòng*]

2. Wind-heat headache [风热型头痛 *fēng rè xíng tóu tòng*]

3. Wind-damp headache [风湿型头痛 *fēng shī xíng tóu tòng*]

4. Liver yáng headache [肝阳型头痛 *gān yáng xíng tóu tòng*]

5. Kidney vacuity headache [肾虚型头痛 *shèn xū xíng tóu tòng*]

6. Qì vacuity headache [气虚型头痛 *qì xū xíng tóu tòng*]

7. Blood vacuity headache [血虚型头痛 *xuè xū xíng tóu tòng*]

8. Phlegm turbidity headache [痰浊型头痛 *tán zhuó xíng tóu tòng*]

9. Blood stasis headache [瘀血型头痛 *yū xuè xíng tóu tòng*]

4.1 POINTS OF ATTENTION FOR HEADACHE

4.1.1 Physiology

Generally, headaches, like other pain syndromes, are specifically brought about by disease giving rise to obstruction of qì and blood flow. However, due to the location of the head and its specific physiology, the causes of headaches and their pathomechanisms bear certain special characteristics that are explained below.

The head is the uppermost part of the body.

Because the head is the uppermost part of the body, it is easily affected by wind evil assailing the exterior [风邪袭表 *fēng xié xí biǎo*]. Wind evil is a yáng evil and as such tends to affect the yáng parts of the body, i.e., the upper part and the exterior. Other external evils, such as cold, damp, and heat, tend to attach themselves to wind evil to invade the head.

When wind evil assails the head it obstructs clear yáng qì [清阳之气 *qīng yáng zhī qì*], congeals and obstructs qì and blood, and results in stoppage in the channels and network vessels [脉络不通 *mài luò bù tōng*], thus causing pain.

▪ Wind evil assailing the head and combining with cold evil causes cold congealing blood stagnation [寒凝血滞 *hán níng xuè zhì*], giving rise to pain.

▪ Wind evil assailing the head and combining with heat evil causes wind-heat flaming upward [风热上炎 *fēng rè shàng yán*], giving rise to pain.

▪ Wind evil assailing the head and combining with dampness evil clouds the clear orifices [湿蒙清窍 *shī méng qīng qiào*] and obstructs clear yáng [清阳 *qīng yáng*], giving rise to pain.

▪ The head is the confluence of the yáng channels [头为诸阳之会 *tóu wéi zhū yáng zhī huì*], and the brain is the sea of marrow [脑为髓之海 *nǎo wéi suǐ zhī hǎi*].

Clear yáng qì moves upward to nourish the head and brain, including the five senses. The remainder turns into turbid yīn [浊阴 *zhuó yīn*], which is a combination of used yáng qì and waste. Turbid yīn must descend, otherwise it can obstruct clear yáng, giving rise to pain.

The brain is the sea of marrow and the kidney engenders marrow [肾生髓 *shèn shēng suǐ*], hence they are closely related and kidney vacuity may bring about an insufficiency of the sea of marrow, giving rise to pain.

4.1.2   Considerations for Diagnosis of Headache

Pain Location (Indication of the Affected Channel)

The head is the confluence of the yáng channels [头为诸阳之会 *tóu wéi zhū yáng zhī huì*], and the three yáng channels and the reverting yīn channel flow to the head. By determining the location of the pain, one can establish which channel is affected.

▪ Pain in the posterior of the head (vertex, occipital region, neck, back) indicates blockage of the greater yáng [太阳 *tài yáng*] channel.

▪ Pain in the forehead (forehead, eyebrows) indicates blockage of the yáng brightness [阳明 *yáng míng*] channel.

▪ Pain of the lateral sides indicates blockage of the lesser yáng [少阳 *shào yáng*] channel.

▪ Pain just at the vertex indicates blockage of the reverting yīn [厥阴 *jué yīn*] channel.

Channel Conductors [引经药 *yǐn jīng yào*]

Channel conductor medicinals conduct the action of the other medicinals in the prescription to certain channels. The following channel conductors are relevant to the treatment of headaches.

greater yáng [太阳 *tài yáng*] channel	Chinese lovage [藁本 *gǎo běn*, Ligustici Rhizoma]
yáng brightness [阳明 *yáng míng*] channel	angelica [白芷 *bái zhǐ*, Angelicae Dahuricae Radix]
lesser yáng [少阳 *shào yáng*] channel	bupleurum [柴胡 *chái hú*, Bupleuri Radix]; chuanxiong [川芎 *chuān xiōng*, Chuanxiong Rhizoma]
reverting yīn [厥阴 *jué yīn*] channel	asarum [细辛 *xì xīn*, Asari Herba]; chuanxiong [川芎 *chuān xiōng*, Chuanxiong Rhizoma]

External Contraction Headache and Internal Damage Headache

Headache can be divided into external contraction headaches and internal damage headaches.

▪ *External Contraction Headaches* [外感头痛 *wài gǎn tóu tòng*]

External contraction headaches are characterized by recent and rapid onset, with the patient showing signs and symptoms of an exterior pattern [表证 *biǎo zhèng*]. The course of disease is usually of short duration.

Pain characteristics: The pain, which tends to be intense and uninterrupted, is mostly pulling pain [掣痛 *chè tòng*], scorching pain [灼痛 *zhuó tòng*], distending pain [胀痛 *zhàng tòng*], or heavy pain [重痛 *zhòng tòng*].

▪ *Internal Damage Headaches* [内伤头痛 *nèi shāng tóu tòng*]

Patients with internal damage headache commonly suffer from chronic headache and do not show any signs of an exterior pattern. The course of disease tends to be of long duration.

Pain characteristics: The pain tends to periodically appear and disappear, and it is mostly dull pain [隐痛 *yǐn tòng*], empty pain [空痛 *kōng tòng*], or, in the case of blood stagnation, stabbing pain [刺痛 *cì tòng*] with fixed location. Pain usually gets worse with taxation [劳 *láo*] (meaning mental or physical exhaustion) or affect damage [内伤七情 *nèi shāng qī qíng*] (excessive or lasting emotions or mental activities).

Vacuity and Repletion Patterns

Vacuity patterns include kidney vacuity headache, qì vacuity headache, and blood vacuity headache. Repletion patterns include external contraction headaches and liver yáng headache. Mixed patterns tend to be phlegm turbidity headache or blood stasis headache.

4.2   CAUSES AND PATHOMECHANISM OF HEADACHE; IDENTIFYING PATTERNS

4.2.1   Wind-Cold Headache [风寒型头痛 *fēng hán xíng tóu tòng*]

Causes and Pathomechanism of Wind-Cold Headache

"Wind damage first affects the upper part of the body" [伤于风者，上先受之 *shāng yú fēng zhě, shàng xiān shòu zhī*].

Externally contracted wind-cold evil enters the greater yáng channel (the greater yáng channel governs the exterior of the body), causing obstruction of clear yáng qì [清阳之气 *qīng yáng zhī qì*]. This gives rise to pain along the foot greater yáng channel (the vertex, occipital region, neck, and back) and pain in the joints. If the wind-evil lodges and is not removed, the headache recurs in irregular intervals and can appear both as hemilateral and medial headache. This is called head wind [头风 *tóu fēng*].

Important Signs of Wind-Cold Headache

- Pain along the vertex, occipital region, and neck.
- Aversion to cold and wind.
- Pain exacerbated by cold.
- The patient likes to cover his head (such as with a hat or scarf).
- No thirst, painful joints.
- Thin tongue and white fur.
- Tight floating pulse.

4.2.2 Wind-Heat Headache [风热型头痛 *fēng rè xíng tóu tòng*]

Causes and Pathomechanism of Wind-Heat Headache

Wind-heat headache is caused by either unresolved wind-cold that transforms into heat [化热 *huà rè*] or by wind combined with heat evil that strikes the yáng network vessels. Heat, a yáng evil, has the tendency to bear upward [升 *shēng*] and dissipate [散 *sàn*]; hence, the headache is characterized by distending pain [胀痛 *zhàng tòng*].

Important Signs of Wind-Heat Headache

This kind of headache is characterized by distending pain that worsens with heat to the point where the head feels like it is going to split apart. Heat effusion and aversion to cold [发热恶寒 *fā rè wù hán*], red face and eyes, swollen and painful throat and cough, dry mouth and thirst. The tongue has a red tip and a thin yellow coating. Rapid and floating pulse.

4.2.3 Wind-Damp Headache [风湿型头痛 *fēng shī xíng tóu tòng*]

Causes and Pathomechanism of Wind-Damp Headache

Wind evil combined with dampness evil harasses the upper body. Dampness evil, a clammy, viscous, and lingering evil, obstructs the clear orifices [清窍 *qīng qiào*], and thus the head feels heavy—like it is covered with a bag—and hurts.

Important Signs of Wind-Damp Headache
- Heavy-headedness (bag-over-the-head sensation).
- Dazed feeling.
- The headache is aggravated by rainy, damp, overcast weather.
- Feeling of oppression in the chest and fullness in the stomach duct.
- Heavy limbs and fatigue.
- Sloppy stool, short voidings of scant urine.
- White slimy tongue fur.
- Soggy [濡 *rú*] or slippery [滑 *huá*] pulse.

4.2.4 Liver Yáng Headache [肝阳型头痛 *gān yáng xíng tóu tòng*]

Causes and Pathomechanism of Liver Yáng Headache

Liver yáng headache is considered an internal damage [内伤 *nèi shāng*] headache. Emotional imbalance and anger damage the liver. This produces liver fire harassing the upper body [肝火上扰 *gān huǒ shàng rǎo*], which results in headache that is made worse by anger. Alternatively, liver-kidney yīn depletion leads to ascendant hyperactivity of liver yáng [肝阳上亢 *gān yáng shàng kàng*], which in turn leads to liver wind stirring internally [肝风内动 *gān fēng nèi dòng*]. If wind yáng harasses the upper body and results in an abnormal upward flow of qì-blood, the result is dizzy head and headache.

Important Signs of Liver Yáng Headache

- Dizziness.
- Headache that tends to be located on the sides or at the vertex of the head.
- Vexation, agitation, and irascibility [烦躁易怒 *fán zào yì nù*].
- Anger that worsens the headache.
- Tinnitus, sleeplessness, or rib-side pain.
- Dry mouth, red face.

The characteristics of liver yáng headache are headache with dizziness that worsens or is set off by anger and often tinnitus and/or rib-side pain.

Chronic liver yáng headache is often accompanied by limp aching lumbus and legs, night sweats, and headache that is not severe but continuous. These are signs of the liver disease reaching the kidney. The tongue is red with thin coating that may be yellow, and there is a stringlike pulse [弦脉 *xián mài*] or a fine rapid pulse [脉细数 *mài xì shuò*].

4.2.5 Kidney Vacuity Headache [肾虚型头痛 *shèn xū xíng tóu tòng*]

Causes and Pathomechanism of Kidney Vacuity Headache

A weak congenital constitution, taxation fatigue (e.g., overwork), excessive sexual activity, or drug abuse may lead to kidney essence depletion (kidney essence is an aspect of kidney yīn). The kidney engenders marrow [肾生髓 *shèn shēng suǐ*] and the brain is the sea of marrow [脑为髓之海 *nǎo wéi suǐ zhī hǎi*]. Brain marrow depends on the supply of marrow engendered by kidney essence. Thus, if kidney essence is depleted for some time and cannot engender marrow, brain marrow will be vacuous [虚 *xū*], giving rise to headache.

If kidney yīn is depleted for a long time, the depletion will also involve kidney yáng, since yīn and yáng are rooted in each other [阴阳互根 *yīn yáng hù gēn*]. Kidney yáng may also be depleted due to a long severe illness. This leads to clear yáng not spreading to the head properly, which gives rise to headache.

In clinical practice, headache due to kidney yīn (essence) depletion is far more common than headache due to depletion of both kidney yīn and yáng.

Important Signs of Kidney Vacuity Headache

- Headache characterized by empty pain [空痛 *kōng tòng*].
- Dizziness [眩晕 *xuàn yūn*], tinnitus.
- Weak, aching, and painful lumbus [腰痛酸软 *yāo tòng suān ruǎn*].
- Fatigued spirit and lack of strength [神疲乏力 *shén pí fá lì*].
- Seminal emission [遗精 *yí jīng*]
- Vaginal discharge [带下 *dài xià*].
- Sleeplessness.
- Red tongue with scant fur [少苔 *shǎo tāi*].
- Forceless fine pulse [脉细无力 *mài xì wú lì*].

4.2.6 Qì Vacuity Headache [气虚型头痛 *qì xū xíng tóu tòng*]

Causes and Pathomechanism of Qì Vacuity Headache

Taxation fatigue (from overworking), dietary irregularities, or enduring sickness can damage qì [伤气 *shāng qì*] and cause spleen vacuity and insufficiency of center qì [中气不足 *zhōng qì bù zú*]. When qì is vacuous, clear yáng fails to bear upward [清阳不升 *qīng yáng bù shēng*] and turbid yīn fails to bear downward [浊阴不降 *zhuó yīn bú jiàng*]; this inhibits the clear orifices [清窍 *qīng qiào*] and causes enduring headache.

Important Signs of Qì Vacuity Headache

- Empty pain [空痛 *kōng tòng*] in the head.
- Enduring headache that gets worse with fatigue.
- Fatigue and lack of strength in the limbs.
- Shortness of breath [气短 *qì duǎn*] and faint voice.
- Poor appetite and sloppy stool.
- Thin white tongue coating [舌苔薄白 *shé tāi bó bái*].
- Vacuous and forceless pulse [脉虚无力 *mài xū wú lì*].

4.2.7 Blood Vacuity Headache [血虚型头痛 *xuè xū xíng tóu tòng*]

Causes and Pathomechanism of Blood Vacuity Headache

Blood vacuity can result from insufficient blood formation caused by spleen vacuity or impairment of splenic movement and transformation, excessive blood loss, postpartum weakness [产后体弱 *chǎn hòu tǐ ruò*], or prolonged illness. When blood is vacuous and fails to nourish the upper body, the result may be dull pain [隐痛 *yǐn tòng*] in the head.

Important Signs of Blood Vacuity Headache

- Dull pain [隐痛 *yǐn tòng*] in the head.
- Dizzy head, bright white facial complexion.
- Heart palpitations, insomnia.
- Flowery vision and dry eyes.
- Pale tongue and lips.
- Fine and weak pulse [脉细而弱 *mài xì ér ruò*].

4.2.8   Phlegm Turbidity Headache [痰浊型头痛 *tán zhuó xíng tóu tòng*]

Causes and Pathomechanism of Phlegm Turbidity Headache

Phlegm is often due to dietary irregularities (e.g., eating too much raw, cold, sweet, or fatty foods) that weaken the spleen and impair the movement and transformation of fluids [运化失调 *yùn huà shī tiáo*]. Dampness develops from untransformed fluids and forms phlegm turbidity [痰浊 *tán zhuó*]. Phlegm turbidity is a yīn evil that obstructs clear yáng qì; it harasses the upper body [痰浊上扰 *tán zhuó shàng rǎo*], clouding the clear orifices [蒙清窍 *méng qīng qiào*] and causing headache, dizziness, and heavy headedness.

Important Signs of Phlegm Turbidity Headache

- Headache, dizziness, and heavy headedness.
- Oppression and fullness in the chest, abdominal distention, retching (the sound of vomiting without actually vomiting matter), and nausea.
- Indigestion and poor appetite.
- White slimy tongue fur [舌苔白腻 *shé tāi bái nì*].
- Stringlike and slippery pulse [脉弦滑 *mài xián huá*].

4.2.9   Blood Stasis Headache [瘀血型头痛 *yū xuè xíng tóu tòng*]

Causes and Pathomechanism of Blood Stasis Headache

Enduring pain, usually enduring wind-cold-damp impediment, may enter the network vessels [久痛入络 *jiǔ tòng rù luò*] and cause blood stasis. Blood stasis may also be caused by external injury or enduring sickness. It obstructs the network vessels and inhibits blood flow, thus creating stoppage. When there is stoppage, there is pain [不通则痛 *bù tōng zé tòng*].

Important Signs of Blood Stasis Headache

- Enduring headache, stabbing pain, pain of fixed location.
- Purple tongue, possibly with stasis macules [舌质紫或有瘀斑 *shé zhì zǐ huò yǒu yū bān*].
- Rough pulse [涩脉 *sè mài*].

4.3 TREATMENT OF HEADACHE USING CHINESE MEDICINALS

4.3.1 Wind-Cold Headache [风寒型头痛 *fēng hán xíng tóu tòng*]

Method of Treatment

Course wind, dissipate cold, and check pain [疏风散寒止痛 *shū fēng sàn hán zhǐ tòng*].

Tea-Blended Chuanxiong Powder [川芎茶调散 *chuān xiōng chá tiáo sǎn*]	
chuanxiong [川芎 *chuān xiōng*, Chuanxiong Rhizoma]	120g
schizonepeta [荆芥 *jīng jiè*, Schizonepetae Herba]	120g
angelica [白芷 *bái zhǐ*, Angelicae Dahuricae Radix]	60g
notopterygium [羌活 *qiāng huó*, Notopterygii Rhizoma et Radix]	60g
licorice [甘草 *gān cǎo*, Glycyrrhizae Radix]	60g
asarum [细辛 *xì xīn*, Asari Herba]	30g
saposhnikovia [防风 *fáng fēng*, Saposhnikoviae Radix]	45g
mint [薄荷叶 *bò hé [yè]*, Menthae Herba]	240g

Directions: Grind all ingredients to fine powder.

Dosage: 6g, twice a day. Take warm with Chinese tea [清茶 *qīng chá*, Camelliae Sinensis Folium]. If taken as a decoction, proportionally reduce the quantity of the medicinals.

Prescription Analysis

Tea-Blended Chuanxiong Powder is the principal prescription for wind-cold headache. It is mainly a combination of acrid-dissipating and wind-dispelling medicinals which courses wind, dissipates cold, and checks pain.

Because this prescription contains many medicinals with acrid [辛 *xīn*] and warm properties which course wind and dissipate cold; it is suitable for external contraction headache [外感头痛 *wài gǎn tóu tòng*] and head wind [头风 *tóu fēng*] attributed to wind-cold.

Chief Medicinals

Chuanxiong especially treats lesser yáng [少阳 *shào yáng*] (lateral side) headaches and reverting yīn [厥阴 *jué yīn*] (vertex) headaches.

Notopterygium treats greater yáng [太阳 *tài yáng*] headaches (posterior side — vertex, occipital region, neck, back).

Angelica treats yáng brightness [阳明 *yáng míng*] headache (forehead, eyebrows).

Support Medicinals

Asarum, mint, schizonepeta, and saposhnikovia are all acrid-dissipating medicinals that conduct the action of the medicinals upwards and course and dissipate wind. These medicinals assist the chief medicinals. They increase the action of coursing wind and dissipating cold, and they resolve the exterior.

Assistant and Conductor Medicinals

Licorice harmonizes the properties of all the medicinals [调和药性 *tiáo hé yào xìng*]. When Chinese tea [清茶 *qīng chá*, Camelliae Sinensis Folium] is added to the prescription, it prevents the other medicinals from being overly warming and drying or too upbearing and dissipating. This effect is achieved because of the cold and bitter properties of Chinese tea, which are both clearing and downbearing. This effect is known as "downbearing within upbearing."

Variation According to Signs

If aversion to cold [恶寒 *wù hán*] is especially strong, or if the patient is also vomiting, add ingredients such as fresh ginger [*shēng jiāng*], perilla leaf [*sū yè*], or cinnamon twig [*guì zhī*] to enforce the dissipation of cold and stop the vomiting.

4.3.2   Wind-Heat Headache [风热型头痛 *fēng rè xíng tóu tòng*]

Method of Treatment for Wind-Heat Headache

Course and dissipate wind-heat, clear heat and resolve toxins [疏散风热，清热解毒 *shū sàn fēng rè, qīng rè jiě dú*].

Lonicera and Forsythia Powder [银翘散 *yín qiào sǎn*]	
forsythia [连翘 *lián qiào*, Forsythiae Fructus]	30g (9g)
lonicera [金银花 *jīn yín huā*, Lonicerae Flos]	30g (9g)
platycodon [桔梗 *jié gěng*, Platycodonis Radix]	18g (6g)
mint [薄荷 *bò hé*, Menthae Herba]	18g (6g)
bamboo leaf [淡竹叶 *dàn zhú yè*, Lophatheri Folium]	12g (4g)
raw licorice [生甘草 *shēng gān cǎo*, Glycyrrhizae Radix Cruda]	15g (5g)
schizonepeta [荆芥 *jīng jiè*, Schizonepetae Herba]	12g (4g)
fermented soybean [淡豆豉 *dàn dòu chǐ*, Sojae Semen Praeparatum]	15g (5g)
arctium [牛蒡子 *niú bàng zǐ*, Arctii Fructus]	18g (6g)

Directions: The original prescription is taken in the form of a powder [散 *sǎn*] at a dosage of 9g each time. Nowadays, the formula is decocted with an appropriate amount of phragmites [芦根 *lú gēn*, Phragmitis Rhizoma].

Dosage: elect doses for the medicinals according to their relative proportion in the original prescription, taking the circumstances into consideration. The quantity suggested in parentheses may be appropriate.

Prescription Analysis

When wind-heat is dispelled and heat toxin is cleared, wind-heat headache will naturally stop.

Chief Medicinals

Used as the chief medicinals, lonicera and forsythia course and dissipate wind-heat, clear heat and resolve toxins [疏散风热，清热解毒 *shū sàn fēng rè, qīng rè jiě dú*].

Support Medicinals

Schizonepeta, mint, and fermented soybean course and dissipate exterior evil [疏散表邪 *shū sàn biǎo xié*] and force the evil through the exterior out of the body [透邪外出 *tòu xié wài chū*].

Although schizonepeta is considered acrid-warm [辛温 *xīn wēn*], it is warming but not drying. The combination of lonicera, forsythia, bamboo leaf, and phragmites restrains the warm property of schizonepeta. Thus, schizonepeta enhances the acrid-dissipating and exterior-resolving properties of the prescription.

Assistant Medicinals

The combination of arctium, platycodon, and raw licorice resolves toxins [解毒 *jiě dú*], disinhibits the throat [利咽 *lì yān*], dissipates bind (a concentration of evils in a specific location) [散结 *sàn jié*], diffuses lung qì [宣肺 *xuān fèi*], and dispels phlegm.

Bamboo leaf and phragmites are sweet and cool, light and clear [甘凉轻清 *gān liáng qīng qīng*]. They clear heat, engender liquid [生津 *shēng jīn*], and stop thirst.

Raw licorice harmonizes all the medicinals in the prescription.

Variation According to Signs

In case of oppression in the chest and diaphragm, add 9g/3qián [钱 *qián*] of agastaches [*huò xiāng*] and 9g/3qián of curcuma [*jiāng huáng*]. In the case of strong thirst, add trichosanthes root [*tiān huā fěn*]. In case of a swollen neck and painful throat, add puffball [*mǎ bó*] and scrophularia [*xuán shēn*]. In case of spontaneous external bleeding, take away schizonepeta and fermented soybean and add 9g/3qián of imperata [*bái máo gēn*], 9g/3qián of charred biota leaf [*cè bǎi tàn*] and 9g/3qián of charred gardenia [*zhī zǐ tàn*]. In case of cough, add apricot kernel [*xìng rén*] to disinhibit lung qì [利肺气 *lì fèi qì*].

If after two or three days the illness harasses the lungs and the heat gradually enters the interior [入里 *rù lǐ*], add dried/fresh rehmannia [*shēng dì huáng*] and ophiopogon [*mài dōng*] to protect the fluids [津液 *jīn yè*]. If it still isn't resolved, or if there are only short voidings of urine [小便短 *xiǎo biàn duǎn*], add the bitter-cold combination of anemarrhena [*zhī mǔ*], scutellaria [*huáng qín*], and gardenia [*zhī zǐ*], which together with the sweet-cool properties of dried/fresh rehmannia and ophiopogon engender yīn [生阴 *shēng yīn*] that has been damaged by heat.[5]

This prescription can also be used to treat the beginning stages of welling-abscess [痈 *yōng*] and sores [疮 *chuāng*] when signs of wind-heat exterior pattern are observed. In this case, medicinals such as dandelion [*pú gōng yīng*], isatis leaf [*dà qīng yè*], and violet [*zǐ huā dì dīng*] may be added to enhance the properties of clearing heat, resolving toxins, and dissipating binds [散结 *sàn jié*] of the welling-abscess or sore.

4.3.3   Wind-Damp Headache [风湿型头痛 *fēng shī xíng tóu tòng*]

Method of Treatment for Wind-Damp Headache

Dispel wind, overcome dampness, and check pain [祛风胜湿止痛 *qū fēng shèng shī zhǐ tòng*].

Notopterygium Dampness-Overcoming Decoction **[羌活胜湿汤 *qiāng huó shèng shī tāng*]**	
notopterygium [羌活 *qiāng huó*, Notopterygii Rhizoma et Radix]	6g
pubescent angelica [独活 *dú huó*, Angelicae Pubescentis Radix]	6g
Chinese lovage [藁本 *gǎo běn*, Ligustici Rhizoma]	4g
saposhnikovia [防风 *fáng fēng*, Saposhnikoviae Radix]	4g
honey-fried licorice [炙甘草 *zhì gān cǎo*, Glycyrrhizae Radix Preparata]	4g
chuanxiong [川芎 *chuān xiōng*, Chuanxiong Rhizoma]	4g
vitex [蔓荆子 *màn jīng zǐ*, Viticis Fructus]	2g
Directions: Take decocted with water [水煎服 *shuǐ jiān fú*].	

---

[5] From *Systematized Identification of Warm Diseases* [温病条辨 *Wēn Bìng Tiáo Biàn*], by Wú Táng [吴瑭].

Prescription Analysis

This combination of medicinals dispels wind, overcomes dampness, and checks pain [祛风胜湿止痛 *qū fēng shèng shī zhǐ tòng*]. When wind-damp is dispelled, headache and heavy-headedness naturally disappear.

Chief Medicinal

As the chief medicinal, notopterygium dispels wind, overcomes dampness, and checks pain; this treats the root [治本 *zhì běn*] of wind-damp headache.

Support Medicinals

Pubescent angelica helps notopterygium dispel wind and overcome dampness.

Chinese lovage dispels wind and overcomes dampness. It is commonly used for both vertex and occipital headaches.

Vitex dispels wind and is an excellent medicinal to check pain in the head caused by external contraction [外感 *wài gǎn*]. It is commonly used for dizziness, headache, and hemilateral headache [偏头痛 *piān tóu tòng*].

Chuanxiong quickens blood and checks pain [活血止痛 *huó xuè zhǐ tòng*], and also dispels wind and overcomes dampness. It is the principal medicinal for the treatment of headache because of its capacity to both upbear and dissipate.

Assistant Medicinals

Saposhnikovia [防风 *fáng fēng*] dispels wind and overcomes dampness.

Honey-fried licorice [炙甘草 *zhì gān cǎo*] harmonizes the properties of all the other medicinals, relaxes tension [缓急 *huǎn jí*], and checks pain.

Variation of Use

This prescription can also be used for common cold or for wind-damp arthritis where headache with heavy headedness is observed, or for other patterns of wind-damp in the fleshy exterior [肌表 *jī biǎo*].

4.3.4 Liver Yáng Headache [肝阳型头痛 *gān yáng xíng tóu tòng*]

Method of Treatment for Liver Yáng Headache

Calm the liver and subdue yang, settle the liver and extinguish wind [平肝潜阳，镇肝熄风 *píng gān qián yáng, zhèn gān xī fēng*].

Liver-Settling Wind-Extinguishing Decoction [镇肝熄风汤 *zhèn gān xī fēng tāng*]	
achyranthes [牛膝 *niú xī*, Achyranthis Bidentatae Radix]	30g
crude hematite [生赭石 *shēng zhě shí*, Haematitum Crudum]	30g
crude dragon bone [生龙骨 *shēng lóng gǔ*, Mastodi Ossis Fossilia Cruda]	15g
crude oyster shell [生牡蛎 *shēng mǔ lì*, Ostreae Concha Cruda]	15g
tortoise plastron [龟版 *guī bǎn*, Testudinis Plastrum]	15g
raw white peony [生白芍 *shēng bái sháo*, Paeoniae Radix Alba Cruda]	15g
scrophularia [玄参 *xuán shēn*, Scrophulariae Radix]	15g
asparagus tuber [天冬 *tiān dōng*, Asparagi Tuber]	15g
toosendan [川楝子 *chuān liàn zǐ*, Toosendan Fructus]	6g
raw barley sprout [生麦芽 *shēng mài yá*, Hordei Fructus Germinatus Crudus]	6g
capillaris [茵陈蒿 *yīn chén hāo*, Artemisiae Capillaris Herba]	6g
licorice [甘草 *gān cǎo*, Glycyrrhizae Radix]	4g
Directions: Take decocted with water.	

Prescription Analysis

This combination of medicinals calms liver yáng, thus stopping pain.

Chief Medicinals

Achyranthes is used as the chief medicinal because it conducts blood downwards [引血下行 *yǐn xuè xià xíng*] and restricts the ascendant hyperactivity of yang; it also supplements liver and kidney yīn.

Crude hematite downbears qì [降气 *jiàng qì*], settles counterflow [镇逆 *zhèn nì*], and calms the liver and subdues yáng [平肝潜阳 *píng gān qián yáng*].

Support Medicinals

Crude dragon bone and crude oyster shell strongly settle and subdue yáng.

Tortoise plastron, raw white peony, scrophularia, and asparagus tuber moisten yīn and extinguish wind.

The support medicinals help the chief medicinals to restrict the ascendant hyperactivity of yáng.

Assistant Medicinals

Capillaris, toosendan, and raw barley sprout assist the chief medicinals in clearing and discharging [清泄 *qīng xiè*] the surplus of liver yáng and in coursing depressed and stagnant liver qì. This helps calm the liver and downbear ascendant hyperactivity of yáng.

Licorice in combination with raw barley sprout harmonizes the stomach, regulates the middle burner, and protects stomach qì. This serves to lessen the unsettling effect that metal or stone medicinals (in this case, crude hematite, crude dragon bone, and crude oyster shell) can have on the stomach. Licorice harmonizes the properties of all the medicinals [调和药性 *tiáo hé yào xìng*].

Variation According to Signs

For severe headache and dizziness, add prunella [*xià kū cǎo*] and chrysanthemum [*jú huā*]. For heat in the chest [胸中热 *xiōng zhōng rè*], add crude gypsum. For copious phlegm, add bile arisaema [*dǎn nán xīng*], Sìchuān fritillaria [*chuān bèi mǔ*], and pinellia [*bàn xià*].

4.3.5　Kidney Vacuity Headache [肾虚型头痛 *shèn xū xíng tóu tòng*]

Method of Treatment for Kidney Vacuity Headache

Enrich and supplement kidney yīn [滋补肾阴 *zī bǔ shèn yīn*].

Six-Ingredient Rehmannia Pill [六味地黄丸 *liù wèi dì huáng wán*]	
cooked rehmannia [熟地黄 *shú dì huáng*, Rehmanniae Radix Conquita]	24g
cornus [山茱萸 *shān zhū yú*, Corni Fructus]	120g
dioscorea [山药 *shān yào*, Dioscoreae Rhizoma]	120g
alisma [泽泻 *zé xiè*, Alismatis Rhizoma]	90g
moutan [牡丹皮 *mǔ dān pí*, Moutan Cortex]	90g
poria [茯苓 *fú líng*, Poria]	90g

Directions: Grind the above medicinals into a powder. Mix the ground medicinals with honey or water and form them into small pills. Take 2–3 times daily, 6–9g each time. Or take as a decoction, proportionally reducing the quantity of the medicinals in the original prescription.

Prescription Analysis

Chief Medicinal

Cooked rehmannia strongly supplements kidney yīn, boosts essence, and fills the depletion of marrow [益精填髓 *yì jīng tián suǐ*]; this treats the root [治本 *zhì běn*] of kidney vacuity headache.

Support Medicinals

Cornus nourishes both liver and kidney yīn and astringes essence [涩精 *sè jīng*]. Dioscorea nourishes yīn, supplements the spleen, and secures essence [固精 *gù jīng*]. This pair of medicinals supports cooked rehmannia and nourishes kidney yīn.

Assistant Medicinals

Poria disinhibits dampness by bland percolation [淡渗利湿 *dàn shèn lì shī*] and fortifies the spleen. It helps dioscorea to supplement later heaven [补后天 *bǔ hòu tiān*], the acquired constitution. The spleen governs later heaven, and proper spleen function is the basis for assimilation and transformation of nutrients that are then used by all the other organs. Also, the production of kidney yīn depends on movement and transformation of the spleen.

Alisma clears and drains kidney fire and counteracts the slimy [腻 *nì*] quality of cooked rehmannia.

Moutan clears and drains liver fire and controls the hot quality of cornus. The cold quality of alisma and moutan also prevents vacuity fire caused by yīn vacuity (depletion of kidney yīn).

This combination of medicinals strongly supplements kidney yīn and does not allow evils to linger and become lodged, because within supplementation there is drainage. Kidney yīn is supplemented, brain marrow recovers its fullness, and the headache stops.

Variation According to Signs

To reinforce the enriching [滋 *zī*] and supplementing [补 *bǔ*] effects on the liver and kidney, add gastrodia [*tiān má*], lycium berry [*gǒu qǐ zǐ*], or chrysanthemum [*jú huā*].

4.3.6   Qì Vacuity Headache [气虚型头痛 *qì xū xíng tóu tòng*]

Method of Treatment for Qì Vacuity Headache

Boost qì and upbear yáng, regulate and supplement spleen and stomach [益气升阳，调补脾胃 *yì qì shēng yáng, tiáo bǔ pí wèi*].

Center-Supplementing Qì-Boosting Decoction [补中益气汤 *bǔ zhōng yì qì tāng*]	
astragalus [黄芪 *huáng qí*, Astragali Radix]	15g
licorice [甘草 *gān cǎo*, Glycyrrhizae Radix]	5g
ginseng [人参 *rén shēn*, Ginseng Radix]	10g
Chinese angelica [当归 *dāng guī*, Angelicae Sinensis Radix]	10g
tangerine peel [橘皮 *jú pí*, Citri Reticulatae Pericarpium]	6g
cimicifuga [升麻 *shēng má*, Cimicifugae Rhizoma]	3g
bupleurum[柴胡 *chái hú*, Bupleuri Radix]	3g
white atractylodes [白术 *bái zhú*, Atractylodis Macrocephalae Rhizoma]	10g

> **Directions:** Take decocted with water [水煎服 *shuǐ jiān fú*]. Alternatively, prepare as pills (grind medicinals into powder, mix with water, and form into pills) and take 2–3 times daily, 6g each time, with warm water.

Prescription Analysis

This combination of medicinals supplements the center, boosts qì, and upbears yáng [升阳 *shēng yáng*]. Once center qì is supplemented and clear yáng bears upward [清阳得升 *qīng yáng dé shēng*], the headache will cease.

Chief Medicinal

Astragalus is used to supplement qì and upbear yáng [补气升阳 *bǔ qì shēng yáng*] and to boost blood and secure the exterior [益血固表 *yì xuè gù biǎo*].

Support Medicinals

Ginseng and white atractylodes boost qì and fortify the spleen [益气健脾 *yì qì jiàn pí*]; they also help astragalus to supplement and reinforce center qì [中气 *zhōng qì*].

Assistant Medicinals

Tangerine peel rectifies qì and regulates the center [理气调中 *lǐ qì tiáo zhōng*]. Chinese angelica supplements blood and constrains qì [敛气 *liǎn qì*]. Cimicifuga and bupleurum upbear yáng. Licorice harmonizes the properties of all the other medicinals.

Variation According to Signs

This prescription is used to treat center qì fall [中气下陷 *zhōng qì xià xiàn*]. If the patient's most distinct symptom is empty pain [空痛 *kōng tòng*] in the head and the other signs and symptoms of center qì insufficiency are not equally apparent, add gastrodia [*tiān má*], chuanxiong [*chuān xiōng*], and vitex [*màn jīng zǐ*].

4.3.7 Blood Vacuity Headache [血虚型头痛 *xuè xū xíng tóu tòng*]

Method of Treatment for Blood Vacuity Headache

Supplement and regulate blood [补血调血 *bǔ xuè tiáo xuè*].

Four Agents Decoction [四物汤 *sì wù tāng*]	
Chinese angelica [当归 *dāng guī*, Angelicae Sinensis Radix]	10g
chuanxiong [川芎 *chuān xiōng*, Chuanxiong Rhizoma]	6g
cooked rehmannia [熟地黄 *shú dì huáng*, Rehmanniae Radix Conquita]	15g
white peony [白芍 *bái sháo*, Paeoniae Radix Alba]	10g
Directions: Take decocted with water [水煎服 *shuǐ jiān fú*].	

Prescription Analysis

This combination of medicinals supplements and harmonizes blood. When yīn-blood is supplemented, the brain marrow regains its proper fullness [脑髓得充 *nǎo suǐ dé chōng*] and headache will naturally stop.

Chief Medicinals

Sweet-warm cooked rehmannia is used as the chief medicinal because its properties enrich and moisten [滋润 *zī rùn*] to strongly enrich yīn and nourish blood.

Support Medicinal

Chinese angelica supplements and harmonizes blood and nourishes the liver. Its acrid and dry properties control the enriching and moistening properties of cooked rehmannia so that the decoction does not impair digestion.

Assistant Medicinal

White peony nourishes blood, boosts yīn, and nourishes the liver.

Conductor Medicinals

Chuanxiong quickens the blood [活血 *huó xuè*] and moves stagnation [行滞 *xíng zhì*]; it allows the decoction to be supplementing and also prevents the enriching and moistening properties of cooked rehmannia from causing stagnation and impairing digestion. Chuanxiong is thus said to "supplement yet not stagnate" [补而不滞 *bǔ ér bú zhì*].

Variation According to Signs

Four Agents Decoction [四物汤 *sì wù tāng*] is the basic prescription to supplement blood and can be used to treat any kind of blood vacuity. To reinforce its ability to treat blood vacuity headache, add lycium berry [*gǒu qǐ zǐ*], chrysanthemum [*jú huā*], vitex [*màn jīng zǐ*], and/or gastrodia [*tiān má*].

4.3.8   Phlegm Turbidity Headache [痰浊型头痛 tán zhuó xíng tóu tòng]

Method of Treatment for Phlegm Turbidity Headache

Transform phlegm and extinguish wind, fortify the spleen and dispel dampness [化痰熄风，健脾祛湿 *huà tán xī fēng, jiàn pí qū shī*].

Pinellia, White Atractylodes, and Gastrodia Decoction **[半夏白术天麻汤 *bàn xià bái zhú tiān má tāng*]**	
pinellia [半夏 *bàn xià*, Pinelliae Rhizoma]	9g
gastrodia [天麻 *tiān má*, Gastrodiae Rhizoma]	6g
poria [茯苓 *fú líng*, Poria]	6g

red tangerine peel [橘红 *jú hóng*, Citri Reticulatae Exocarpium Rubrum]	6g
white atractylodes [白术 *bái zhú*, Atractylodis Macrocephalae Rhizoma]	9g
licorice [甘草 *gān cǎo*, Glycyrrhizae Radix]	2g
fresh ginger [生姜 *shēng jiāng*, Zingiberis Rhizoma Recens]	1 thin slice
jujube [大枣 *dà zǎo*, Jujubae Fructus]	2 pc

Directions: Take decocted with water [水煎服 *shuǐ jiān fú*].

Prescription Analysis

This combination of medicinals transforms phlegm and extinguishes wind, fortifies the spleen and dispels dampness [化痰熄风，健脾祛湿 *huà tán xī fēng, jiàn pí qū shī*]. When dampness is dispelled and splenic movement and transformation is restored, then phlegm turbidity headache will cease.

Chief Medicinals

Pinellia dries dampness and transforms phlegm [燥湿化痰 *zào shī huà tán*] and thus treats the root [治本 *zhì běn*]. Gastrodia extinguishes wind [熄风 *xī fēng*] and checks headache and dizziness.

This is a combination of the principal medicinals for the treatment of wind-phlegm headache and dizziness. In *Treatise on the Spleen & Stomach* by Lǐ Dōng-Yuán [李东垣*脾胃论 *pí wèi lùn*], there is a commentary on this formula in book 3, chapter 10:

> This kind of tormenting headache is referred to as a foot *tài yīn* phlegm inversion headache. Nothing but Rhizoma Pinelliae Ternatae [半夏 *bàn xià*] can cure it. Dark vision with spinning head is due to internal attack of wind vacuity (evils). Nothing but Rhizoma Gastrodiae Elatae [天麻 *tiān má*] can relieve it.[6]

Thus, Pinellia, White Atractylodes, and Gastrodia Decoction uses pinellia and gastrodia as its chief medicinals.

Support Medicinals

The spleen is the source of phlegm formation [脾为生痰之源 *pí wéi shēng tán zhī yuán*]; white atractylodes and poria fortify the spleen and dispel dampness [健脾祛湿 *jiàn pí qū shī*].

---

[6] Lǐ Dōng-Yuán's *Treatise on the Spleen & Stomach,* translated by Yang Shou-Zhong and Li Jian-Yong, Blue Poppy Press, p. 178.

Assistant Medicinal

Red tangerine peel rectifies qì and regulates the middle burner [理气调中 *lǐ qì tiáo zhōng*] and also dries dampness and transforms phlegm [燥湿化痰 *zào shī huà tán*].

Conductor Medicinals

Licorice, fresh ginger, and jujube harmonize the spleen and stomach.

Variation According to Signs

Pinellia, White Atractylodes, and Gastrodia Decoction treats wind-phlegm dizziness and headache, with the main signs and symptoms being headache, dizziness, a white slimy tongue fur [舌苔白腻 *shé tāi bái nì*], and a stringlike slippery pulse [脉弦滑 *mài xián huá*].

If there is strong dizziness, add silkworm [*bái jiāng cán*] and bile arisaema [*dǎn nán xīng*] to increase the capacity to transform phlegm and extinguish wind.

If the patient shows sign of qì vacuity, one may add codonopsis [*dǎng shēn*] and astragalus [*huáng qí*] to supplement qì.

4.3.9   Blood Stasis Headache [瘀血型头痛 *yū xuè xíng tóu tòng*]

Treatment Method for Blood Stasis Headache

Quicken blood and transform stasis [活血祛瘀 *huó xuè qū yū*], free the orifices and check pain [通窍止痛 *tōng qiào zhǐ tòng*].

Orifice-Freeing Blood-Quickening Decoction [通窍活血汤 *tōng qiào huó xuè tāng*]	
red peony [赤芍 *chì sháo*, Paeoniae Radix Rubra]	10g
chuanxiong [川芎 *chuān xiōng*, Chuanxiong Rhizoma]	10g
peach kernel [桃仁 *táo rén*, Persicae Semen]	10g
carthamus [红花 *hóng huā*, Carthami Flos]	6g
scallion white [葱白 *cōng bái*, Allii Fistulosi Bulbus]	10g
fresh ginger [生姜 *shēng jiāng*, Zingiberis Rhizoma Recens]	3 thin slices
jujube [大枣 *dà zǎo*, Jujubae Fructus]	6 pieces
musk [麝香 *shè xiāng*, Moschus]	0.1g
yellow wine [黄酒 *huáng jiǔ*, Vinum Aureum]	as needed
Directions: Decoct all ingredients [水煎服 *shuǐ jiān fú*], except the musk and yellow wine, which should be added to the decoction just before drinking.	

Prescription Analysis

This combination of medicinals quickens blood and dispels stasis [活血祛瘀 *huó xuè qū yū*] and also frees the orifices and checks pain [通窍止痛 *tōng qiào zhǐ tòng*]. When blood stasis is dispelled and the clear orifices are freed, the headache will stop.

Chief Medicinal

The aromatic quality of musk tends to move and penetrate blockages and to quicken the blood and free the orifices, thus treating the root.

Support Medicinals

When there is stoppage, there is pain [不通则痛 *bù tōng zé tòng*]. Red peony, chuanxiong, peach kernel, and carthamus help to quicken the blood and transform stasis and to free the channels and check pain.

Assistant Medicinals

Yellow wine warms and frees the channels. The acrid quality of scallion white dissipates [散 *sàn*] and frees the orifices.

Conductor Medicinals

Fresh ginger and jujube harmonize qì and blood.

Variation According to Signs

Add corydalis [*yán hú suǒ*] or scorpion [*quán xiē*] to increase the capacity to quicken blood and check pain.

The main indication for Orifice-Freeing Blood-Quickening Decoction is headache caused by blood stasis. The prescription can also be used for hair loss, green-blue or purplish face color, childhood gān disease [小儿疳积 *xiǎo ér gān jī*] (emaciation, abdominal distention with bluish superficial veins, and heat effusion), or dry blood consumption [干血痨 *gān xuè láo*] in women.

4.4 TREATMENT OF HEADACHE USING ACUPUNCTURE

4.4.1 Acupuncture Points for Wind-Cold Headache [风寒型头痛 *fēng hán xíng tóu tòng*]

Treatment Method for Wind-Cold Headache

Dispel wind and dissipate cold, quicken the network vessels and check pain [祛风散寒，活络止痛 *qū fēng sàn hán, huó luò zhǐ tòng*].

Points for Wind-Cold Headache [风寒型头痛 *fēng hán xíng tóu tòng*]
TB-5 Outer Pass [外关 *wài guān*]
LI-4 Union Valley [合谷 *hé gǔ*]
GB-20 Wind Pool [风池 *fēng chí*]
GV-16 Wind Mansion [风府 *fēng fǔ*]
M-HN-9 (Extra Point) Greater Yang [太阳 *tài yáng*]

Prescription Analysis

GB-20, the intersection point [交会穴 *jiāo huì xué*] of the foot lesser yáng gallbladder channel and the yáng linking vessel [阳维脉 *yáng wéi mài*], dispels wind. GV-16, a point where wind tends to gather, dispels both interior wind and exterior wind-cold. TB-5 is the network point [络穴 *luò xué*] of the hand lesser yáng triple burner channel. Combining TB-5 with LI-4 and M-HN-9 quickens the network vessels and checks pain.

4.4.2 Acupuncture Points for Wind-Heat Headache [风热型头痛 *fēng rè xíng tóu tòng*]

Treatment Method for Wind-Heat Headache

Clear heat and dissipate wind, quicken the network vessels and check pain [清热散风，活络止痛 *qīng rè sàn fēng, huó luò zhǐ tòng*].

Points for Wind-Heat Headache [风热型头痛 *fēng rè xíng tóu tòng*]
GV-14 Great Hammer [大椎 *dà zhuī*]
LI-4 Union Valley [合谷 *hé gǔ*]
GV-16 Wind Mansion [风府 *fēng fǔ*]
TB-5 Outer Pass [外关 *wài guān*]
LI-11 Pool at the Bend [曲池 *qū chí*]

Prescription Analysis

TB-5 is the network point [络穴 *luò xué*] of the hand lesser yáng triple burner channel. Combining TB-5 with GV-16 dispels wind. Combining LI-4, LI-11, and GV-14 clears heat.

4.4.3 Acupuncture Points for Wind-Damp Headache [风湿型头痛 *fēng shī xíng tóu tòng*]

Treatment Method for Wind-Damp Headache

Dispel wind and eliminate dampness, quicken the network vessels and check pain [祛风除湿，活络止痛 *qū fēng chú shī, huó luò zhǐ tòng*].

> ### Points for Wind-Damp Headache [风湿型头痛 *fēng shī xíng tóu tòng*]
>
> TB-5 Outer Pass [外关 *wài guān*]
> GV-16 Wind Mansion [风府 *fēng fǔ*]
> SP-9 Yīn Mound Spring [阴陵泉 *yīn líng quán*]

Prescription Analysis

The combination of TB-5 and GV-16 dispels wind. SP-9 is the uniting point [合穴 *hé xué*] of the foot greater yīn spleen channel. The *Classic of Difficult Issues* says: "Uniting points are indicated in cases of counterflow qì and diarrhea" [《难经八十八难 *nán jīng bā shí bā nán*》* 合主逆气而泄 *hé zhǔ nì qì ér xiè*]. In this type of headache, the channels and collaterals are obstructed by damp evil, which leads to an upward attack [上攻 *shàng gōng*] of qì, and causes headache. Needling the above points will eliminate dampness, thus stopping the pain.

4.4.4 Acupuncture Points for Liver Yáng Headache [肝阳型头痛 *gān yáng xíng tóu tòng*]

Treatment Method for Liver Yáng Headache

Calm the liver and subdue yáng [平肝潜阳 *píng gān qián yáng*].

> ### Points for LiverYáng Headache [肝阳型头痛 *gān yáng xíng tóu tòng*]
>
> LR-3 Supreme Surge [太冲 *tài chōng*]
> **joining** KI-1 Gushing Spring [涌泉 *yǒng quán*]
> M-HN-1 (Extra Point) Alert Spirit Quartet [四神聪 *sì shén cōng*]

Prescription Analysis

LR-3 is the source point [原穴 *yuán xué*] of the foot reverting yīn liver channel; it soothes and calms the liver [舒肝平肝 *shū gān píng gān*]. KI-1 is the well point [井穴 *jǐng xué*] of the foot lesser yīn kidney channel; from the saying "When the disease is in the upper body, select points in the lower body" [上病下取 *shàng bìng xià qǔ*], it follows that when the disease is in the head one should select points on the feet. KI-1 calms the liver, downbears fire, and subdues yáng [降火潜阳 *jiàng huǒ qián yáng*]. Alert Spirit Quartet is a local point that checks pain.

4.4.5 Acupuncture Points for Kidney Vacuity Headache [肾虚型头痛 *shèn xū xíng tóu tòng*]

Treatment Method for Kidney Vacuity Headache

Supplement the kidney and replenish marrow [补肾填髓 *bǔ shèn tián suǐ*].

Points for Kidney Vacuity Headache [肾虚型头痛 *shèn xū xíng tóu tòng*]
KI-3 Great Ravine [太溪 *tài xī*]
GB-39 Suspended Bell [悬钟 *xuán zhōng*]
CV-4 Pass Head [关元 *guān yuán*]

Prescription Analysis

CV-4 is located three body-inches *(cùn)* below the umbilicus, at the center of an area called cinnabar field [丹田 *dān tián*]. According to the Daoists, the cinnabar field corresponds with the chamber of essence in men and the uterus in women. CV-4 strongly supplements [大补 *dà bǔ*] original yáng [元阳 *yuán yáng*] and is a principal point for invigorating yáng [壮阳 *zhuàng yáng*]. KI-3, the source point [原穴 *yuán xué*] of the foot lesser yīn kidney channel, regulates and supplements kidney qì. GB-39, the meeting point of marrow [髓会 *suǐ huì*], supplements essence and replenishes marrow. This combination of points supplements the kidney and replenishes marrow, thus the headache will stop.

4.4.6   Acupuncture Points for Qì Vacuity Headache
[气虚型头痛 *qì xū xíng tóu tòng*]

Treatment Method for Qì Vacuity Headache

Boost qì and upbear yáng [益气升阳 *yì qì shēng yáng*].

Points for Qì Vacuity Headache [气虚型头痛 *qì xū xíng tóu tòng*]
GV-20 Hundred Convergences [百会 *bǎi huì*]
LU-9 Great Abyss [太渊 *tài yuān*]
CV-11 Interior Strengthening [建里 *jiàn lǐ*]
CV-6 Sea of Qì [气海 *qì hǎi*] joining [透 *tòu*]
CV-4 Pass Head [关元 *guān yuán*]

Prescription Analysis

LU-9, the source point [原穴 *yuán xué*] of the hand greater yīn lung channel, supplements lung qì. CV-11 fortifies the center [健中 *jiàn zhōng*] and boosts qì. CV-6 joining CV-4 boosts lower burner original qì [元气 *yuán qì*]. GV-20 is the meeting point of all the yáng channels and is thus a powerful point to upbear yáng and boost qì [升阳益气 *shēng yáng yì qì*]; it upbears clear qì and checks headache caused by qì vacuity.

4.4.7 Acupuncture Points for Blood Vacuity Headache
[血虚型头痛 *xuè xū xíng tóu tòng*]

Treatment Method for Blood Vacuity Headache

Supplement qì and nourish blood, quicken the network vessels and check pain [补气养血，活络止痛 *bǔ qì yǎng xuè, huó luò zhǐ tòng*].

Points for Blood Vacuity Headache [血虚型头痛 *xuè xū xíng tóu tòng*]
CV-6 Sea of Qì [气海 *qì hǎi*] **joining** [透 *tòu*] CV-4 Pass Head [关元 *guān yuán*]
BL-15 Heart Transport [心俞 *xīn shū*]
BL-20 Spleen Transport [脾俞 *pí shū*]
SP-6 Three Yīn Intersections [三阴交 *sān yīn jiāo*]
ST-36 Leg Three Lǐ [足三里 *zú sān lǐ*]
GB-39 Suspended Bell [悬钟 *xuán zhōng*]
SI-3 Back Ravine [后溪 *hòu xī*]

Prescription Analysis

CV-6 joining CV-4 boosts and supplements original qì [元气 *yuán qì*]. BL-15, BL-20, and SP-6 fortify the spleen and nourish blood. ST-36 fortifies the spleen and harmonizes the stomach, thus fortifying the source of qì and blood engenderment and transformation [气血生化之源 *qì xuè shēng huà zhī yuán*]. GB-39 supplements and boosts [补益 *bǔ yì*] essence and marrow. Essence and blood are of the same source [精血同源 *jīng xuè tóng yuán*], and essence can engender blood [精能生血 *jīng néng shēng xuè*]. SI-3 frees the governing vessel [督脉 *dū mài*], and the governing vessel nets [络 *luò*] to the brain. SI-3 thus quickens network vessels and checks headaches.

4.4.8 Acupuncture Points for Phlegm Turbidity Headache
[痰浊型头痛 *tán zhuó xíng tóu tòng*]

Treatment Method for Phlegm Turbidity Headache

Dispel dampness and transform phlegm, upbear the clear and downbear the turbid [祛湿化痰,升清降浊 *qū shī huà tán, shēng qīng jiàng zhuó*].

Points for Phlegm Turbidity Headache [痰浊型头痛 *tán zhuó xíng tóu tòng*]
CV-12 Center Stomach Duct [中脘 *zhōng wǎn*]
ST-40 Bountiful Bulge [丰隆 *fēng lóng*]
SP-9 Yīn Mound Spring [阴陵泉 *yīn líng quán*]
GV-20 Hundred Convergences [百会 *bǎi huì*]

Prescription Analysis

The stomach alarm point [募穴 *mù xué*], CV-12, and the stomach network point [络穴 *luò xué*], ST-40, dispel dampness and transform phlegm. GV-20 upbears clear qì, while SP-9 disinhibits dampness [利湿 *lì shī*] and downbears turbid.

4.4.9 Acupuncture Points for Blood Stasis Headache [瘀血型头痛 *yū xuè xíng tóu tòng*]

Treatment Method for Blood Stasis Headache

Quicken blood, transform stasis, and check pain [活血化瘀止痛 *huó xuè huà yū zhǐ tòng*].

Points for Blood Stasis Headache [瘀血型头痛 *yū xuè xíng tóu tòng*]
BL-17 Diaphragm Transport [膈俞 *gé shū*]
BL-40 Bend Center [委中 *wěi zhōng*]
PC-6 Inner Pass [内关 *nèi guān*]
Ouch point [阿是穴 *ā shì xué*]

Prescription Analysis

BL-17, the meeting point [会穴 *huì xué*] for blood, treats all blood diseases. BL-40 is also called Blood Cleft Point [血郄 *xuè xī*], a point where blood gathers, suggesting that BL-40 possesses the qualities of a cleft point [郄穴 *xī xué*]. Cleft points are very effective in treating pain—especially the cleft points of the yáng channels. BL-40 treats any stagnation pattern; it frees the channels, dissipates stasis [散瘀 *sàn yū*], and checks pain. PC-6 regulates the qì dynamic [气机 *qì jī*]. When qì moves, the blood moves with it [气行血行 *qì xíng xuè xíng*]. Thus, the above points regulate qì and blood and check pain.

CHAPTER 5
Trigeminal Neuralgia

Searing, paroxysmal pain in the area of one or more trigeminal nerve branches, caused by a malfunction of the trigeminal nerve, is called trigeminal neuralgia.

There are seven main forms of trigeminal neuralgia:

- wind-cold assailing the exterior [风寒外袭 *fēng hán wài xí*]
- liver-gallbladder depression heat [肝胆郁热 *gān dǎn yù rè*]
- stomach heat attacking upward [胃热上攻 *wèi rè shàng gōng*]
- yīn vacuity with yáng hyperactivity [阴虚阳亢 *yīn xū yáng kàng*]
- qì and blood depletion [气血亏虚 *qì xuè kuī xū*]
- wind-phlegm obstructing the network vessels [风痰阻络 *fēng tán zǔ luò*]
- static blood obstructing the network vessels [瘀血阻络 *yū xuè zǔ luò*]

5.1 POINTS OF ATTENTION FOR TRIGEMINAL NEURALGIA

5.1.1 Pathomechanism of Trigeminal Neuralgia

The essential qì [精气 *jīng qì*] of the five viscera and six bowels meets in the head, including the face. If external evil is invading [犯 *fàn*], or if internal fire is flaming upwards, or if wind, phlegm, and heat are binding and congesting [壅 *yōng*] the channels and network vessels, then the flow of qì-blood in the channels will be obstructed. When there is stoppage, there is pain [不通则痛 *bù tōng zé tòng*]. Alternatively, in the case of vacuity, impaired nourishment of the channels and network vessels gives rise to pain.

5.1.2   Establishing the Nature of the Pain

Repletion

Repletion pain is marked by severe pain [疼痛剧烈 *téng tòng jù liè*] that could be pulling pain [掣痛 *chè tòng*], distending pain [胀痛 *zhàng tòng*], or scorching pain [灼痛 *zhuó tòng*]. Other signs include a short course of disease; the cause is an external evil.

Vacuity

Vacuity pain usually involves frequent attacks of pain that are relatively mild. It is often dull pain [隐痛 *yǐn tòng*] or empty pain [空痛 *kōng tòng*]. Other signs include a long course of disease; the cause is internal damage.

Qì

Qì pain is mainly distending pain [胀痛 *zhàng tòng*] or scurrying pain (moving pain) [窜痛 *cuàn tòng*] that is set off or exacerbated by emotional discomfort.

Blood

Blood pain (i.e., blood stasis pain) is usually stabbing pain [刺痛 *cì tòng*] in a fixed location. As blood stasis is an evil that has a physical form and is thus considered yīn [属阴 *shǔ yīn*], the pain caused by blood stasis is lighter during daytime and gets worse during nighttime. Another sign of blood stasis is dark purple tongue [舌质紫暗 *shé zhì zǐ àn*]

5.2   Causes and Pathomechanism of Trigeminal Neuralgia; Identifying Patterns

5.2.1   Wind-Cold Assailing the Exterior [风寒外袭 *fēng hán wài xí*]

Causes and Pathomechanism of Wind-Cold Assailing the Exterior

Wind-cold assailing the body. Wind is a yáng evil and mostly invades the upper part of the body, e.g., the face. Cold governs congealing [凝滞 *níng zhì*] and contracture and tautness [收引 *shōu yǐn*], which inhibits the normal flow of qì and blood and thereby blocks the channels, causing pain.

Important Signs of Wind-Cold Assailing the Exterior

Rapid onset of disease, brief bouts of recurrent severe pain in the area of one or more trigeminal nerve branches. During a pain attack the cheek muscles feel taut. Pain is relieved by warmth and exacerbated or set off by wind-cold. There may be a runny nose (clear mucus). No thirst. The tongue has a thin white fur [薄

白苔 *bò bái tāi*], and the pulse is floating tight or stringlike tight [脉浮紧或弦紧 *mài fú jǐn huò xián jǐn*].

5.2.2 Liver-Gallbladder Depression Heat [肝胆郁热 *gān dǎn yù rè*]

Causes and Pathomechanism of Liver-Gallbladder Depression Heat

The liver and gallbladder stand in interior-exterior relationship [肝胆相表里 *gān dǎn xiāng biǎo lǐ*]. The gallbladder channel starts at the outside corner of the eye and runs along the side of the head. If there is emotional damage [情志内伤 *qíng zhì nèi shāng*] and enduring liver depression, or excessive anger, then qì depression develops and transforms into fire. The fire harasses the upper body along the path of the gallbladder channel and obstructs the clear orifices [清窍 *qīng qiào*]. Qì-blood then flows abnormally and obstructs the channels and network vessels, causing pain.

Important Signs of Liver-Gallbladder Depression Heat

Bouts of severe scorching pain [灼痛 *zhuó tòng*] in the area of one or more trigeminal nerve branches. The pain spreads to the corner of the forehead and periodically causes spasms. It is often set off by emotional upset. The patient may also have vexation and irascibility [心烦易怒 *xīn fán yì nù*], red face and bloodshot eyes, and a bitter taste in the mouth. The tongue has red sides and tip, with yellow fur [舌边尖红苔黄 *shé biān jiān hóng tāi huáng*]; the pulse is stringlike and rapid [脉弦数 *mài xián shuò*].

5.2.3 Stomach Heat Attacking Upward [胃热上攻 *wèi rè shàng gōng*]

Causes and Pathomechanism of Stomach Heat Attacking Upward

Stomach heat is caused by eating too many hot spicy foods or by externally contracted wind-heat and heat evil invading the stomach. Stomach fire swelters [熏蒸 *xūn zhēng*] and attacks upwards [上攻 *shàng gōng*] along the channel to the head.

Important Signs of Stomach Heat Attacking Upward

Bouts of severe pain in the area of one or more trigeminal nerve branches. Pain is set off or exacerbated by heat and feels like fire burning in the muscle. Swollen gums, bad breath. Vexation and agitation [烦躁 *fán zào*]. Thirst with desire to drink cold drinks [口渴喜冷饮 *kǒu kě xǐ lěng yǐn*]. Dry bound stool [大便干结 *dà biàn gān jié*], yellow or reddish urine. Red tongue with thick or slimy yellow fur [舌质红，苔黄厚或腻 *shé zhì hóng, tāi huáng hòu huò nì*]. Slippery rapid pulse [脉滑数 *mài huá shuò*].

5.2.4   Yīn Vacuity with Yáng Hyperactivity [阴虚阳亢 *yīn xū yáng kàng*]

Causes and Pathomechanism of Yīn Vacuity with Yáng Hyperactivity

The liver and kidney are of the same source [肝肾同源 *gān shèn tóng yuán*]. If sexual taxation [房劳 *fáng láo*] gradually damages kidney essence or if an enduring febrile disease [热病 *rè bìng*] damages true yīn [真阴 *zhēn yīn*], this may eventually lead to water failing to moisten wood [水不涵木 *shuǐ bù hán mù*] and yīn not controlling yáng [阴不制阳 *yīn bú zhì yáng*]. This causes hyperactivity of liver yáng, or liver yáng transforms into wind and harasses the upper body [上扰 *shàng rǎo*], causing pain.

Important Signs of Yīn Vacuity with Yáng Hyperactivity

Distending pain [胀痛 *zhàng tòng*] in the area of one or more trigeminal nerve branches. Occasional spasms or numbness and tingling [麻木 *má mù*] in the affected side. Pain is exacerbated by frustration or anger. Baking heat [effusion] in the face [面部烘热 *miàn bù hōng rè*]. Dizziness, dizzy vision. Rib-side distention. Vexation and irascibility [心烦易怒 *xīn fán yì nù*]. Sleeplessness, profuse dreaming. Limp aching lumbus and knees [腰膝酸软 *yāo xī suān ruǎn*]. Dry throat, red eyes. Red tongue with scant fur [舌质红少苔 *shé zhì hóng shǎo tāi*]. Stringlike fine or rapid pulse [脉弦细而数 *mài xián xì ér shuò*].

5.2.5   Qì and Blood Depletion [气血亏虚 *qì xuè kuī xū*]

Causes and Pathomechanism of Qì and Blood Depletion

The spleen is the source of qì and blood formation [脾为生化气血之源 *pí wéi shēng huà qì xuè zhī yuán*]. When the spleen is damaged by dietary irregularities, taxation fatigue, or an enduring illness that weakens the body, then qì of the middle burner is depleted and clear yáng does not bear upwards [清阳不升 *qīng yáng bù shēng*]. The result is impaired nourishment of the clear orifices [清窍 *qīng qiào*], which causes pain.

Important Signs of Qì and Blood Depletion

Dull pain [隐痛 *yǐn tòng*] and empty pain [空痛 *kōng tòng*] in the area of one or more trigeminal nerve branches. Pain is exacerbated by standing up and relieved by lying down. Pain tends to be set off by taxation. Shortness of breath and disinclination to speak. Fatigue. Pale face. Reduced food intake. Pale tongue with white fur [舌质淡苔白 *shé zhì dàn tāi bái*]. Fine and weak pulse [脉细弱 *mài xì ruò*].

5.2.6 Wind-Phlegm Obstructing the Network Vessels [风痰阻络 *fēng tán zǔ luò*]

Causes and Pathomechanism of Wind-Phlegm Obstructing the Network Vessels

The spleen is the source of phlegm formation [脾为生痰之源 *pí wéi shēng tán zhī yuán*]. When the spleen is vacuous, dampness accumulates, and phlegm is engendered from dampness. Repeated contraction of wind-evil allows phlegm turbidity and wind to combine; wind-phlegm obstructs the channels and network vessels of the head and face, and clouds clear yáng [清阳 *qīng yáng*].

Important Signs of Wind-Phlegm Obstructing the Network Vessels

Oppressive pain [闷痛 *mèn tòng*] in the area of one or more trigeminal nerve branches. The affected side may be numb and tingling [麻木 *má mù*]. Dizziness, nausea. Occasional vomiting of phlegm-drool [痰涎 *tán xián*]. Fullness and oppression in the stomach duct and chest [胸脘满闷 *xiōng wǎn mǎn mèn*]. Fatigue, heavy feeling in the limbs. The tongue has white slimy fur [苔白腻 *tāi bái nì*], and there is a stringlike and slippery pulse [脉弦滑 *mài xián huá*].

5.2.7 Static Blood Obstructing the Network Vessels [瘀血阻络 *yū xuè zǔ luò*]

Causes and Pathomechanism of Static Blood Obstructing the Network Vessels

Blood stasis results from enduring illness entering the network vessels and blood, from qì stagnating and not being able to move blood, from vacuous qì not being able to command [帅 *shuài*] blood, or from phlegm obstruction [痰阻 *tán zǔ*]. Blood stasis obstructs the network vessels, creating stoppage and pain [不通则痛 *bù tōng zé tòng*].

Important Signs of Static Blood Obstructing the Network Vessels

Severe, stabbing pain [刺痛 *cì tòng*] of fixed location in the area of one or more trigeminal nerve branches. Frequent recurrence of pain attacks. Pain is more intense during the night and relieved during the day. Pain attacks are persistent. Dark purple tongue that may have stasis macules [紫暗或有瘀斑 *zǐ àn huò yǒu yū bān*]. Stringlike rough or fine rough pulse [脉弦涩或细涩 *mài xián sè huò xì sè*].

5.3 TREATMENT OF TRIGEMINAL NEURALGIA USING CHINESE MEDICINALS

5.3.1 Wind-Cold Assailing the Exterior [风寒外袭 *fēng hán wài xí*]

Method of Treatment for Wind-Cold Assailing the Exterior

Course wind and check pain [疏风止痛 *shū fēng zhǐ tòng*].

Tea-Blended Chuanxiong Powder [川芎茶调散 *chuān xiōng chá tiáo sǎn*]	
chuanxiong [川芎 *chuān xiōng*, Chuanxiong Rhizoma]	120g
schizonepeta [荆芥 *jīng jiè*, Schizonepetae Herba]	120g
angelica [白芷 *bái zhǐ*, Angelicae Dahuricae Radix]	60g
notopterygium [羌活 *qiāng huó*, Notopterygii Rhizoma et Radix]	60g
licorice [甘草 *gān cǎo*, Glycyrrhizae Radix]	60g
asarum [细辛 *xì xīn*, Asari Herba]	30g
saposhnikovia [防风 *fáng fēng*, Saposhnikoviae Radix]	45g
mint [薄荷叶 *bò hé [yè]*, Menthae Herba]	240g

Directions: Grind all ingredients to a fine powder.

Dosage: 6g, twice a day. Take warm with Chinese tea [清茶 *qīng chá*, Camelliae Sinensis Folium]. If taken as a decoction, proportionally reduce the quantities of the medicinals.

Prescription Analysis

Tea-Blended Chuanxiong Powder [川芎茶调散 *chuān xiōng chá tiáo sǎn*] treats pain caused by wind-cold assailing the exterior. It is mainly a combination of acrid-dissipating and wind-dispelling medicinals.

Chief Medicinal

Chuanxiong has acrid-warm dissipating properties. It quickens blood and moves qì [活血行气 *huó xuè xíng qì*], rises to the head, and checks pain.

Support Medicinals

Notopterygium and angelica help chuanxiong dissipate wind-cold. Furthermore, notopterygium is indicated for headache along the greater yáng [太阳 *tài yáng*] channel, and angelica is indicated for headache along the yáng brightness [阳明 *yáng míng*] channel; thus, both medicinals help chuanxiong check pain.

Assistant and Conductor Medicinals

Schizonepeta, saposhnikovia, asarum, and mint are all acrid-dissipating medicinals that conduct the action of the medicinals upwards. These medicinals assist the chief medicinal in dispelling evil [祛邪 *qū xié*].

Licorice harmonizes the properties of all the medicinals [调和药性 *tiáo hé yào xìng*]. The cold and bitter properties of Chinese tea prevent excessive warming and drying by the other acrid-warm medicinals.

This combination of medicinals courses wind and checks pain. When wind-evil is dispelled, the pain will stop.

Variation According to Signs

Most warm acrid medicinals [温辛药 *wēn xīn yào*] that course wind and dissipate cold are concentrated within this one prescription, which is rather strong for coursing and dissipating and effectively treats the root [本 *běn*].

Medicinals that check pain are used in rather small quantities. If the patient experiences pain that is hard to bear, it is advisable to also treat the tip [标 *biāo*] by adding medicinals that extinguish wind and check pain such as corydalis [*yán hú suǒ*], scorpion [*quán xiē*], centipede [*wú gōng*], and gastrodia [*tiān má*].

5.3.2 Liver-Gallbladder Depression Heat [肝胆郁热 *gān dǎn yù rè*]

Method of Treatment for Liver-Gallbladder Depression Heat

Clear and disinhibit liver-gallbladder depression heat [清利肝胆郁热 *qīng lì gān dǎn yù rè*].

Chinese Angelica, Gentian, and Aloe Pill [当归龙荟丸 *dāng guī lóng huì wán*]	
Chinese angelica [当归 *dāng guī*, Angelicae Sinensis Radix]	30g
gentian [龙胆草 *lóng dǎn cǎo*, Gentianae Radix]	15g
aloe [芦荟 *lú huì*, Aloe]	30g
gardenia [栀子 *zhī zǐ*, Gardeniae Fructus]	30g
coptis [黄连 *huáng lián*, Coptidis Rhizoma]	30g
scutellaria [黄芩 *huáng qín*, Scutellariae Radix]	30g
phellodendron [黄柏 *huáng bǎi*, Phellodendri Cortex]	30g
rhubarb [大黄 *dà huáng*, Rhei Rhizoma et Radix]	15g
costusroot [木香 *mù xiāng*, Aucklandiae Radix]	8g
musk [麝香 *shè xiāng*, Moschus]	2g
Directions: Grind the above medicinals into powder. Mix the ground medicinals with honey, and form them into small pills. Take 2 times daily, 6g each time.	

Prescription Analysis

Chief Medicinal

Gentian, which is extremely bitter and cold [大苦大寒 *dà kǔ dà hán*], is used to clear liver-gallbladder repletion fire [实火 *shí huǒ*].

Support Medicinals

Coptis, scutellaria, and phellodendron clear the exuberant fire [火盛 *huǒ shèng*] of the triple burner. Gardenia clears heart fire. Aloe and rhubarb clear stomach fire. All of these support medicinals help gentian drain fire [泻火 *xiè huǒ*].

Assistant and Conductor Medicinals

Chinese angelica supplements and quickens the blood [补血活血 *bǔ xuè huó xuè*]. Costusroot rectifies qì [理气 *lǐ qì*] and checks pain. Musk, a mobile and penetrating [走窜 *zǒu cuàn*] aromatic medicinal, opens the orifices and arouses the spirit [开窍醒神 *kāi qiào xǐng shén*] to dissipate depressed fire [郁火 *yù huǒ*].

This combination of medicinals clears repletion fire. Once the fire is cleared, the pain will stop.

Variation According to Signs

For excruciating pain and twitching face, add medicinals such as earthworm [*dì lóng*], silkworm [*bái jiāng cán*], scorpion [*quán xiē*], and gastrodia [*tiān má*] to reinforce the capacity to extinguish wind [熄风 *xī fēng*] and check pain.

5.3.3 Stomach Heat Attacking Upward [胃热上攻 *wèi rè shàng gōng*]

Method of Treatment for Stomach Heat Attacking Upward

Clear and drain stomach fire [清泻胃火 *qīng xiè wèi huǒ*].

Stomach-Clearing Powder [清胃散 *qīng wèi sǎn*]	
Chinese angelica [当归 *dāng guī*, Angelicae Sinensis Radix]	6g
coptis [黄连 *huáng lián*, Coptidis Rhizoma]	5g[7]
dried/fresh rehmannia [生地黄 *shēng dì huáng*, Rehmanniae Radix seu Recens]	12g
moutan [牡丹皮 *mǔ dān pí*, Moutan Cortex]	6g
cimicifuga [升麻 *shēng má*, Cimicifugae Rhizoma]	6g
Directions: Take decocted with water [水煎服 *shuǐ jiān fú*].	

Prescription Analysis

Chief Medicinals

Coptis, bitter and cold [苦寒 *kǔ hán*], clears stomach fire.

Support Medicinals

Dried/fresh rehmannia and moutan clear heat and cool blood [清热凉血 *qīng rè liáng xuè*] and also resolve toxicity [解毒 *jiě dú*]. They help coptis clear and drain stomach fire.

---

[7] Use more than 5g of this during summer months.

Assistant and Conductor Medicinals

Chinese angelica supplements and quickens the blood [补血活血 *bǔ xuè huó xuè*], disperses swelling [消肿 *xiāo zhǒng*], and checks pain. Fire depression is treated by effusing [火郁发之 *huǒ yù fā zhī*].

Cimicifuga dissipates fire [散火 *sàn huǒ*] and resolves toxicity; it also functions as a yáng brightness [阳明 *yáng míng*] channel conductor medicinal.

The Stomach-Clearing Powder [清胃散 *qīng wèi sǎn*] mentioned in the classic *Medical Formulas Gathered and Explained* [医方集解 *Yī Fāng Jí Jiě*] also includes gypsum [*shí gāo*], which increases the power to clear and drain stomach fire.

This combination of medicinals clears and drains stomach fire [清泻胃火 *qīng xiè wèi huǒ*]. When stomach fire is cleared, the pain will stop.

Variation According to Signs

If the patient is constipated, add rhubarb [*dà huáng*] and mirabilite [*máng xiāo*]. If there is painful swelling of the gums, add cyathula [*chuān niú xī*] to conduct the heat downwards. If there is headache with red eyes, add gentian [*lóng dǎn cǎo*], chrysanthemum [*jú huā*], and mint [*bò hé*] to clear and drain liver-gallbladder repletion fire.

5.3.4   Yīn Vacuity with Yáng Hyperactivity [阴虚阳亢 *yīn xū yáng kàng*]

Method of Treatment for Yīn Vacuity with Yáng Hyperactivity

Enriching and supplementing the liver and kidney, and calming the liver and extinguishing wind [滋补肝肾，平肝熄风 *zī bǔ gān shèn, píng gān xī fēng*].

Gastrodia and Uncaria Beverage [天麻钩藤饮 *tiān má gōu téng yǐn*]	
gastrodia [天麻 *tiān má*, Gastrodiae Rhizoma]	9g
uncaria [钩藤 *gōu téng*, Uncariae Ramulus cum Uncis]	12g
abalone shell [石决明 *shí jué míng*, Haliotidis Concha]	18g
gardenia [栀子 *zhī zǐ*, Gardeniae Fructus]	9g
scutellaria [黄芩 *huáng qín*, Scutellariae Radix]	9g
cyathula [川牛膝 *chuān niú xī*, Cyathulae Radix]	15g
eucommia [杜仲 *dù zhòng*, Eucommiae Cortex]	9g
leonurus [益母草 *yì mǔ cǎo*, Leonuri Herba]	15g
mistletoe [桑寄生 *sāng jì shēng*, Taxilli Herba]	20g
flowery knotweed stem [夜交藤 *yè jiāo téng*, Polygoni Multiflori Caulis]	20g
root poria [茯神 *fú shén*, Poria cum Pini Radice]	12g
Directions: Take decocted with water [水煎服 *shuǐ jiān fú*].	

Prescription Analysis

Chief Medicinals

Gastrodia and uncaria extinguish wind [熄风 *xī fēng*], check tetany [止痉 *zhǐ jìng*], and check pain.

Support Medicinals

Mistletoe, flowery knotweed stem, cyathula, and eucommia enrich and supplement the liver and kidney, thus treating the root [治本 *zhì běn*].

Assistant and Conductor Medicinals

Abalone shell settles the liver and extinguishes wind [镇肝熄风 *zhèn gān xī fēng*]; gardenia clears and drains heart fire; scutellaria clears and drains lung fire; root poria quiets the spirit and stabilizes the mind [安神定志 *ān shén dìng zhì*]; and leonurus quickens the blood [活血 *huó xuè*].

This combination of medicinals is used to extinguish wind [熄风 *xī fēng*] and check tetany [止痉 *zhǐ jìng*] and to clear heat and nourish yīn.

Variation According to Signs

The original prescription is primarily used to clear heat, calm the liver [平肝 *píng gān*], and check pain. If there is extreme vacuity of liver and kidney yīn, add dried/fresh rehmannia [*shēng dì huáng*], cooked rehmannia [*shú dì huáng*], lycium berry [*gǒu qǐ zǐ*], flowery knotweed [*hé shǒu wū*], tortoise plastron [*guī bǎn*], and turtle shell [*biē jiǎ*]; this enriches water to moisten wood [滋水涵木 *zī shuǐ hán mù*]. If the patient is suffering from severe dizziness and headache, add tribulus [*bái jí lí*], crude dragon bone [*shēng lóng gǔ*], and crude oyster shell [*shēng mǔ lì*]. For mild heat [effusion] and heart vexation [心烦热 *xīn fán rè*], add medicinals such as lycium root bark [*dì gǔ pí*], moutan [*mǔ dān pí*], and baiwei [*bái wēi*].

5.3.5   Qì and Blood Depletion [气血亏虚 *qì xuè kuī xū*]

Method of Treatment for Qì and Blood Depletion

Dual supplementation of qì and blood [气血双补 *qì xuè shuāng bǔ*].

Eight Gem Decoction [八珍汤 *bā zhēn tāng*]	
ginseng [人参 *rén shēn*, Ginseng Radix]	6g
white atractylodes [白术 *bái zhú*, Atractylodis Macrocephalae Rhizoma]	9g
poria [茯苓 *fú líng*, Poria]	10g
Chinese angelica [当归 *dāng guī*, Angelicae Sinensis Radix]	10g

chuanxiong [川芎 *chuān xiōng*, Chuanxiong Rhizoma]	6g
white peony [白芍 *bái sháo*, Paeoniae Radix Alba]	10g
cooked rehmannia [熟地黄 *shú dì huáng*, Rehmanniae Radix Conquita]	9g
licorice [甘草 *gān cǎo*, Glycyrrhizae Radix]	6g
fresh ginger [生姜 *shēng jiāng*, Zingiberis Rhizoma Recens]	6g
jujube [大枣 *dà zǎo*, Jujubae Fructus]	3 fruits

Directions: Take decocted with water [水煎服 *shuǐ jiān fú*].

Prescription Analysis

Chief Medicinals

Ginseng and cooked rehmannia supplement qì and nourish blood.

Support Medicinals

White atractylodes and poria fortify the spleen and boost qì [健脾益气 *jiàn pí yì qì*] to strengthen the source of qì and blood formation [气血生化之源 *qì xuè shēng huà zhī yuán*].

Chinese angelica and white peony help cooked rehmannia supplement blood.

Assistant and Conductor Medicinals

Chuanxiong quickens blood and moves qì; and fresh ginger and jujube harmonize the spleen and stomach to stimulate the production of qì and blood.

Licorice boosts qì and supplements the center [补中 *bǔ zhōng*].

This combination of medicinals supplements both qì and blood.

Variation According to Signs

For spontaneous sweating, aversion to wind, and wilting, add astragalus [*huáng qí*]. For severe pain, add peach kernel [*táo rén*] and carthamus [*hóng huā*]. If the patient feels dizzy and heavy-headed, add acorus [*shí chāng pú*] and vitex [*màn jīng zǐ*]. If the pain is aggravated by cold, add dried ginger [*gān jiāng*] and asarum [*xì xīn*] to warm and free [通 *tōng*] the exterior and interior.

5.3.6 Wind-Phlegm Obstructing the Network Vessels
[风痰阻络 *fēng tán zǔ luò*]

Method of Treatment for Wind-Phlegm Obstructing the Network Vessels

Dry dampness and transform phlegm, free the network vessels and check pain [燥湿化痰, 通络止痛 *zào shī huà tán, tōng luò zhǐ tòng*].

Pinellia, White Atractylodes, and Gastrodia Decoction
[半夏白术天麻汤 *bàn xià bái zhú tiān má tāng*]

pinellia [半夏 *bàn xià*, Pinelliae Rhizoma]	9g
gastrodia [天麻 *tiān má*, Gastrodiae Rhizoma]	6g
poria [茯苓 *fú líng*, Poria]	6g
red tangerine peel [橘红 *jú hóng*, Citri Reticulatae Exocarpium Rubrum]	6g
white atractylodes [白术 *bái zhú*, Atractylodis Macrocephalae Rhizoma]	9g
licorice [甘草 *gān cǎo*, Glycyrrhizae Radix]	2g

Directions: Take decocted with water [水煎服 *shuǐ jiān fú*].

Prescription Analysis

Chief Medicinal

Pinellia dries dampness and transforms phlegm [燥湿化痰 *zào shī huà tán*] and thus treats the root [治本 *zhì běn*].

Support Medicinals

White atractylodes fortifies the spleen and dispels dampness [健脾祛湿 *jiàn pí qū shī*], as the spleen is the source of phlegm formation [脾为生痰之源 *pí wéi shēng tán zhī yuán*]. Gastrodia extinguishes wind [熄风 *xī fēng*] and checks pain.

Assistant Medicinals

Red tangerine peel dries dampness and transforms phlegm [燥湿化痰 *zào shī huà tán*]. Poria disinhibits dampness by bland percolation [淡渗利湿 *dàn shèn lì shī*] and fortifies the spleen.

Conductor Medicinal

Licorice harmonizes all the medicinals in the prescription.

This combination of medicinals dries dampness and transforms phlegm, frees the network vessels and checks pain. When phlegm-damp is dispelled and when the channels and network vessels are freed, the pain stops.

Variation According to Signs

This prescription has a great capacity to dry dampness and transform phlegm. If the face muscles are numb, add white mustard [*bái jiè zǐ*] and vaccaria [*wáng bù liú xíng*] to increase the actions of freeing the channels and quickening the network vessels.

5.3.7 Static Blood Obstructing the Network Vessels
[瘀血阻络 *yū xuè zǔ luò*]

Method of Treatment

Quicken the blood and free the orifices [活血通窍 *huó xuè tōng qiào*].

Orifice-Freeing Blood-Quickening Decoction
[通窍活血汤 *tōng qiào huó xuè tāng*]

red peony [赤芍 *chì sháo*, Paeoniae Radix Rubra]	6g
chuanxiong [川芎 *chuān xiōng*, Chuanxiong Rhizoma]	6g
peach kernel [桃仁 *táo rén*, Persicae Semen]	6g
carthamus [红花 *hóng huā*, Carthami Flos]	6g
scallion white [葱白 *cōng bái*, Allii Fistulosi Bulbus]	10g
musk [麝香 *shè xiāng*, Moschus]	0.1g
fresh ginger [生姜 *shēng jiāng*, Zingiberis Rhizoma Recens]	10g
jujube [大枣 *dà zǎo*, Jujubae Fructus]	6 pieces
yellow wine [黄酒 *huáng jiǔ*, Vinum Aureum]	as needed

Directions: Prepare decoction as follows: Using equal parts of medicinal wine and water, cook all medicinals except the musk. Remove the dregs, add the musk, and take while still warm.

Prescription Analysis

Chief Medicinal

Musk, a mobile and penetrating [走窜 *zǒu cuàn*] aromatic medicinal, is used to quicken blood and free the channels and to free the orifices and check pain.

Support Medicinals

Red peony, chuanxiong, peach kernel, and carthamus quicken the blood, transform stasis, and check pain.

Assistant and Conductor Medicinals

Scallion white, a warm acrid [辛温 *xīn wēn*] medicinal, is mobile and penetrating [走窜 *zǒu cuàn*]. Yellow wine warms and frees the channels. Fresh ginger and jujube harmonize construction and defense [营卫 *yíng wèi*] and support quickening blood and freeing channels.

This combination of medicinals quickens the blood, frees the orifices, and checks pain. When the channels and network vessels are freed and qì and blood are regulated, the pain will naturally stop.

Variation According to Signs

If the patient's constitution tends towards yáng vacuity, add aconite [*fù zǐ*] and cinnamon bark [*ròu guì*] to warm yáng and free the vessels. If there is qì stagnation [气滞 *qì zhì*], add cyperus [*xiāng fù*] and unripe tangerine peel [*qīng pí*] to move qì and transform phlegm.

5.4   ACUPUNCTURE TREATMENTS FOR TRIGEMINAL NEURALGIA

5.4.1   Base Acupuncture Prescription for Trigeminal Neuralgia

This base prescription should be modified according to the identified patterns that are discussed below and according to the condition of the individual patient.

Treatment Method for Trigeminal Neuralgia

Course the three yáng channels [疏通三阳 *shū tōng sān yáng*], quicken the network vessels and settle pain [活络镇痛 *huó luò zhèn tòng*].

Base Acupuncture Prescription for Trigeminal Neuralgia
TB-1 Passage Hub [关冲 *guān chōng*]
SI-1 Lesser Marsh [少泽 *shào zé*]
LI-1 Shāng Yáng [商阳 *shāng yáng*]
Ouch Point [阿是穴 *ā shì xué*]
ST-45 Severe Mouth [厉兑 *lì duì*]
GB-44 Foot Orifice Yīn [足窍阴 *zú qiào yīn*]
BL-67 Reaching Yīn [至阴 *zhì yīn*]

Prescription Analysis

The distribution of the trigeminal nerve branches in the face overlaps with the three yáng channels of the hand (large intestine, small intestine, triple burner channels), the foot lesser yáng gallbladder channel, and the foot yáng brightness stomach channel. Although the foot greater yáng bladder channel does not overlap with the trigeminal nerve branches, it intersects with the foot yáng brightness stomach channel at BL-1.

All of the points in the prescription are well points [井穴 *jǐng xué*] (one of the five transport points [五输穴 *wǔ shū xué*]). Well points are often used in clinical practice to treat acute pain. Stimulating local ouch points reinforces the effect of settling pain.

5.4.2   Points to Add to the Base Prescription

Points for Wind-Cold Assailing the Exterior [风寒外袭 *fēng hán wài xí*]
TB-5 Outer Pass [外关 *wài guān*]

TB-5 connects to the yáng linking vessel [阳维脉 *yáng wéi mài*], which nets all the yáng channels and governs the exterior of the body [主一身之表 *zhǔ yì shēn zhī biǎo*]. Thus, TB-5 resolves the exterior [解表 *jiě biǎo*].

Points for Liver-Gallbladder Depression Heat [肝胆郁热 *gān dǎn yù rè*]

GB-34 Yáng Mound Spring [阳陵泉 *yáng líng quán*]

GB-34 courses the liver and disinhibits the gallbladder, soothes the sinews and quickens the network vessels.

Points for Stomach Heat Attacking Upward 胃热上攻 *wèi rè shàng gōng*]

ST-44 Inner Court [内庭 *nèi tíng*]
LI-2 Second Space [二间 *èr jiān*]

ST-44 is used to clear and discharge stomach fire and to check pain. LI-2 is the spring point [荥穴 *yíng xué*] of the hand yáng brightness large intestine channel [手阳明大肠经 *shǒu yáng míng dà cháng jīng*]. Because water restrains fire, spring points govern heat in the body [荥主身热 *yíng zhǔ shēn rè*]; thus, LI-2 has a strong ability to clear heat and discharge fire.

Points for Yīn Vacuity with Yáng Hyperactivity 阴虚阳亢 *yīn xū yáng kàng*]

KI-7 Recover Flow [复溜 *fù liū*]

KI-7 supplements the kidney and boosts yīn.

Points for Qì and Blood Depletion [气血亏虚 *qì xuè kuī xū*]

CV-6 Sea of Qì [气海 *qì hǎi*]
SP-6 Three Yīn Intersection [三阴交 *sān yīn jiāo*]

CV-6 supplements original qì [元气 *yuán qì*]. SP-6 Three Yīn Intersections nourishes and harmonizes blood [养血和血 *yǎng xuè hé xuè*]. It is a principal point for treating blood patterns because it is the intersection point of the spleen, liver, and kidney channels. The liver stores blood, the kidney stores essence, and the spleen manages the blood [脾统血 *pí tǒng xuè*] and is the source of qì and blood formation [脾为生化气血之源 *pí wéi shēng huà qì xuè zhī yuán*]. As essence and blood are of the same source [精血同源 *jīng xuè tóng yuán*], their replenishment depends on a common source (i.e., acquired essence provided by the spleen and stomach) and they are closely related physiologically and pathologically. SP-6 is thus an important point for treating blood-essence depletion.

Points for Wind-Phlegm Obstructing the Network Vessels [风痰阻络 *fēng tán zǔ luò*]
GB-20 Wind Pool [风池 *fēng chí*] ST-40 Bountiful Bulge [丰隆 *fēng lóng*]

GB-20 dispels wind. ST-40 harmonizes the stomach and fortifies the spleen, transforms phlegm and disinhibits dampness.

Points for Static Blood Obstructing the Network Vessels [瘀血阻络 *yū xuè zǔ luò*]
BL-40 Bend Center [委中 *wěi zhōng*] (needling or bloodletting [放血 *fàng xuè*])

BL-40 is used to free the channels and quicken the network vessels and to move blood and transform stasis.

CHAPTER 6

Cervical Spondylosis

Cervical spondylosis is a result of degeneration of the disks and vertebrae in the neck, which constricts the spinal canal. Symptoms are a painful neck and other symptoms resulting from compression of the spinal cord or spinal nerve roots.

There are five main forms of cervical spondylosis:

- External evil bì obstruction [外邪痹阻 *wài xié bì zǔ*]
- Phlegm-damp obstruction [痰湿阻滞 *tán shī zǔ zhì*]
- Qì stagnation and blood stasis [气滞血瘀 *qì zhì xuè yū*]
- Qì-blood vacuity [气血虚弱 *qì xuè xū ruò*]
- Liver-kidney depletion [肝肾亏虚 *gān shèn kuī xū*]

6.1   POINTS OF ATTENTION FOR CERVICAL SPONDYLOSIS

6.1.1   Physiology

The kidney stores essence and governs the bones [肾藏精而主骨 *shèn cáng jīng ér zhǔ gǔ*]; the liver stores blood and governs the sinews [肝藏血而主筋 *gān cáng xuè ér zhǔ jīn*]. When liver and kidney are depleted, the sinews and bones do not receive proper nourishment and are debilitated. The structure of the neck is relatively delicate, has a wide range of movement, and is often unprotected by clothing; thus, the bones and sinews of the neck easily suffer from the effects of liver-kidney depletion.

A certain degree of liver-kidney depletion is part of the aging process. If people age well, this depletion is slow and not severe. If people do not age well, the depletion is quick and gives rise to weakness in the bones and sinews, including the cervical spine. This is why cervical spondylosis tends to occur at age 40 and above.

6.1.2   Pathomechanism

Internal causes [内因 *nèi yīn*] of cervical spondylosis are liver-kidney depletion and qì-blood vacuity; external causes [外因 *wài yīn*] are wind-cold-damp evil assailing the body and long-term taxation detriment [劳损 *láo sǔn*].

The disease tends to start with wind-cold-damp evil that exploits [乘 *chéng*] vacuity and assails the body, obstructing the channels and network vessels. The disease is located in the exterior of the body, the skin and muscle, and channels and network vessels.

When the disease endures it tends to develop into a vacuity repletion complex [虚实错杂 *xū shí cuò zá*], with phlegm turbidity and blood stasis obstruction reaching deep into the sinews, bones, and marrow.

6.2   CAUSES AND PATHOMECHANISM OF CERVICAL SPONDYLOSIS; IDENTIFYING PATTERNS

6.2.1   External Evil Bì Obstruction [外邪痹阻 *wài xié bì zǔ*]

Causes and Pathomechanism of External Evil Bì Obstruction

This pattern is seen in the beginning stage of the disease. Constitutional issues such as liver-kidney depletion in patients above 40 years of age with deteriorating health, qì-blood vacuity, and insecurity of defense qì [卫气不固 *wèi qì bú gù*] allow wind-cold-damp evil to exploit [乘 *chéng*] vacuity and assail [侵袭 *qīn xí*] the governing vessel [督脉 *dū mài*]. The external evil gets lodged in the neck and shoulders, obstructs the channels and network vessels, and inhibits the free flow of qì-blood.

Important Signs of External Evil Bì Obstruction

Pain in the neck, head, shoulders, and back. Pain is in a fixed location. Aversion to cold and liking for warmth. Stiffness and inhibited movement in the neck. Painful pressure points in the back of the neck. One or both arms feel heavy and weak. Head feels heavy. Oppression in the chest [胸闷 *xiōng mèn*]. The tongue is pale with thin white fur [舌质淡苔薄白 *shé zhì dàn tāi bó bái*]. The pulse is stringlike and tight [弦紧 *xián jǐn*].

6.2.2   Phlegm-Damp Obstruction [痰湿阻滞 *tán shī zǔ zhì*]

Causes and Pathomechanism of Phlegm-Damp Obstruction

Kidney yáng vacuity can lead to weak qì transformation [气化 *qì huà*] and to water that does not transform and that starts collecting [水停 *shuǐ tíng*], which forms phlegm-rheum [痰饮 *tán yǐn*]. As the patient's body is vacuous and easily contracts wind-evil, the wind and phlegm combine, obstruct the channels and network vessels in the neck region, and harass the head.

Important Signs of Phlegm-Damp Obstruction

Severe pain in the head and neck. Distention and soreness in the shoulder and arms. The limbs feel heavy. No strength to lift objects. Heavy headedness, dizziness. Oppression and fullness in the chest and stomach duct. Reduced food intake. Increased need for sleep. The tongue has a white slimy coating [苔白腻 *tāi bái nì*], while the pulse is deep and slippery [脉沉滑 *mài chén huá*].

6.2.3   Qì Stagnation and Blood Stasis [气滞血瘀 *qì zhì xuè yū*]

Causes and Pathomechanism of Qì Stagnation and Blood Stasis

External injury [外伤 *wài shāng*] or taxation detriment [劳损 *láo sǔn*] causes bleeding and formation of blood stasis in the cervical spine. Blood stasis obstructs the channels and network vessels, causing stoppage and pain.

Important Signs of Qì Stagnation and Blood Stasis

Numbness and tingling [麻木 *má mù*] in the neck, head, shoulders, back, and limbs. Stabbing pain [刺痛 *cì tòng*] in a fixed location. The pain refuses pressure [拒按 *jù àn*] and is exacerbated during the night. Dizziness and dizzy vision. Lusterless facial complexion [面色不华 *miàn sè bù huá*]. Dark purple tongue, or tongue with stasis macules [舌质紫暗或有瘀斑 *shé zhì zǐ àn huò yǒu yū bān*]. Fine rough pulse or stringlike rough pulse [脉细涩或弦涩 *mài xì sè huò xián sè*].

6.2.4   Qì-Blood Vacuity [气血虚弱 *qì xuè xū ruò*]

Causes and Pathomechanism of Qì-Blood Vacuity

Qì-blood vacuity, which often occurs in old age, results in impaired nourishment of the channel sinews [经筋 *jīng jīn*] and bones. Qì-blood vacuity brings about insecurity of defense qì [卫气不固 *wèi qì bú gù*] and allows wind-cold-damp evil to repeatedly exploit [乘 *chéng*] vacuity and assail [侵袭 *qīn xí*] the body, obstructing the channels and inhibiting the smooth flow of qì.

Important Signs of Qì-Blood Vacuity

Aching pain [酸痛 *suān tòng*]. Numbness and tingling in the shoulders and arms. Spontaneous sweating [自汗 *zì hàn*]. Dizziness and dizzy vision. Palpitations and shortness of breath. Sleeplessness and dream-disturbed sleep. Lusterless facial complexion. Female patients experience an exacerbation of such symptoms after menstruation. Pale tongue with thin white coating [舌质淡苔薄白 *shé zhì dàn tāi bó bái*]; thin weak pulse [脉细弱 *mài xì ruò*].

6.2.5 Liver-Kidney Depletion [肝肾亏虚 *gān shèn kuī xū*]

Causes and Pathomechanism of Liver-Kidney Depletion

Liver-kidney depletion, which often occurs in old age, causes the sinews and bones to lack nourishment.

Important Signs of Liver-Kidney Depletion

Discomfort in neck and shoulders. Distending pain [胀痛 *zhàng tòng*] in the head. Dizziness and tinnitus [耳鸣 *ěr míng*]. Lassitude of spirit [神疲 *shén pí*] and lack of strength [乏力 *fá lì*]. Aching lumbus and limp knees [腰膝酸软 *yāo xī suān ruǎn*]. Forgetfulness [键忘 *jiàn wàng*]. Sleeplessness. Shrunken crimson tongue with scant fur or no fur [舌质瘦绛，少苔或无苔 *shé zhì shòu jiàng, shǎo tāi huò wú tāi*]. Stringlike fine pulse [脉弦细 *mài xián xì*].

6.3 TREATMENT OF CERVICAL SPONDYLOSIS USING CHINESE MEDICINALS

6.3.1 External Evil Bì Obstruction [外邪痹阻 *wài xié bì zǔ*]

Method of Treatment for External Evil Bì Obstruction

Dispel wind and eliminate dampness, alleviate impediment and check pain [祛风除湿，蠲痹止痛 *qū fēng chú shī, juān bì zhǐ tòng*].

Impediment-Alleviating Decoction [蠲痹汤 *juān bì tāng*]	
Chinese angelica [当归 *dāng guī*, Angelicae Sinensis Radix]	45g
notopterygium [羌活 *qiāng huó*, Notopterygii Rhizoma et Radix]	45g
turmeric [姜黄 *jiāng huáng*, Curcumae Longae Rhizoma]	45g
white peony [白芍 *bái sháo*, Paeoniae Radix Alba]	45g
mix-fried astragalus [炙黄芪 *zhì huáng qí*, Astragali Radix cum Liquido Fricta]	45g
saposhnikovia [防风 *fáng fēng*, Saposhnikoviae Radix]	45g
honey-fried licorice [炙甘草 *zhì gān cǎo*, Glycyrrhizae Radix Preparata]	15g

> **Directions:** Grind the above medicinals into a fine powder. Boil 10g of the powder with 3 slices of fresh ginger [生姜 *shēng jiāng*, Zingiberis Rhizoma Recens]; drink warm.

Prescription Analysis

Chief Medicinal

Notopterygium dispels wind and eliminates dampness, alleviates impediment and checks pain, thus treating the root.

Support Medicinals

Turmeric quickens blood, moves qì and checks pain; it is also particularly effective in treating shoulder and back pain. Chinese angelica and mix-fried astragalus supplement qì and nourish blood. Saposhnikovia dispels wind and eliminates dampness.

Assistant Medicinals

White peony supplements blood and prevents damage to yīn [伤阴 *shāng yīn*] by the acrid-dissipating [辛散 *xīn sàn*] medicinals (i.e., notopterygium and saposhnikovia). White peony and honey-fried licorice are the ingredients of Peony and Licorice Decoction [芍药甘草汤 *sháo yào gān cǎo tāng*], which relaxes tension and checks pain [缓急止痛 *huǎn jí zhǐ tòng*].

Conductor Medicinals

Licorice harmonizes the properties of all the medicinals [调和药性 *tiáo hé yào xìng*].

This combination of medicinals is used to dispel wind and eliminate dampness and to alleviate impediment and check pain.

Variation According to Signs

If pain is more severe than numbness and tingling, add cinnamon twig [*guì zhī*] to warm and free the network vessels, asarum [*xì xīn*] to dissipate cold and check pain, and corydalis [*yán hú suǒ*] to quicken blood and check pain.

If numbness and tingling are quite severe, add chaenomeles [*mù guā*] and clematis [*wēi líng xiān*] to quicken blood and free the network vessels.

6.3.2   Phlegm-Damp Obstruction [痰湿阻滞 *tán shī zǔ zhì*]

Method of Treatment for Phlegm-Damp Obstruction

Dry dampness and transform phlegm, rectify qì and free the network vessels [燥湿化痰，理气通络 *zào shī huà tán, lǐ qì tōng luò*].

Poria Pill [茯苓丸 *fú líng wán*][8]	
pinellia [半夏 *bàn xià*, Pinelliae Rhizoma]	60g
poria [茯苓 *fú líng*, Poria]	30g
bitter orange [枳壳 *zhǐ ké*, Aurantii Fructus]	15g
mirabilite efflorescence [风化硝 *fēng huà xiāo*, Mirabilitum Efflorescentia]	8g

Directions: Grind the above medicinals into a fine powder. Use ginger paste to form into pills. Take 30g of the pills, and drink ginger decoction to swallow the pills. Take twice a day.

Prescription Analysis

Chief Medicinal

Pinellia dries dampness and transforms phlegm to treat the root [治本 *zhì běn*].

Support Medicinals

Poria disinhibits dampness by bland percolation [淡渗利湿 *dàn shèn lì shī*], fortifies the spleen [健脾 *jiàn pí*], and transforms phlegm; it thus treats the source of phlegm formation, for "the spleen is the source of phlegm formation" [脾为生痰之源 *pí wéi shēng tán zhī yuán*].

Assistant Medicinals

Bitter orange rectifies qì and transforms phlegm. Mirabilite efflorescence frees the intestine and softens hardness [软坚 *ruǎn jiān*]. Fresh ginger warms and transforms phlegm and dampness; it also resolves the toxicity of pinelliae.

This combination of medicinals is used to dry dampness and transform phlegm, and to rectify qì and free the network vessels.

Variation According to Signs

If there are also signs of blood stasis, add pangolin scales [*chuān shān jiǎ*], chuanxiong, and earthworm [*dì lóng*] to quicken blood and transform stasis, free the network vessels and check pain. If there are also signs of cold-damp impediment, add cinnamon twig [*guì zhī*], notopterygium [*qiāng huó*], and clematis [*wēi líng xiān*], to dispel wind-damp and relieve impediment pain. If the patient feels dizzy, add gastrodia [*tiān má*] and white atractylodes [*bái zhú*] to transform phlegm and extinguish wind.

---

[8] This prescription is from *Principles and Prohibitions of the Medical Profession* [医门法律 *Yī Mén Fǎ Lù*].

6.3.3　Qì Stagnation and Blood Stasis [气滞血瘀 *qì zhì xuè yū*]

Method of Treatment for Qì Stagnation and Blood Stasis

Quicken blood and transform stasis, course and free the channels and network vessels [活血化瘀，疏通经络 *huó xuè huà yū, shū tōng jīng luò*].

<table>
<tr><td colspan="2" align="center">Stasis-Transforming Impediment-Freeing Decoction
[化瘀通痹汤 huà yū tōng bì tāng]</td></tr>
<tr><td>Chinese angelica [当归 dāng guī, Angelicae Sinensis Radix]</td><td>18g</td></tr>
<tr><td>salvia [丹参 dān shēn, Salviae Miltiorrhizae Radix]</td><td>30g</td></tr>
<tr><td>spatholobus [鸡血藤 jī xuè téng, Spatholobi Caulis]</td><td>20g</td></tr>
<tr><td>frankincense [乳香 rǔ xiāng, Olibanum]</td><td>9g</td></tr>
<tr><td>myrrh [没药 mò yào, Myrrha]</td><td>9g</td></tr>
<tr><td>corydalis [延胡索 yán hú suǒ, Corydalis Rhizoma]</td><td>12g</td></tr>
<tr><td>pueraria [葛根 gé gēn, Puerariae Radix]</td><td>18g</td></tr>
<tr><td>turmeric [姜黄 jiāng huáng, Curcumae Longae Rhizoma]</td><td>12g</td></tr>
<tr><td colspan="2">Directions: Take decocted with water [水煎服 shuǐ jiān fú].</td></tr>
</table>

Prescription Analysis

Chief Medicinal

Salvia quickens blood, transforms stasis, and checks pain.

Support Medicinals

Frankincense, Chinese angelica,肝主运动 spatholobus, and turmeric help salvia in quickening blood and transforming stasis to treat the root.

Assistant Medicinals

Corydalis quickens blood and moves qì. Pueraria resolves the flesh and checks pain [解肌止痛 *jiě jī zhǐ tòng*].

This combination of medicinals is used to quicken blood and transform stasis and to course and free the channels and network vessels.

Variation According to Signs

If the patient also shows symptoms of cold, add cinnamon twig [*guì zhī*] and asarum [*xì xīn*]; if there are stronger signs of cold, add aconite main tuber [*chuān wū tóu*] and wild aconite [*cǎo wū tóu*] to warm the channels and dissipate cold. If the patient shows signs of phlegm damp, add white mustard [*bái jiè zǐ*], pinellia [*bàn xià*], and arisaema [*tiān nán xīng*] to dry dampness and transform phlegm.

6.3.4   Qì-Blood Vacuity [气血虚弱 *qì xuè xū ruò*]

Method of Treatment for Qì-Blood Vacuity

Boost qì, quicken blood, free the network vessels [益气 活血 通络 *yì qì huó xuè tōng luò*].

Astragalus and Cinnamon Twig Five Agents Decoction [黄芪桂枝五物汤 *huáng qí guì zhī wǔ wù tāng*]	
astragalus [黄芪 *huáng qí*, Astragali Radix]	10g
cinnamon twig [桂枝 *guì zhī*, Cinnamomi Ramulus]	10g
white peony [白芍 *bái sháo*, Paeoniae Radix Alba]	6g
fresh ginger [生姜 *shēng jiāng*, Zingiberis Rhizoma Recens]	10g
jujube [大枣 *dà zǎo*, Jujubae Fructus]	6g
Directions: Take decocted with water [水煎服 *shuǐ jiān fú*].	

Prescription Analysis

Chief Medicinal

Astragalus supplements qì [补气 *bǔ qì*].

Support Medicinals

White peony supplements and quickens blood [补血活血 *bǔ xuè huó xuè*]. Cinnamon twig warms and frees the channels.

Assistant Medicinals

Fresh ginger and jujube harmonize construction and defense [调和营卫 *tiáo hé yíng wèi*].

This combination of medicinals boosts qì, quickens blood, and frees the network vessels.

Variation According to Signs

Add Chinese angelica [*dāng guī*], cooked rehmannia [*shú dì huáng*], and codonopsis [*dǎng shēn*] to reinforce the function of supplementing qì and nourishing blood.

If there is pronounced numbness and tingling, add chaenomeles [*mù guā*], pueraria [*gé gēn*], notopterygium [*qiāng huó*], clematis [*wēi líng xiān*], chuanxiong [*chuān xiōng*], pangolin scales [*chuān shān jiǎ*], and vaccaria [*wáng bù liú xíng*]. If there is a tendency to aching pain [酸痛 *suān tòng*], add turmeric [*jiāng huáng*] and corydalis [*yán hú suǒ*] to reinforce the action of the formula.

6.3.5 Liver-Kidney Depletion [肝肾亏虚 *gān shèn kuī xū*]

Method of Treatment for Liver-Kidney Depletion

Enrich and supplement the true yīn of liver and kidney [滋补肝肾真阴 *zī bǔ gān shèn zhēn yīn*].

Left-Restoring (Kidney Yīn) Pill [左归丸 *zuǒ guī wán*]	
cooked rehmannia [熟地黄 *shú dì huáng*, Rehmanniae Radix Conquita]	240g
dioscorea [山药 *shān yào*, Dioscoreae Rhizoma]	120g
cornus [山茱萸 *shān zhū yú*, Corni Fructus]	120g
lycium berry [枸杞子 *gǒu qǐ zǐ*, Lycii Fructus]	120g
cuscuta [菟丝子 *tù sī zǐ*, Cuscutae Semen]	120g
deerhorn glue [鹿角胶 *lù jiǎo jiāo*, Cervi Cornus Gelatinum]	120g
tortoise plastron glue [龟版胶 *guī bǎn jiāo*, Testudinis Plastri Gelatinum]	120g
cyathula [川牛膝 *chuān niú xī*, Cyathulae Radix]	90g

Directions: Grind the medicinals into a fine powder, bind the powder with a small quantity of honey, and form the medicinals into small pills of not more than 0.5 cm in diameter. Take 30 pills at a time with warm water, twice daily.

This prescription can also be taken as a decoction with modified quantities of the ingredients.

Prescription Analysis

Chief Medicinal

Cooked rehmannia powerfully supplements true yīn of the liver and kidney.

Support Medicinals

Cornus, deerhorn glue, tortoise plastron glue, and lycium berry help the chief medicinal enrich and supplement kidney yīn.

Assistant Medicinals

Dioscorea fortifies the spleen [健脾 *jiàn pí*], and the spleen is the source of qì and blood formation [脾为生化气血之源 *pí wéi shēng huà qì xuè zhī yuán*]. Cuscuta enriches and supplements the liver and kidney. Cyathula supplements liver and kidney and also quickens blood.

This combination of medicinals enriches and supplements the true yīn of the liver and kidney.

Variation According to Signs

If there are also signs of wind-damp, add clematis [*wēi líng xiān*]. If the patient also has sinew and bone weakness, add eucommia [*dù zhòng*], acanthopanax [*wǔ jiā pí*], and mistletoe [*sāng jì shēng*] to strengthen the sinews and bones.

6.4   ACUPUNCTURE TREATMENTS FOR CERVICAL SPONDYLOSIS

6.4.1   Base Acupuncture Prescription for Cervical Spondylosis

This base prescription should be modified according to the identified patterns that are discussed below and according to the condition of the individual patient.

Treatment Method for Cervical Spondylosis

Free yáng and move bì [通阳行痹 *tōng yáng xíng bì*], transform phlegm and eliminate dampness [化痰除湿 *huà tán chú shī*], transform stasis, and check pain [祛瘀止痛 *qū yū zhǐ tòng*].

Base Acupuncture Prescription for Cervical Spondylosis
GV-14 Great Hammer [大椎 *dà zhuī*]
M-BW-35 Huá Tuó's Paravertebral Points [华佗夹脊穴 *huá tuó jiā jǐ xué*]
LU-7 Broken Sequence [列缺 *liè quē*]
SI-7 Branch to the Correct [支正 *zhī zhèng*]
BL-58 Taking Flight [飞扬 *fēi yáng*]
ST-40 Bountiful Bulge [丰隆 *fēng lóng*]
LR-5 Woodworm Canal [蠡沟 *lǐ gōu*]

Prescription Analysis

GV-14 is the meeting point of the yáng qì of all yáng channels. Thus, GV-14 frees [宣通 *xuān tōng*] the yáng qì of all yáng channels, dispels evil, and eliminates bì [祛邪除痹 *qū xié chú bì*].

The Huá Tuó paravertebral points (at the neck) points are local points [局部取穴 *jú bù qǔ xué*]. Select the ones that are painful.

LU-7, SI-7, BL-58, ST-40, and LR-5 are all network points [络穴 *luò xué*]. Network points are often used to treat the network vessels themselves rather than internal diseases. Thus, in this case, they are used to quicken the network vessels and settle pain [活络镇痛 *huó luò zhèn tòng*].

LU-7 is one of the four command points [四总穴 *sì zǒng xué*]. The area of the body that LU-7 commands is the "head and neck."

SI-7 and BL-58 course and free the greater yáng channel [太阳经 *tài yáng jīng*] of the hand and foot.

ST-40 and LR-5 transform phlegm and eliminate dampness [化痰除湿 *huà tán chú shī*].

6.4.2   Points to Add to the Base Prescription

Points for External Evil Bì Obstruction [外邪痹阻 *wài xié bì zǔ*]
TB-5 Outer Pass [外关 *wài guān*]

Use this point to dissipate wind [散风 *sàn fēng*], quicken the network vessels [活络 *huó luò*], and dispel evil [祛邪 *qū xié*].

Points for Phlegm-Damp Obstruction [痰湿阻滞 *tán shī zǔ zhì*]
CV-12 Center Stomach Duct [中脘 *zhōng wǎn*]

The combination of CV-12 with ST-40 Bountiful Bulge [丰隆 *fēng lóng*] from the base prescription transforms phlegm and eliminates dampness [化痰除湿 *huà tán chú shī*].

Points for Qì Stagnation and Blood Stasis [气滞血瘀 *qì zhì xuè yū*]
PC-6 Inner Pass [内关 *nèi guān*]

PC-6 regulates the qì dynamic [调畅气机 *tiáo chàng qì jī*]. When the qì dynamic is restored, qì is able to move blood and the blood stasis dissipates.

Qì-Blood Vacuity [气血虚弱 *qì xuè xū ruò*]
CV-6 Sea of Qì [气海 *qì hǎi*]
SP-6 Three Yīn Intersections [三阴交 *sān yīn jiāo*]

This pair of points supplements and boosts qì-blood [补益气血 *bǔ yì qì xuè*].

Points for Liver-Kidney Depletion [肝肾亏虚 *gān shèn kuī xū*]
KI-3 Great Ravine [太溪 *tài xī*]
LR-3 Supreme Surge [太冲 *tài chōng*]
GB-39 Suspended Bell [悬钟 *xuán zhōng*]

KI-3 and LR-3 are points on the kidney and liver channels, respectively. They stimulate the qì of both channels and regulate and supplement liver and kidney.

GB-39 is one of the eight meeting points [八会穴 *bā huì xué*] and treats diseases of the marrow (GB-39 is the meeting point of marrow [髓会 *suǐ huì*]). GB-39 can therefore be used to supplement essence-marrow [精髓 *jīng suǐ*], moisten the sinews and bones, and check pain [止痛 *zhǐ tòng*].

CHAPTER 7
Stiff Neck *(Lào Zhěn)*

Stiff neck, or lào zhěn [落枕 *lào zhěn*], manifests as spasm, rigidity, and pain on one side of the sternocleidomastoid and/or trapezius muscles.

There are two main forms of stiff neck:

- muscle sprain [肌肉扭伤 *jī ròu niǔ shāng*]
- external evil invading [外邪侵袭 *wài xié qīn xí*]

7.1   POINTS OF ATTENTION FOR STIFF NECK

7.1.1   Treatment

Stiff neck is caused by pathological changes in the greater yáng channel [太阳 经 *tài yáng jīng*] if the pain spreads to the nape and back, if the nape and back are especially painful to the touch, and if there is inhibited movement of the head either backward and forward or right and left.

The pathological changes are in the lesser yáng channel [少阳经 *shào yáng jīng*] if the pain spreads along the side of the neck and arm, if the sides of the neck are especially painful to the touch, and if there is inhibited movement of the neck (inclining the head) either backward and forward or right and left.

The common factor is the local obstruction of the channels and network vessels; thus, freeing [通 *tōng*] the channels and network vessels is the main treatment principle. If there is external evil, relieve the exterior and dispel evil.

7.2 Causes and Pathomechanism of Stiff Neck; Identifying Patterns

7.2.1 Muscle Sprain [肌肉扭伤 *jī ròu niǔ shāng*]

Causes and Pathomechanism of Muscle Sprain

Stiff neck can result from sleeping in an unsuitable position in which the neck is overstretched, e.g., as the result of an unsuitable cushion or pillow. This obstructs the qì-blood flow on one side of the neck, causing pain.

Important Signs

No discomfort in the neck before going to sleep, but when rising the next morning, there is sudden onset of pain and discomfort in the neck that extends towards the back or towards the arm. Impaired movement of the neck. In severe cases, the head will be inclined towards the painful side.

7.2.2 External Evil Invading [外邪侵袭 *wài xié qīn xí*]

Causes and Pathomechanism of External Evil Invading

External evils result in stiff neck when cold evil assails the neck during sleep, when the patient is exposed to wind while sweating, or if a patient has long-term exposure to a damp living environment. When the above external evils assail the neck, they cause local congealing and stagnation of qì-blood and impediment obstruction of the channels and network vessels.

Important Signs

Wind-Cold

Painful neck and impaired movement of the neck. Headache and generalized pain. Aversion to cold and heat effusion. Pale tongue with thin white fur [舌质淡, 苔薄白 *shé zhì dàn, tāi bó bái*]. Floating tight pulse [脉浮紧 *mài fú jǐn*].

Wind-Cold-Damp

Painful neck and impaired movement of the neck. Heavy pain in the head [头重痛 *tóu zhòng tòng*] and aching joints. White tongue with slimy fur [苔白腻 *tāi bái nì*]. Floating moderate pulse [脉浮缓 *mài fú huǎn*].

7.3 TREATMENT OF STIFF NECK USING CHINESE MEDICINALS

7.3.1 Muscle Sprain [肌肉扭伤 *jī ròu niǔ shāng*]

Method of Treatment

Quicken blood and soothe sinews, free the network vessels and check pain [活血舒筋, 通络止痛 *huó xuè shū jīn, tōng luò zhǐ tòng*].

Generalized Pain Stasis-Expelling Decoction **[身痛逐瘀汤 *shēn tòng zhú yū tāng*]**	
peach kernel [桃仁 *táo rén*, Persicae Semen]	10g
carthamus [红花 *hóng huā*, Carthami Flos]	10g
chuanxiong [川芎 *chuān xiōng*, Chuanxiong Rhizoma]	6g
large gentian [秦艽 *qín jiāo*, Gentianae Macrophyllae Radix]	6g
notopterygium [羌活 *qiāng huó*, Notopterygii Rhizoma et Radix]	6g
Chinese angelica [当归 *dāng guī*, Angelicae Sinensis Radix]	6g
myrrh [没药 *mò yào*, Myrrha]	10g
flying squirrel's droppings [五灵脂 *wǔ líng zhī*, Trogopteri Faeces]	6g
cyperus [香附 *xiāng fù*, Cyperi Rhizoma]	6g
achyranthes [牛膝 *niú xī*, Achyranthis Bidentatae Radix]	10g
earthworm [地龙 *dì lóng*, Pheretima]	6g
licorice [甘草 *gān cǎo*, Glycyrrhizae Radix]	6g
Directions: Take decocted with water [水煎服 *shuǐ jiān fú*].	

Prescription Analysis

Chief Medicinals

The chief medicinals, peach kernel and carthamus, are used to quicken blood and transform stasis and to free the network vessels and check pain.

Support Medicinals

Chuanxiong, Chinese angelica, earthworm, myrrh, and flying squirrel's droppings assist the chief medicinals in quickening blood and dispelling stasis, freeing the network vessels and checking pain.

Assistant Medicinals

Notopterygium and large gentian dispel wind, eliminate [除 *chú*] dampness, and check pain. Cyperus moves qì [行气 *xíng qì*] and quickens blood. Achyranthes supplements and boosts [补益 *bǔ yì*] the liver and kidney.

Licorice harmonizes the properties of all medicinals in the prescription.

This combination of medicinals is used to quicken blood and soothe sinews and to free the network vessels and check pain. When the stasis is dispelled and the channels and network vessels are freed, the pain stops.

Variation According to Signs

If the patient feels aversion to wind and cold [恶风寒 *wù fēng hán*], add schizonepeta [*jīng jiè*] and saposhnikovia [*fáng fēng*] to resolve the exterior. If the patient suffers from headaches, add Chinese lovage [*gǎo běn*], angelica [*bái zhǐ*], and asarum [*xì xīn*] to dissipate cold [散寒 *sàn hán*] and check pain.

7.3.2   External Evil Invading [外邪侵袭 *wài xié qīn xí*]

Method of Treatment for External Evil Invading

Course and dissipate wind-cold, free the channels and check pain [疏散风寒，通络止痛 *shū sàn fēng hán, tōng luò zhǐ tòng*].

Bupleurum and Pueraria Flesh-Resolving Decoction [柴葛解肌汤 *chái gé jiě jī tāng*]	
bupleurum [柴胡 *chái hú*, Bupleuri Radix]	9g
pueraria [葛根 *gé gēn*, Puerariae Radix]	9g
scutellaria [黄芩 *huáng qín*, Scutellariae Radix]	9g
white peony [白芍 *bái sháo*, Paeoniae Radix Alba]	3g
notopterygium [羌活 *qiāng huó*, Notopterygii Rhizoma et Radix]	3g
angelica [白芷 *bái zhǐ*, Angelicae Dahuricae Radix]	3g
platycodon [桔梗 *jié gěng*, Platycodonis Radix]	3g
licorice [甘草 *gān cǎo*, Glycyrrhizae Radix]	3g
gypsum [石膏 *shí gāo*, Gypsum Fibrosum]	3g
fresh ginger [生姜 *shēng jiāng*, Zingiberis Rhizoma Recens]	3 slices
jujube [大枣 *dà zǎo*, Jujubae Fructus]	2 fruits
Directions: Take decocted with water [水煎服 *shuǐ jiān fú*].	

Prescription Analysis

Chief Medicinals

Bupleurum and pueraria are used as the chief medicinals to resolve the flesh and outthrust evil [解肌透邪 *jiě jī tòu xié*], thus treating the root.

Support Medicinals

Notopterygium and angelica are acrid and dissipating [辛散 *xīn sàn*] and warm and freeing [温通 *wēn tōng*]. They resolve the exterior [解表 *jiě biǎo*] and diffuse impediment [宣痹 *xuān bì*]. Scutellaria and gypsum clear and drain [清泻 *qīng xiè*] internal heat.

Assistant Medicinals

White peony and licorice together harmonize construction and discharge heat [和营泄热 *hé yíng xiè rè*] as well as relax tension [缓急 *huǎn jí*] to check pain. Platycodon diffuses the lung [宣肺 *xuān fèi*] and assists in dispelling evil. Fresh ginger and jujube harmonize construction and defense [调和营卫 *tiáo hé yíng wèi*].

Licorice harmonizes the properties of all medicinals in the prescription.

This combination of medicinals courses and dissipates wind-cold while simultaneously clearing internal heat. The channels are freed and the pain stops.

Variation According to Signs

The strong point of this prescription is its capacity to resolve the flesh and check pain. If the pain spreads to the shoulders and back, add chaenomeles [*mù guā*], loofah [*sī guā luò*], and asarum [*xì xīn*]. If the patient also shows signs of blood stasis, add chuanxiong [*chuān xiōng*], curcuma [*yù jīn*], and corydalis [*yán hú suǒ*] to quicken blood and check pain.

7.4 ACUPUNCTURE TREATMENTS FOR STIFF NECK

7.4.1 Base Acupuncture Prescription for Stiff Neck

This base prescription should be modified according to the identified patterns that are discussed below and according to the condition of the individual patient.

Treatment Method for Stiff Neck

Free the channels and check pain [通经止痛 *tōng jīng zhǐ tòng*].

Base Acupuncture Prescription Points for Stiff Neck
GB-39 Suspended Bell [悬钟 *xuán zhōng*]
BL-62 Extending Vessel [申脉 *shēn mài*]

Prescription Analysis

BL-62 is one of the confluence points of the eight vessels [八脉交会穴 *bā mài jiāo huì xué*] and is linked to the yáng springing vessel [阳跷脉 *yáng qiāo mài*]. The yáng springing vessel controls muscular movement and nimbleness and heavily influences the head and neck.

GB-39 is one of the eight meeting points [八会穴 *bā huì xué*] and is the meeting point of marrow. Its main functions are nourishing essence and marrow and moistening the sinews and bones.

Both points can therefore be used for any kind of stiff neck.

7.4.2   Points to Add to the Base Prescription

Points for Muscle Sprain [肌肉扭伤 *jī ròu niǔ shāng*]
SI-7 Branch to the Correct [支正 *zhī zhèng*]

This point has a strong capacity to soothe the sinews and free the network vessels. It is often used to treat sinew and muscle pain along the hand greater yáng small intestine channel [手太阳小肠经 *shǒu tài yáng xiǎo cháng jīng*].

Points for External Evil Invading [外邪侵袭 *wài xié qīn xí*]
SI-3 Back Ravine [后溪 *hòu xī*]
GB-20 Wind Pool [风池 *fēng chí*]

SI-3 frees the network vessels and soothes the sinews. It is on the hand greater yáng small intestine channel [手太阳小肠经 *shǒu tài yáng xiǎo cháng jīng*], and the greater yáng governs the exterior [太阳主表 *tài yáng zhǔ biǎo*]. SI-3 courses wind, frees the channels, soothes the sinews, and checks pain. GB-20 dispels wind and resolves the exterior.

CHAPTER 8
Periarthritis of the Shoulder

Periarthritis of the shoulder refers to inflammation of the tissue around the shoulder joint that causes pain and stiffness of the shoulder. It is also called "leaky shoulder wind" [漏肩风 *lòu jiān fēng*], "fifty-year-old's shoulder" [五十肩 *wǔ shí jiān*] (often seen in people around the age of 50), or "frozen shoulder" [肩凝 *jiān níng*].

There are three main forms:

- invasion of wind-cold-damp [风寒湿侵袭 *fēng hán shī qīn xí*]

- qì stagnation and blood stasis [气滞血瘀 *qì zhì xuè yū*]

- qì-blood vacuity [气血亏虚 *qì xuè kuī xū*]

8.1   POINTS OF ATTENTION FOR PERIARTHRITIS OF THE SHOULDER

Internal causes [内因 *nèi yīn*], an insufficiency of construction, defense, qì, and blood [营卫气血 *yíng wèi qì xuè*], are the most important causes of scapulohumeral periarthritis. This also accounts for the frequent occurrence around the age of 50.

Vacuity and weakness of right qì [正气虚弱 *zhèng qì xū ruò*] is the underlying condition that allows external evil to enter the body and cause scapulohumeral periarthritis. Invasion of wind-cold-damp [风寒湿侵袭 *fēng hán shī qīn xí*] tends to be the beginning stage of scapulohumeral periarthritis. If wind-cold-damp is not removed but stays lodged in the channels, this gives rise to qì stagnation and blood stasis [气滞血瘀 *qì zhì xuè yū*], the middle stage of scapulohumeral periarthritis. Qì-blood vacuity [气血亏虚 *qì xuè kuī xū*] tends to occur in the late stage of the disease.

8.1.1 Physiology

The spleen governs the four limbs [脾主四肢 *pí zhǔ sì zhī*]. The back is the house of the yáng brightness [背为阳明之府 *bèi wéi yáng míng zhī fǔ*].

8.1.2 Treatment

The basis of acupuncture treatment lies in treating the three yáng channels of the hand.

8.2 CAUSES AND PATHOMECHANISM OF PERIARTHRITIS OF THE SHOULDER; IDENTIFYING PATTERNS

8.2.1 Invasion of Wind-Cold-Damp [风寒湿侵袭 *fēng hán shī qīn xí*]

Causes and Pathomechanism of Invasion of Wind-Cold-Damp

Fatigue in combination with conditions such as exposure to wind-cold (e.g., while sleeping) or living in a damp environment allows wind-cold-damp to assail the body, invade the sinews and vessels, and create stoppage.

Important Signs of Wind-Cold-Damp

Aching cold pain [酸冷痛 *suān lěng tòng*] in the shoulder area that is exacerbated by wind-cold and relieved by warmth. Aversion to wind-cold [畏风寒 *wèi fēng hán*]. Feeling of heaviness, tightness, or numbness and tingling in the shoulder. Pale tongue, thin white or slimy white coating [舌质淡，苔薄白或白腻 *shé zhì dàn, tāi bó bái huò bái nì*]. Stringlike and tight or stringlike and slippery pulse [脉弦紧或弦滑 *mài xián jǐn huò xián huá*].

8.2.2 Qì Stagnation and Blood Stasis [气滞血瘀 *qì zhì xuè yū*]

Causes and Pathomechanism of Qì Stagnation and Blood Stasis

Qì stagnation and blood stasis [气滞血瘀 *qì zhì xuè yū*] result from chronic overstrain that damages the sinews, from recent trauma, or from knocks and falls that cause sprain and bruising [闪挫 *shǎn cuò*] which does not heal for a long time. When there is stoppage, there is pain [不通则痛 *bù tōng zé tòng*].

Important Signs of Qì Stagnation and Blood Stasis

Swelling of the shoulder joint. Distending pain [胀痛 *zhàng tòng*] or stabbing pain [刺痛 *cì tòng*] that refuses pressure [拒按 *jù àn*]. Pain gets worse with movement. Severe restriction of movement. As blood stasis is an evil that has a physical form and is thus considered yīn [属阴 *shǔ yīn*], the pain caused by blood stasis is lighter during daytime and worse during nighttime. Dark purple tongue, or tongue with stasis macules [舌暗紫或有瘀斑 *shé àn zǐ huò yǒu yū bān*]. Rough pulse [涩脉 *sè mài*].

8.2.3 Qì-Blood Vacuity [气血亏虚 *qì xuè kuī xū*]

Causes and Pathomechanism of Qì-Blood Vacuity

Qì-blood vacuity is the result of enduring illness that damages qì-blood and leads to qì-blood vacuity and inhibited movement of construction [营 *yíng*]. It can also result from constitutional vacuity brought on by old age [年老体虚 *nián lǎo tǐ xū*], or taxation, which lead to qì-blood vacuity and liver-kidney insufficiency and to sinews and bones losing nourishment.

Important Signs of Qì-Blood Vacuity

Enduring aching pain [酸痛 *suān tòng*] in the shoulder region, which is exacerbated by exertion. Local muscles are decreased in size. Aching lumbus and limp knees. Dizziness and dizzy vision [目眩 *mù xuàn*]. Sleeplessness and palpitations, lack of strength in the four limbs [四肢乏力 *sì zhī fá lì*]. Torpid intake [纳呆 *nà dāi*], distention in the abdomen. Pale tongue, white fur [舌淡，苔白 *shé dàn, tāi bái*]. Weak and fine or deep pulse [脉细弱或沉 *mài xì ruò huò chén*].

8.3 TREATMENT OF PERIARTHRITIS OF THE SHOULDER USING CHINESE MEDICINALS

8.3.1 Invasion of Wind-Cold-Damp [风寒湿侵袭 *fēng hán shī qīn xí*]

Method of Treatment for Invasion of Wind-Cold-Damp

Boost the liver and kidney, supplement qì and blood, dispel wind-damp, check impediment pain [益肝肾，补气血，祛风湿，止痹痛 *yì gān shèn, bǔ qì xuè, qū fēng shī, zhǐ bì tòng*].

Three Impediment Decoction [三痹汤 *sān bì tāng*]	
pubescent angelica [独活 *dú huó*, Angelicae Pubescentis Radix]	10g
large gentian [秦艽 *qín jiāo*, Gentianae Macrophyllae Radix]	10g
chuanxiong [川芎 *chuān xiōng*, Chuanxiong Rhizoma]	10g
cooked rehmannia [熟地黄 *shú dì huáng*, Rehmanniae Radix Conquita]	15g
white peony [白芍 *bái sháo*, Paeoniae Radix Alba]	10g
cinnamon bark [肉桂 *ròu guì*, Cinnamomi Cortex]	6g
poria [茯苓 *fú líng*, Poria]	10g

saposhnikovia [防风 *fáng fēng*, Saposhnikoviae Radix]	10g
asarum [细辛 *xì xīn*, Asari Herba]	3g
Chinese angelica [当归 *dāng guī*, Angelicae Sinensis Radix]	10g
eucommia [杜仲 *dù zhòng*, Eucommiae Cortex]	10g
achyranthes [牛膝 *niú xī*, Achyranthis Bidentatae Radix]	10g
ginseng [人参 *rén shēn*, Ginseng Radix]	6g
astragalus [黄芪 *huáng qí*, Astragali Radix]	15g
dipsacus [续断 *xù duàn*, Dipsaci Radix]	10g
fresh ginger [生姜 *shēng jiāng*, Zingiberis Rhizoma Recens]	3 slices
licorice [甘草 *gān cǎo*, Glycyrrhizae Radix]	6g

Directions: Take decocted with water [水煎服 *shuǐ jiān fú*].

Prescription Analysis

Chief Medicinals

Pubescent angelica and large gentian are used to dispel wind and overcome dampness and to alleviate impediment and check pain [祛风胜湿，蠲痹止痛 *qū fēng shèng shī, juān bì zhǐ tòng*].

Support Medicinals

Cooked rehmannia, Chinese angelica, white peony, and chuanxiong supplement and boost yīn-blood of the liver and kidney [补益肝肾之阴血 *bǔ yì gān shèn zhī yīn xuè*], thus banking up the root [培本 *péi běn*].

Ginseng, poria, and astragalus boost qì and supplement the center. Thus, later heaven [后天 *hòu tiān*] is supplemented by supplementing the spleen, the source of qì and blood formation [脾为生化气血之源 *pí wéi shēng huà qì xuè zhī yuán*].

Eucommia, achyranthes, and dipsacus are used to supplement and boost the liver and kidney and to strengthen the sinews and invigorate the bones [强筋壮骨 *qiáng jīn zhuàng gǔ*].

Assistant Medicinals

Saposhnikovia dispels wind and overcomes dampness. Cinnamon bark and asarum warm the channels, dissipate wind, and check pain. Fresh ginger warms the center and dissipates cold.

Licorice harmonizes the properties of all the medicinals [调和药性 *tiáo hé yào xìng*], and it combines with white peony to form Peony and Licorice Decoction [芍药甘草汤 *sháo yào gān cǎo tāng*], which relaxes tension and checks pain [缓急止痛 *huǎn jí zhǐ tòng*].

This combination of medicinals dispels wind and overcomes dampness, supplements and boosts the liver and kidney, and alleviates impediment and checks pain.

Variation According to Signs

Three Impediment Decoction [三痹汤 *sān bì tāng*] treats the root [治本 *zhì běn*]. It strongly supplements qì-blood and boosts liver and kidney. To strengthen its function of treating the tip [治标 *zhì biāo*] and stop pain, add notopterygium [*qiāng huó*], corydalis [延胡索 *yán hú suǒ*], turmeric [*jiāng huáng*], or even aconite main tuber [*chuān wū tóu*] or wild aconite [*cǎo wū tóu*].

8.3.2 Qì Stagnation and Blood Stasis [气滞血瘀 *qì zhì xuè yū*]

Method of Treatment for Qì Stagnation and Blood Stasis

Move qì, quicken blood, and check pain [行气 活血 止痛 *xíng qì huó xuè zhǐ tòng*].

Generalized Pain Stasis-Expelling Decoction [身痛逐瘀汤 *shēn tòng zhú yū tāng*]	
large gentian [秦艽 *qín jiāo*, Gentianae Macrophyllae Radix]	3g
chuanxiong [川芎 *chuān xiōng*, Chuanxiong Rhizoma]	6g
peach kernel [桃 仁 *táo rén*, Persicae Semen]	9g
carthamus [红花 *hóng huā*, Carthami Flos]	9g
licorice [甘草 *gān cǎo*, Glycyrrhizae Radix]	6g
notopterygium [羌活 *qiāng huó*, Notopterygii Rhizoma et Radix]	3g
myrrh [没药 *mò yào*, Myrrha]	6g
Chinese angelica [当归 *dāng guī*, Angelicae Sinensis Radix]	9g
flying squirrel's droppings [五灵脂 *wǔ líng zhī*, Trogopteri Faeces]	6g
cyperus [香附 *xiāng fù*, Cyperi Rhizoma]	3g
achyranthes [牛膝 *niú xī*, Achyranthis Bidentatae Radix]	9g
earthworm [地龙 *dì lóng*, Pheretima]	6g

Directions: Take decocted with water [水煎服 *shuǐ jiān fú*].

Prescription Analysis

Chief Medicinals

Peach kernel and carthamus quicken blood, transform stasis, and check pain.

Support Medicinals

Chinese angelica supplements and quickens blood.

Myrrh and flying squirrel's droppings quicken blood and check pain.

Earthworm quickens blood and frees the channels.

Assistant Medicinals

Notopterygium and large gentian dispel wind, overcome dampness, and check pain.

Cyperus moves qì and quickens blood.

Achyranthes strengthens the sinews and invigorates the bones [强筋壮骨 *qiáng jīn zhuàng gǔ*].

Licorice harmonizes the properties of all the medicinals [调和药性 *tiáo hé yào xìng*].

This combination of medicinals quickens blood and checks pain. When blood stasis is dispelled and qì-blood is freed, the pain stops.

Variation According to Signs

Generalized Pain Stasis-Expelling Decoction powerfully quickens blood and dispels stasis. When qì moves blood then blood will also move [气行则血行 *qì xíng zé xuè xíng*]; based on this rule one may add bupleurum [*chái hú*], unripe bitter orange [*zhǐ shí*], and unripe tangerine peel [*qīng pí*] to move qì in order to help move blood.

If the pain is severe, add scorpion [*quán xiē*], corydalis [延胡索 *yán hú suǒ*], and frankincense [*rǔ xiāng*] to reinforce the capacity to quicken blood and check pain.

8.3.3   Qì-Blood Vacuity [气血亏虚 *qì xuè kuī xū*]

Method of Treatment for Qì-Blood Vacuity

Boost qì and nourish blood, soothe the sinews and free the network vessels [益气养血，舒筋通络 *yì qì yǎng xuè, shū jīn tōng luò*].

Astragalus and Cinnamon Twig Five Agents Decoction [黄芪桂枝五物汤 *huáng qí guì zhī wǔ wù tāng*]	
astragalus [黄芪 *huáng qí*, Astragali Radix]	10g
cinnamon twig [桂枝 *guì zhī*, Cinnamomi Ramulus]	10g
white peony [白芍 *bái sháo*, Paeoniae Radix Alba]	10g
fresh ginger [生姜 *shēng jiāng*, Zingiberis Rhizoma Recens]	6g
jujube [大枣 *dà zǎo*, Jujubae Fructus]	6 pieces
Directions: Take decocted with water [水煎服 *shuǐ jiān fú*].	

Prescription Analysis

Chief Medicinal

Astragalus supplements qì [补气 *bǔ qì*].

Support Medicinals

Cinnamon twig warms and frees the channels [温通经脉 *wēn tōng jīng mài*]. White peony supplements and quickens blood [补血活血 *bǔ xuè huó xuè*].

Assistant Medicinals

Fresh ginger and jujube harmonize construction and defense [调和营卫 *tiáo hé yíng wèi*] in order to help blood move.

This combination of medicinals regulates qì-blood and frees the channels and collaterals, thus stopping pain and numbness.

Variation According to Signs

Astragalus and Cinnamon Twig Five Agents Decoction is an excellent traditional prescription from *Essential Prescriptions of the Golden Coffer* [金匮要略 *jīn guì yào lüè*] that treats blood impediment pattern [血痹证 *xuè bì zhèng*]. When the above impediment is caused by qì-blood vacuity, one may add Chinese angelica [*dāng guī*], cooked rehmannia [*shú dì huáng*], and chuanxiong [*chuān xiōng*], or even pangolin scales [*chuān shān jiǎ*], vaccaria [*wáng bù liú xíng*], frankincense [*rǔ xiāng*], and myrrh [*mò yào*] to supplement and quicken blood and to free the channels and alleviate impediment.

8.4 ACUPUNCTURE TREATMENTS FOR PERIARTHRITIS OF THE SHOULDER

8.4.1 Invasion of Wind-Cold-Damp [风寒湿侵袭 *fēng hán shī qīn xí*]

Treatment Method for Invasion of Wind-Cold-Damp

Dissipate cold and eliminate dampness, dispel wind and free the network vessels [散寒除湿，祛风通络 *sàn hán chú shī, qū fēng tōng luò*].

Points for Invasion of Wind-Cold Damp
GV-14 Great Hammer [大椎 *dà zhuī*]
TB-5 Outer Pass [外关 *wài guān*]
LI-2 Second Space [二间 *èr jiān*] joining [透 *tòu*]
LI-3 Third Space [三间 *sān jiān*]
LI-15 Shoulder Bone [肩髃 *jiān yú*]
ST-38 Ribbon Opening [条口 *tiáo kǒu*]
joining [透 *tòu*] BL-57 Mountain Support [承山 *chéng shān*]

Prescription Analysis

Yáng qì of all the yáng channels meets in point GV-14; thus, it is indicated for external contraction [外感 *wài gǎn*]. GV-14 frees [宣通 *xuān tōng*] the yáng qì of all yáng channels.

TB-5 is the opening point for the yáng linking vessel [阳维脉 *yáng wéi mài*], one of the eight extraordinary vessels which connects all yáng channels and influences the sides of the body. TB-5 is an important point for releasing the exterior and treating pain induced by wind. LI-15 courses wind, quickens the network vessels, and frees and disinhibits the joints [通利关节 *tōng lì guān jié*]. Together, TB-5 and LI-15 dispel wind-cold-damp evil.

LI-2 joining LI-3 and ST-38 joining BL-57 are points validated by experience in clinical practice [经验穴 *jīng yàn xué*] for the treatment of periarthritis of the shoulder.

8.4.2   Qì Stagnation and Blood Stasis [气滞血瘀 *qì zhì xuè yū*]

Treatment Method for Qì Stagnation and Blood Stasis

Move qi, quicken the blood, and settle pain [行气活血镇痛 *xíng qì huó xuè zhèn tòng*].

Points for Qì Stagnation and Blood Stasis [气滞血瘀 *qì zhì xuè yū*]
PC-6 Inner Pass [内关 *nèi guān*]
LI-11 Pool at the Bend [曲池 *qū chí*]

Prescription Analysis

PC-6 regulates the qì dynamic [调畅气机 *tiáo chàng qì jī*].

LI-11 is the uniting point [合穴 *hé xué*] of the hand yáng brightness channel (LI). As mentioned in the *Classic of Difficult Issues* (68) [《难经八十八难 *nán jīng bā shí bā nán*》* 合主逆气而泄 *hé zhǔ nì qì ér xiè*], uniting points are indicated in cases of upward counterflow or downward draining of the qì dynamic [合穴主治气机上逆和下泄 *hé xué zhǔ zhì qì jī shàng nì hé xià xiè*]. Thus, LI-11 can be used in all cases of inhibited qì flow of the large intestine channel.

8.4.3   Addendum: Trauma [外伤 *wài shāng*]

Treatment Method

Local network vessel pricking [刺络 *cì luò*] (also called bloodletting [放血 *fàng xuè*]), disperses the stasis caused by trauma and thus checks pain.

8.4.4 Qì-Blood Vacuity [气血亏虚 *qì xuè kuī xū*]

Treatment Method for Qì-Blood Vacuity

Supplement and boost qì-blood [补益气血 *bǔ yì qì xuè*].

Points for Qì-Blood Vacuity 气血亏虚 *qì xuè kuī xū*]
CV-6 Sea of Qi [气海 *qì hǎi*]
SP-6 Three Yīn Intersections [三阴交 *sān yīn jiāo*]
GV-14 Great Hammer [大椎 *dà zhuī*]

Prescription Analysis

CV-6 is a principal point for treating qì diseases. It strongly supplements [大补 *dà bǔ*] original qì [元气 *yuán qì*]. The combination of GV-14 and CV-6 frees yáng [通阳 *tōng yáng*] and supplements qì [补气 *bǔ qì*].

SP-6 nourishes and harmonizes blood [养血和血 *yǎng xuè hé xuè*]. As explained in Section 5.4.2, SP-6 is a principal point for treating blood patterns and for treating blood-essence depletion.

This prescription is ideal for patients suffering from periarthritis of the shoulder who have a weak constitution and/or are suffering from long-term illnesses.

CHAPTER 9
Tennis Elbow

Tennis elbow refers to painful inflammation of the tendon at the outer side of the elbow (the lateral epicondyle of the humerus) that results from excessive strain on the forearm muscles.

There are two main forms of tennis elbow:

- channel sinew taxation damage [经筋劳伤 *jīng jīn láo shāng*]
- external contraction wind-cold [外感风寒 *wài gǎn fēng hán*]

9.1   POINTS OF ATTENTION FOR TENNIS ELBOW

9.1.1   Physiology

Tennis elbow is a pathological change in the channel sinew [经筋 *jīng jīn*] of the hand lesser yīn heart channel [手少阴心经 *shǒu shào yīn xīn jīng*].

9.2   CAUSES AND PATHOMECHANISM OF TENNIS ELBOW; IDENTIFYING PATTERNS

9.2.1   Channel Sinew Taxation Damage [经筋劳伤 *jīng jīn láo shāng*]

Causes and Pathomechanism of Channel Sinew Taxation Damage

Taxation damage that results from overstraining the forearm over a period of time gives rise to qì stagnation and blood stasis [气滞血瘀 *qì zhì xuè yū*]; this causes the channel sinews [经筋 *jīng jīn*] to be deprived of nourishment.

Important Signs for Channel Sinew Taxation Damage

History of taxation damage. Painful outer side of the elbow. Pain is exacerbated by taxation, twisting of the forearm, and by pressure [拒按 *jù àn*].

The pain can extend into the forearm. Dark red or pale red tongue and thin white coating [舌暗红或淡红，苔薄白 *shé àn hóng huò dàn hóng, tāi bó bái*]. Deep and rough or deep and fine pulse [脉沉涩或沉细 *mài chén sè huò chén xì*].

9.2.2 External Contraction of Wind-Cold [外感风寒 *wài gǎn fēng hán*]

Causes and Pathomechanism of External Contraction of Wind-Cold

Taxation damage combined with repeated contraction of cold evil can cause congealing cold and stagnating qì [寒凝气滞 *hán níng qì zhì*]. This results in stoppage in the channels and deprivation of nourishment in the channel sinews.

Important Signs for External Contraction of Wind-Cold

Often a history of taxation damage with exposure to cold. Painful outer side of the elbow. Pain is exacerbated by twisting of the forearm and refuses pressure [拒按 *jù àn*]. Pale red tongue with thin white coating [舌淡红，苔薄白 *shé dàn hóng, tāi bó bái*]. Fine or tight pulse [脉细或紧 *mài xì huò jǐn*].

9.3 TREATMENT OF TENNIS ELBOW USING CHINESE MEDICINALS

For tennis elbow, acupuncture is the recommended form of treatment.

9.4 ACUPUNCTURE TREATMENTS FOR TENNIS ELBOW

9.4.1 Base Acupuncture Prescription for Tennis Elbow

This base prescription should be modified according to the identified patterns noted below and according to the patient's individual condition.

Treatment Method for Tennis Elbow

Quicken blood, free the network vessels, and check pain [活血通络止痛 *huó xuè tōng luò zhǐ tòng*].

Base Acupuncture Prescription Points for Tennis Elbow
LI-11 Pool at the Bend [曲池 *qū chí*]
joining [透 *tòu*] HT-3 Lesser Sea [少海 *shào hǎi*]
HT-5 Connecting Li [通里 *tōng lǐ*]

Prescription Analysis

LI-11 is the uniting point [合穴 *hé xué*] of the hand yáng brightness channel [手阳明经 *shǒu yáng míng jīng*]; HT-3 is the uniting point [合穴 *hé xué*] of the hand lesser yīn channel [手少阴经 *shǒu shào yīn jīng*]. Joining LI-11 and HT-3 quickens blood and frees the network vessels. HT-5 is the network point [络穴 *luò xué*] of the hand lesser yīn channel. Network points are often used to treat the network vessels themselves rather than internal diseases. Thus, in this case, HT-5 is used to quicken the network vessels and settle pain [活络镇痛 *huó luò zhèn tòng*].

9.4.2 Points to Add to the Base Prescription for Tennis Elbow

Points for Channel Sinew Taxation Damage [经筋劳伤 *jīng jīn láo shāng*]
LI-10 Arm Three Lǐ [手三里 *shǒu sān lǐ*]

LI-10 is a point on the hand yáng brightness channel [手阳明经 *shǒu yáng míng jīng*], which has copious qì and copious blood [阳明多气多血 *yáng míng duō qì duō xuè*]. Needling LI-10 thus nourishes the channel sinews.

Points for External Contraction of Wind-Cold [外感风寒 *wài gǎn fēng hán*]
Moxibustion at local points expels and dissipates wind-cold [驱散风寒 *qū sàn fēng hán*].

CHAPTER 10
Carpal Tunnel Syndrome

Carpal tunnel syndrome arises when the median nerve is compressed within the carpal tunnel, which causes pain, numbness, and weakness in the thumb, index, and middle fingers. In severe cases, there is atrophy of the affected muscles.

There are two main forms of carpal tunnel syndrome:

- channel sinew taxation damage [经筋劳伤 *jīng jīn láo shāng*]
- invasion of wind-cold [风寒入侵 *fēng hán rù qīn*]

10.1 POINTS OF ATTENTION FOR CARPAL TUNNEL SYNDROME

The syndrome often appears in craftsmen and keyboard users.

10.1.1 Physiology

The pathological changes of carpal tunnel syndrome occur mainly in the hand lesser yáng triple burner channel [手少阳三焦经 *shǒu shào yáng sān jiāo jīng*] and the hand reverting yīn pericardium channel [手厥阴心包经 *shǒu jué yīn xīn bāo jīng*].

10.2 CAUSES OF DISEASE AND PATHOMECHANISM OF CARPAL TUNNEL SYNDROME; IDENTIFYING PATTERNS

10.2.1 Channel Sinew Taxation Damage [经筋劳伤 *jīng jīn láo shāng*]

Causes and Pathomechanism of Channel Sinew Taxation Damage

Taxation damage that results from overstraining the wrist for a long period of time, or knocks and falls that cause sprain and bruising [闪挫 *shǎn cuò*], can give rise to qì stagnation and blood stasis [气滞血瘀 *qì zhì xuè yū*] and cause impaired nourishment of the channel sinews [经筋 *jīng jīn*].

Important Signs of Channel Sinew Taxation Damage

History of taxation damage. The thumb and index and middle fingers are numb and painful. Difficulty in bending and stretching these fingers. Pain is exacerbated by working the hand. Dark red or pale red tongue with a thin white coating [舌暗红或淡红，苔薄白 *shé àn hóng huò dàn hóng, tāi bó bái*]. Deep and rough or deep and fine pulse [脉沉涩或沉细 *mài chén sè huò chén xì*].

10.2.2   Invasion of Wind-Cold [风寒入侵 *fēng hán rù qīn*]

Causes and Pathomechanism of Invasion of Wind-Cold

When an old injury repeatedly contracts cold evil, such as by exposing the hands and forearms to cold water, cold congeals and qì stagnates [寒凝气滞 *hán níng qì zhì*], the channel sinews [经筋 *jīng jīn*] are hypertonic, there is stoppage in the channels, and the result is impaired nourishment of the channel sinews.

Important Signs of Invasion of Wind-Cold

Often a history of taxation damage with exposure to cold. The thumb, index, and middle fingers are weak, numb, and painful. If the symptom has persisted for a long time the abductor muscle of the thumb is atrophied. Pale red tongue with thin white coating [舌淡红，苔薄白 *shé dàn hóng, tāi bó bái*]; fine or tight pulse [脉细或紧 *mài xì huò jǐn*].

10.3   TREATMENT OF CARPAL TUNNEL SYNDROME USING CHINESE MEDICINALS

For carpal tunnel syndrome, acupuncture is the recommended form of treatment.

10.4   ACUPUNCTURE TREATMENT FOR CARPAL TUNNEL SYNDROME

10.4.1   Base Acupuncture Prescription for Carpal Tunnel Syndrome

This base prescription should be modified according to the identified patterns that are discussed below and according to the condition of the individual patient.

Treatment Method for Carpal Tunnel Syndrome

Nourish the blood and soothe the sinews, course and free the channels [养血舒筋，疏通经脉 *yǎng xuè shū jīn, shū tōng jīng mài*].

Base Acupuncture Prescription for Carpal Tunnel Syndrome
TB-4 Yáng Pool [阳池 *yáng chí*]
joining [透 *tòu*] PC-7 Great Mound [大陵 *dà líng*]
LI-5 Yáng Ravine [阳溪 *yáng xī*]
TB-5 Outer Pass [外关 *wài guān*]
joining [透 *tòu*] PC-6 Inner Pass [内关 *nèi guān*]
SI-4 Wrist Bone [腕骨 *wàn gǔ*]

Prescription Analysis

TB-4 is the source point [原穴 *yuán xué*] of the triple burner channel and PC-7 is the source point [原穴 *yuán xué*] of the pericardium channel. Joining both source points of these interior-exterior related channels strongly stimulates the channel qì and frees the channels, causing the pain to stop.

TB-5 joining [透 *tòu*] PC-6 means joining the network points [络穴 *luò xué*] of two channels. This increases the function of freeing the network vessels and improves the ability to check pain.

LI-5 and SI-4 are selected as local points [局部取穴 *jú bù qǔ xué*]; they regulate the flow of qì and blood.

10.4.2   Points to Add to the Base Prescription

Points for Channel Sinew Taxation Damage [经筋劳伤 ***jīng jīn láo shāng***]
LI-11 Pool at the Bend [曲池 *qū chí*]

LI-11 is the uniting point [合穴 *hé xué*] of the hand yáng brightness channel [手阳明经 *shǒu yáng míng jīng*]. Because the yáng brightness channel has copious qì and copious blood [阳明多气多血 *yáng míng duō qì duō xuè*], needling LI-11 nourishes the channel sinews.

Points for Invasion of Wind-Cold [风寒入侵 ***fēng hán rù qīn***]
Moxibustion at local points

Applying moxa at local points will expel and dissipate wind-cold and warm and free yáng qì [驱散风寒，温通阳气 *qū sàn fēng hán, wēn tōng yáng qì*].

CHAPTER 11
Intercostal Neuralgia

Intercostal neuralgia refers to severe pain between the ribs. There are five main forms of intercostal neuralgia:

- evil invading the lesser yáng channel [邪犯少阳 *xié fàn shào yáng*]

- congealing cold-damp [寒湿搏结 *hán shī bó jié*]

- binding depression of liver qì [肝气郁结 *gān qì yù jié*]

- blood stasis collecting [瘀血停着 *yū xuè tíng zhī*]

- insufficiency of liver yīn [肝阴不足 *gān yīn bù zú*]

11.1   POINTS OF ATTENTION FOR INTERCOSTAL NEURALGIA

11.1.1 Physiology

The liver and gallbladder channels travel across the area of the ribs, thus intercostal neuralgia is closely linked with pathological changes of liver and gallbladder functions.

The characteristic pathology of all types of intercostal neuralgia is binding depression of liver qì, which inhibits the coursing and blocks free movement of qì-blood.

11.1.2 Pathology

After some time, repletion patterns [实证 *shí zhèng*], i.e., qì stagnation and blood stasis, tend to transform into heat and damage yīn, and thus change into vacuity-repletion complexes [虚实错杂 *xū shí cuò zá*].

11.1.3 Differentiating the Nature of Pain

Qì Stagnation

When intercostal neuralgia results from qì stagnation, usually there is a scurrying pain [窜痛 *cuàn tòng*] that appears and disappears in waves. Such pain is set off or exacerbated by emotional discomfort.

Blood Stasis

If blood stasis is the cause, the pain tends to be stabbing pain [刺痛 *cì tòng*] that is in a fixed location and that is worse during the night and lighter during the day; the tongue is purple.

Vacuity

Vacuity is marked by dull pain [隐痛 *yǐn tòng*]; there may be a long course of disease, and the pain is exacerbated by fatigue.

11.2 CAUSES AND PATHOMECHANISM OF INTERCOSTAL NEURALGIA; IDENTIFYING PATTERNS

11.2.1 Evil Invading the Lesser Yáng Channel [邪犯少阳 *xié fàn shào yáng*]

Causes and Pathomechanism of Evil Invading the Lesser Yáng Channel

When external evil assails the ribs and gets lodged in the lesser yáng channel [少阳经 *shào yáng jīng*], there is a struggle between right and evil in which the evil can transform into heat. Evil heat stagnates and inhibits the coursing function of the liver-gallbladder, which blocks the movement of channel qì and causes rib-side pain.

Important Signs of Evil Invading the Lesser Yáng Channel

Pain in the rib-side, chest, and back. Pain is strong in the chest and below the armpits. Breathing is not smooth. Alternating heat [effusion] and [aversion to] cold [寒热往来 *hán rè wǎng lái*], fullness in the chest and rib-side [胸胁苦满 *xiōng xié kǔ mǎn*]. Dizziness, dizzy vision. Distention in the corner of the forehead. Bitter taste in the mouth, dry throat. Vexation, retching [呕 *ǒu*]. The tongue has thin white fur [舌苔薄白 *shé tāi bó bái*]. Stringlike pulse [脉弦 *mài xián*].

11.2.2 Congealing Cold-Damp [寒湿搏结 *hán shī bó jié*]

Causes and Pathomechanism of Congealing Cold-Damp

Dampness has a downward tendency and is heavy [重着 *zhòng zhuó*]; cold governs congealing [凝滞 *níng zhì*] and contracture and tautness [收引 *shōu yǐn*].

When cold-damp evil accumulates and binds in the chest, rib-side, and back, it inhibits the normal flow of qì and blood and blocks the channels.

Important Signs of Congealing Cold-Damp

Pain in the rib-side, the chest, and the back. Pain is in a fixed location and may spread to the lumbus. Numbness, tingling [麻木 *má mù*], and feeling of heaviness in the skin and muscles. Pain is exacerbated by yīn-type weather [阴雨天 *yīn yǔ tiān*].[9] The tongue has white slimy fur [苔白腻 *tāi bái nì*]. Soggy and moderate pulse [脉濡缓 *mài rú huǎn*].

11.2.3 Binding Depression of Liver Qì [肝气郁结 *gān qì yù jié*]

Causes and Pathomechanism of Binding Depression of Liver Qì

Affect-mind binding depression [情志郁结 *qíng zhì yù jié*] or sudden bursts of anger damage the liver and cause binding depression of liver qì. The depressed qì dynamic blocks the network vessels in the rib-side, giving rise to pain.

Important Signs of Binding Depression of Liver Qì

Distending pain [胀痛 *zhàng tòng*] in the rib-side. Scurrying pain [窜痛 *cuàn tòng*] that wanders from one location to the other. Pain is exacerbated by emotional discomfort and diminished by emotional balance. Oppression and discomfort in the chest. Reduced food intake, belching. The tongue has thin white fur [薄白苔 *bó bái tāi*]. Stringlike pulse [脉弦 *mài xián*].

11.2.4 Blood Stasis Collecting [瘀血停着 *yū xuè tíng zhì*]

Causes and Pathomechanism of Blood Stasis Collecting

Qì is the commander of blood [气为血之帅 *qì wéi xuè zhī shuài*], and blood relies on the moving force of qì to move in the vessels. Thus, when qì stagnates, blood also stagnates. Enduring binding depression of liver qì with a depressed qì dynamic will, after some time, cause blood stasis. Furthermore, external injury that damages the rib-side network vessels results in blood stasis that gives rise to stoppage and pain.

Important Signs of Blood Stasis Collecting

Stabbing pain [刺痛 *cì tòng*] in the rib-side. Such pain has a fixed location and is exacerbated during the night. There may be palpable lumps under the rib-side. Dark purple tongue [舌紫暗 *shé zǐ àn*]. Deep rough pulse [脉沉涩 *mài chén sè*].

---

[9] Yīn -type weather refers to cloudy, damp, and/or rainy weather. (Ed.)

11.2.5   Insufficiency of Liver Yīn [肝阴不足 *gān yīn bù zú*]

Causes and Pathomechanism of Insufficiency of Liver Yīn

Insufficiency of liver yīn can be caused by enduring liver depression that transforms into fire [化火 *huà huǒ*] and damages yīn. It is also caused by liver-kidney yīn depletion, because the liver and kidney are of the same source [肝肾同源 *gān shèn tóng yuán*]. Sexual taxation [房劳 *fáng láo*] or weakness after an enduring illness leads to kidney essence depletion and wearing [耗 *hào*] of yīn-blood. Essence-blood vacuity can lead to liver yīn insufficiency, for when blood is vacuous it does not properly nourish the liver. As a result, the channels and network vessels lack nourishment, and loss of luxuriance [荣 *róng*] gives rise to pain.

Important Signs of Insufficiency of Liver Yīn

Continuous dull pain [隐痛 *yǐn tòng*] in the rib-side. Pain is exacerbated by fatigue. Dry mouth and throat. Heat vexation [烦热 *fán rè*] in the chest. Dizziness, dizzy vision. Red tongue with scant fur [舌红少苔 *shé hóng shǎo tāi*]. Fine stringlike rapid pulse [脉细弦数 *mài xì xián shuò*].

11.3   TREATMENT OF INTERCOSTAL NEURALGIA USING CHINESE MEDICINALS

11.3.1   Evil Invading the Lesser Yáng Channel [邪犯少阳 *xié fàn shào yáng*]

Method of Treatment for Evil Invading the Lesser Yáng Channel

Harmonize lesser yáng, course the liver, and check pain [和解少阳，疏肝止痛 *hé jiě shào yáng, shū gān zhǐ tòng*].

Minor Bupleurum Decoction [小柴胡汤 *xiǎo chái hú tāng*]	
bupleurum [柴胡 *chái hú*, Bupleuri Radix]	12g
scutellaria [黄芩 *huáng qín*, Scutellariae Radix]	9g
ginseng [人参 *rén shēn*, Ginseng Radix]	9g
licorice [甘草 *gān cǎo*, Glycyrrhizae Radix]	6g
fresh ginger [生姜 *shēng jiāng*, Zingiberis Rhizoma Recens]	9g
pinellia [半夏 *bàn xià*, Pinelliae Rhizoma]	9g
jujube [大枣 *dà zǎo*, Jujubae Fructus]	4 fruits
Directions: Take decocted with water [水煎服 *shuǐ jiān fú*].	

Prescription Analysis

Chief Medicinal

Bupleurum is used as the chief medicinal to harmonize the half-exterior half-interior [半表半里 *bàn biǎo bàn lǐ*] pattern of lesser yáng and to course the liver and resolve depression [疏肝解郁 *shū gān jiě yù*], thus checking pain.

Support Medicinal

Scutellaria helps bupleurum clear the evil of the reverting yīn liver channel and the lesser yáng gallbladder channel.

Assistant Medicinals

Ginseng, pinellia, fresh ginger, and jujube support the middle burner [中焦 *zhōng jiāo*]. This both helps the lesser yáng to expel evil and prevents the evil in lesser yáng from passing further into the body and assailling greater yīn [太阴 *tài yīn*]. This is what is meant by: "When seeing a liver disease, one knows that the liver disease tends to pass to the spleen, and it is appropriate to first strengthen the spleen" [见肝之病，知肝传脾， 当先实脾 *jiàn gān zhī bìng, zhī gān chuán pí, dàng xiān shí pí*].

Licorice serves as conductor medicinal, harmonizes the properties of all the medicinals [调和药性 *tiáo hé yào xìng*], and supports right qì [正气 *zhèng qì*].

This combination of medicinals resolves the lesser yáng [解少阳 *jiě shào yáng*], courses the liver, and checks pain. When the lesser yáng is resolved and liver qì flows uninhibited, then intercostal pain will stop.

Variation According to Signs

To further course the liver and check pain [疏肝止痛 *shū gān zhǐ tòng*], add toosendan [*chuān liàn zǐ*] and corydalis [延胡索 *yán hú suǒ*].

The original indication for this prescription was lesser yáng disease [少阳病 *shào yáng bìng*] with the symptoms of alternating fever and chills [寒热往来 *hán rè wǎng lái*], fullness in the chest and rib-side [胸胁苦满 *xiōng xié kǔ mǎn*], bitter taste in the mouth, and dry pharynx [口苦咽干 *kǒu kǔ yān gān*]. In addition to lesser yáng disease, this prescription may be used for miscellaneous diseases such as malaria or jaundice, or for postpartum common cold or common cold during menstruation when the above symptoms are present; modify the prescription according to the individual patient.

11.3.2 Congealing Cold-Damp [寒湿搏结 *hán shī bó jié*]

Method of Treatment for Congealing Cold-Damp

Dispel wind, overcome dampness, and check pain [祛风胜湿止痛 *qū fēng shèng shī zhǐ tòng*].

Notopterygium Dampness-Overcoming Decoction [羌活胜湿汤 *qiāng huó shèng shī tāng*]	
notopterygium [羌活 *qiāng huó*, Notopterygii Rhizoma et Radix]	6g
pubescent angelica [独活 *dú huó*, Angelicae Pubescentis Radix]	6g
Chinese lovage [藁本 *gǎo běn*, Ligustici Rhizoma]	4g
saposhnikovia [防风 *fáng fēng*, Saposhnikoviae Radix]	4g
honey-fried licorice [炙甘草 *zhì gān cǎo*, Glycyrrhizae Radix Preparata]	4g
chuanxiong [川芎 *chuān xiōng*, Chuanxiong Rhizoma]	4g
vitex [蔓荆子 *màn jīng zǐ*, Viticis Fructus]	2g
Directions: Take decocted with water [水煎服 *shuǐ jiān fú*].	

Prescription Analysis

Chief Medicinal

Notopterygium is used as the chief medicinal because its acrid-dissipating and warm-freeing qualities [辛散温通 *xīn sàn wēn tōng*] dispel wind, overcome dampness, and check pain.

Support Medicinals

Pubescent angelica assists notopterygium in dispelling wind, overcoming dampness, and checking pain. Saposhnikovia dispels wind and dries dampness. Chuanxiong quickens blood, frees the channels, and checks pain.

Assistant Medicinals

Chinese lovage and vitex dispel wind and relieve headaches.

Honey-fried licorice harmonizes the properties of all the medicinals [调和药性 *tiáo hé yào xìng*], relaxes tension [缓急 *huǎn jí*], and checks pain.

This combination of medicinals dispels wind, overcomes dampness, and checks pain. Once wind-damp is dispelled and construction and blood are harmonized, the pain naturally stops.

Variation According to Signs

For generalized heaviness and a sense of heaviness in the lumbus that result from cold-damp in the channels, add fangji [*fáng jǐ*]. For patients with lighter symptoms add aconite [*fù zǐ*], with stronger symptoms add wild aconite [*cǎo wū tóu*]. This is in order to warm the channels and dissipate cold and to reinforce yáng [助阳 *zhù yáng*] and transform dampness.

11.3.3   Binding Depression of Liver Qì [肝气郁结 *gān qì yù jié*]

Method of Treatment for Binding Depression of Liver Qì

Course the liver and move qì, quicken blood and check pain [疏肝行气，活血止痛 *shū gān xíng qì, huó xuè zhǐ tòng*].

Bupleurum Liver-Coursing Powder [柴胡疏肝散 *chái hú shū gān sǎn*]	
bupleurum [柴胡 *chái hú*, Bupleuri Radix]	6g
tangerine peel [陈皮 *chén pí*, Citri Reticulatae Pericarpium]	6g
white peony [白芍 *bái sháo*, Paeoniae Radix Alba]	5g
bitter orange [枳壳 *zhǐ ké*, Aurantii Fructus]	5g
chuanxiong [川芎 *chuān xiōng*, Chuanxiong Rhizoma]	5g
cyperus [香附 *xiāng fù*, Cyperi Rhizoma]	5g
honey-fried licorice [炙甘草 *zhì gān cǎo*, Glycyrrhizae Radix Preparata]	3g
Directions: Take decocted with water [水煎服 *shuǐ jiān fú*].	

Prescription Analysis

Chief Medicinals

Use bupleurum to course the liver, resolve depression [解郁 *jiě yù*], move qì, and check pain.

Support Medicinals

Chuanxiong quickens blood, moves qì, and checks pain; it is considered the qì medicinal amongst the blood medicinals [血中之气药 *xuè zhōng zhī qì yào*] and helps bupleurum move qì, quicken blood, and check pain. Cyperus is considered the "commander in chief of qì diseases," but is equally important in gynecological diseases. It moves qì and quickens blood, and it supports bupleurum in coursing the liver and moving qì.

Assistant Medicinals

Tangerine peel and bitter orange rectify qì [理气 *lǐ qì*] and harmonize the middle burner. White peony emolliates the liver [柔肝 *róu gān*] and checks pain.

Honey-fried licorice harmonizes the properties of all other medicinals. It is combined with white peony to form Peony and Licorice Decoction, which relaxes tension [缓急 *huǎn jí*] and checks pain.

This combination of medicinals is used to course the liver and move qì and to quicken blood and check pain. Once the binding depression of liver qì is removed and qì and blood move freely, the pain will stop.

Variations According to Signs

If liver depression transforms into fire and the patient suffers from vexation and agitation [烦躁 *fán zào*] and has a red tongue, add toosendan [*chuān liàn zǐ*] and corydalis [*yán hú suǒ*] to reinforce the function of coursing the liver and checking pain.

11.3.4 Blood Stasis Collecting [瘀血停着 *yū xuè tíng zhì*]

Method of Treatment for Blood Stasis Collecting

Quicken blood and transform stasis, move qì and check pain [活血祛瘀，行气止痛 *huó xuè qū yū, xíng qì zhǐ tòng*].

House of Blood Stasis-Expelling Decoction [血府逐瘀汤 *xuè fǔ zhú yū tāng*]	
peach kernel [桃仁 *táo rén*, Persicae Semen]	12g
carthamus [红花 *hóng huā*, Carthami Flos]	9g
Chinese angelica [当归 *dāng guī*, Angelicae Sinensis Radix]	9g
dried/fresh rehmannia [生地黄 *shēng dì huáng*, Rehmanniae Radix seu Recens]	9g
chuanxiong [川芎 *chuān xiōng*, Chuanxiong Rhizoma]	9g
red peony [赤芍 *chì sháo*, Paeoniae Radix Rubra]	6g
achyranthes [牛膝 *niú xī*, Achyranthis Bidentatae Radix]	9g
platycodon [桔梗 *jié gěng*, Platycodonis Radix]	5g
bupleurum [柴胡 *chái hú*, Bupleuri Radix]	3g
bitter orange [枳壳 *zhǐ ké*, Aurantii Fructus]	6g
licorice [甘草 *gān cǎo*, Glycyrrhizae Radix]	3g
Directions: Take decocted with water [水煎服 *shuǐ jiān fú*].	

Prescription Analysis

Chief Medicinals

Peach kernel, carthamus, red peony, chuanxiong, Chinese angelica, and achyranthes are used as chief medicinals to quicken blood, transform stasis, and check pain.

Support Medicinals

When qì moves this also causes blood to move [气行则血行 *qì xíng zé xuè xíng*]; thus, moving qì will help to move blood. Bupleurum courses the liver and moves qì. Platycodon opens and diffuses lung qì [开宣肺气 *kāi xuān fèi qì*]. Bitter orange opens the chest and rectifies qì [理气 *lǐ qì*].

Assistant Medicinals

Dried/fresh rehmannia supplements blood and nourishes yīn. This prevents the blood-quickening and stasis-dispelling medicinals from damaging yīn-blood [伤阴血 *shāng yīn xuè*].

Licorice harmonizes the actions of the other medicinals.

This prescription not only moves blood and dispels stasis without damaging blood, but also dispels depression and stagnation of the qì aspect [气分 *qì fēn*]. It dispels stasis and moves qì so that the pain will stop.

Variation According to Signs

House of Blood Stasis-Expelling Decoction is frequently used to treat intercostal neuralgia caused by blood stasis collecting and shows reliable results in clinical practice. For very severe pain, however, add corydalis [*yán hú suǒ*], turmeric [*jiāng huáng*], and scorpion [*quán xiē*] to reinforce the prescription.

11.3.5 Insufficiency of Liver Yīn [肝阴不足 *gān yīn bù zú*]

Method of Treatment for Insufficiency of Liver Yīn

Enrich and nourish the liver and kidney, course the liver and rectify qì [滋养肝肾，疏肝理气 *zī yǎng gān shèn, shū gān lǐ qì*].

All-the-Way-Through Brew [一贯煎 *yī guàn jiān*]	
adenophora/glehnia [沙参 *shā shēn*, Adenophorae Radix][10]	10g
ophiopogon [麦冬 *mài dōng*, Ophiopogonis Radix]	10g
Chinese angelica [当归 *dāng guī*, Angelicae Sinensis Radix]	10g
dried/fresh rehmannia [生地黄 *shēng dì huáng*, Rehmanniae Radix seu Recens]	30g
lycium berry [枸杞子 *gǒu qǐ zǐ*, Lycii Fructus]	12g
toosendan [川楝子 *chuān liàn zǐ*, Toosendan Fructus]	5g
Directions: Take decocted with water [水煎服 *shuǐ jiān fú*].	

Prescription Analysis

Chief Medicinal

Dried/fresh rehmannia is used as the chief medicinal to enrich yīn and nourish blood and thereby supplement the liver and kidney.

---

[10] There are two types of [沙参 *shā shēn*], both of which are used to clear the lungs and nourish yin1 and to boost the stomach and engender liquid. One of them is adenophora [南沙参 *nán shā shēn*, Adenophorae Radix], which also dispels phlegm; the other is glehnia [北沙参 *beǐ shā shēn*, Glehniae Radix], whose strong point lies in enriching yīn.

Support Medicinals

Glehnia, ophiopogon, Chinese angelica, and lycium berry boost yīn and emolliate the liver [益阴柔肝 *yì yīn róu gān*]. Together with the chief medicinal they enrich yīn, nourish blood, and engender liquid [生津 *shēng jīn*].

Assistant Medicinal

A small quantity of toosendan courses the liver and, although bitter and dry in quality, will not damage liquids because it is combined with large quantities of sweet cold medicinals that nourish yīn.

This combination of medicinals nourishes liver yīn and courses liver qì, thus stopping the pain.

Variations According to Signs

This prescription is frequently used to treat intercostal neuralgia caused by insufficiency of liver yīn. Through long clinical experience with this prescription, Dr. Wèi Liǔ-Zhōu [魏柳州] has developed the following variations: If the patient has bitter and dry mouth, add wine-fried Sichuan coptis [*chuān huáng lián*]. If there is vacuity heat or profuse sweating, add lycium root bark [*dì gǔ pí*]. For copious phlegm add fritillaria [*bèi mǔ*]. If the tongue is red and dry and if yīn is extremely depleted [阴亏 *yīn kuī*], add dendrobium [*shí hú*]. If the costal region has distending pain and is hard to the touch, add turtle shell [*biē jiǎ*]. For heat vexation [烦热 *fán rè*] and thirst, add anemarrhena [*zhī mǔ*] and gypsum [*shí gāo*]. For abdominal pain, add white peony [*bái sháo*] and licorice [*gān cǎo*]. For weak legs, add achyranthes [*niú xī*]. For sleeplessness, add spiny jujube kernel [*suān zǎo rén*].

11.4   ACUPUNCTURE TREATMENT FOR INTERCOSTAL NEURALGIA

11.4.1   Evil Invading the Lesser Yáng Channel [邪犯少阳 *xié fàn shào yáng*]

Treatment Method

Harmonize lesser yáng [和解少阳 *hé jiě shào yáng*].

Points for Evil Invading the Lesser Yáng Channel [邪犯少阳 *xié fàn shào yáng*]
LR-3 Supreme Surge [太冲 *tài chōng*] GB-40 Hill Ruins [丘墟 *qiū xū*]

Prescription Analysis

GB-40 is the source point [原穴 *yuán xué*] of the foot lesser yáng gallbladder channel, while LR-3 is the source point of the foot reverting yīn liver channel. The liver and gallbladder stand in exterior-interior relationship. Needling the source points of both channels stimulates the channel qì, harmonizes the lesser yáng, and dispels evil [祛邪 *qū xié*], thus checking pain.

11.4.2 Congealing Cold-Damp [寒湿搏结 *hán shī bó jié*]

Treatment Method for Congealing Cold-Damp

Dispel cold and disinhibit dampness [祛寒利湿 *qū hán lì shī*].

Points for Congealing Cold-Damp [寒湿搏结 *hán shī bó jié*]
LR-5 Woodworm Canal [蠡沟 *lǐ gōu*] Moxibustion at local points

Prescription Analysis

Local moxibustion dispels cold evil. LR-5 clears and disinhibits liver-gallbladder damp evil.

11.4.3 Binding Depression of Liver Qì [肝气郁结 *gān qì yù jié*]

Treatment Method for Binding Depression of Liver Qì

Course the liver and rectify qì [疏肝理气 *shū gān lǐ qì*].

Points for Binding Depression of Liver Qì [肝气郁结 *gān qì yù jié*]
LR-3 Supreme Surge [太冲 *tài chōng*] PC-6 Inner Pass [内关 *nèi guān*] LR-14 Cycle Gate [期门 *qī mén*]

Prescription Analysis

Both LR-3 and PC-6 course the liver and rectify qì [疏肝理气 *shū gān lǐ qì*].

PC-6 is a point of the yīn linking vessel [阴维脉 *yīn wéi mài*], which connects to the foot greater yīn, foot lesser yīn, and foot reverting yīn channels and also meets with the conception vessel and unites with the foot yáng brightness channel. All these channels pass through the chest and ribs, thus the yīn linking vessel strongly influences the chest (and heart). PC-6 is particularly effective in treating pains of the chest and rib-side. It is also a major point for treating obstruction of the qì dynamic.

LR-3 is selected both because of its location on the affected channel [循经取 穴 *xún jīng qǔ xué*] and according to the pattern identified [辨证取穴 *biàn zhèng qǔ xué*]. It is often combined with LR-14 to course the liver and rectify qì.

LR-14 is an alarm point [募穴 *mù xué*] and is located on the ribs. It moves qì [行气 *xíng qì*] and its major indication is rib-side pain, particularly rib-side pain caused by binding depression of liver qì [肝气郁结 *gān qì yù jié*].

11.4.4   Blood Stasis Collecting [瘀血停着 *yū xuè tíng zhì*]

Treatment Method for Blood Stasis Collecting

Quicken the blood and free the vessels [活血通脉 *huó xuè tōng mài*].

Points for Blood Stasis Collecting [瘀血停着 *yū xuè tíng zhì*]
SI-6 Nursing the Aged [养老 *yǎng lǎo*]
Local bloodletting–i.e., network vessel pricking [刺络放血 *cì luò fàng xuè*]–can be performed as well.

Prescription Analysis

Local bloodletting dissipates blood stasis.

SI-6 is the cleft point [郄穴 *xī xué*] of the hand greater yáng small intestine channel. The cleft points are where qì and blood accumulate, and they are mostly used in acute patterns, especially in the treatment of pain. SI-6 is a point validated by clinical experience for the treatment of intercostal neuralgia.

11.4.5   Insufficiency of Liver Yīn [肝阴不足 *gān yīn bù zú*]

Treatment Method for Insufficiency of Liver Yīn

Enrich the liver and kidney [滋养肝肾 *zī yǎng gān shèn*].

Points for Insufficiency of Liver Yīn [肝阴不足 *gān yīn bù zú*]
KI-7 Recover Flow [复溜 *fù liū*]
LR-8 Spring at the Bend [曲泉 *qū quán*]

Prescription Analysis

KI-7 nourishes kidney yīn, and nourishing kidney yīn indirectly nourishes liver yīn; since wood (liver) is engendered by water (kidney) in the five phases [五行 *wǔ xíng*]. This treatment is called "enriching water to moisten wood" [滋水涵木 *zī shuǐ hán mù*].

LR-8 is the uniting point [合穴 *hé xué*] of the liver channel, and the uniting points of the yīn channels correspond to water. According to five-phase correspondences, because the liver corresponds to wood, which is engendered by water, LR-8, which corresponds to water, is therefore able to nourish yīn and moisten the liver [养阴濡肝 *yǎng yīn rú gān*].

CHAPTER 12

Herpes Zoster

Herpes zoster is also known as shingles. According to Western medicine, it is caused by the same virus that causes chickenpox. But in herpes zoster, the virus gives rise to an inflammation of the sensory ganglia of spinal and cranial nerves. This disease starts with pain along the distribution of a nerve in the face, chest, or abdomen, and later there are eruptions of fluid-filled blisters on the area of skin along the distribution of the affected nerve. The afflicted area is extremely sensitive and painful.

There are four main forms:

- liver-gallbladder exuberant heat [肝胆热盛 *gān dǎn rè shèng*]
- damp-heat in the spleen channel [脾经湿热 *pí jīng shī rè*]
- qì stagnation and blood stasis [气滞血瘀 *qì zhì xuè yū*]
- yīn depletion blood stagnation [阴亏血滞 *yīn kuī xuè zhì*]

12.1 POINTS OF ATTENTION FOR HERPES ZOSTER

12.1.1 Pathomechanism

The disease often starts out as a damp-heat pattern and later develops qì-blood stagnation. The pathological changes occur in the liver and spleen. Possible causes are:

- affect-mind internal damage [情志内伤 *qíng zhì nèi shāng*] that gives rise to liver-gallbladder fire
- eating too many spicy, greasy, and/or sweet foods that engender damp-heat
- spleen vacuity that gives rise to dampness which, after enduring depression, transforms into heat

- Liver fire and damp-heat bind and obstruct the channels and network vessels, causing stoppage of qì-blood and pain. While herpes zoster has a damp-heat pathomechanism, it is important to establish whether damp or heat is more pronounced.

Pathomechanism of the Skin Symptoms

Heat-toxin brewing in the blood aspect [血分 *xuè fēn*] is responsible for red patches on the skin. When vacuous spleen does not move dampness, water accumulates in the skin and damp-heat congealing is responsible for the fluid-filled blisters.

12.2 CAUSES AND PATHOMECHANISM OF HERPES ZOSTER; IDENTIFYING PATTERNS

12.2.1 Liver-Gallbladder Exuberant Heat [肝胆热盛 *gān dǎn rè shèng*]

Causes and Pathomechanism of Liver-Gallbladder Exuberant Heat

This pattern may result from emotional disharmony impeding the liver's function of free coursing [疏泄 *shū xiè*]; in this case, liver depression transforms into fire [肝郁化火 *gān yù huà huǒ*] and gives rise to liver-gallbladder fire. Another possibility is toxin evil [毒邪 *dú xié*] assailing the interior, which intensifies the damp-heat brewing in the liver and gallbladder. Here, damp-heat congests in the skin and forms fluid-filled blisters. In this pattern, heat is more pronounced than dampness.

Important Signs of Liver-Gallbladder Exuberant Heat

Red skin, eruption of tight, fluid-filled blisters. Scorching hot pain [灼热痛 *zhuó rè tòng*] or itching of the affected skin. Bitter taste in the mouth, dry throat. Dry stool. The tongue is red with yellow fur [舌质红苔黄 *shé zhì hóng tāi huáng*]. Stringlike rapid pulse [脉弦数 *mài xián shuò*].

12.2.2 Damp-Heat in the Spleen Channel [脾经湿热 *pí jīng shī rè*]

Causes and Pathomechanism of Damp-Heat in the Spleen Channel

Damp-heat in the spleen channel results from eating too many spicy, greasy, sweet, and/or rich foods that damage the spleen and impair its function of movement and transformation [运化 *yùn huà*]. This causes water-damp to collect and, after prolonged brewing [蕴 *yùn*], transform into heat. The result is damp-heat binding internally that obstructs the channels and network vessels. In this pattern, damp is more pronounced than heat.

Important Signs of Damp-Heat in the Spleen Channel

Eruption of soft fluid-filled blisters that burst easily. Pain is not severe. Torpid intake [纳呆 *nà dāi*], distention in the abdomen. Dry stool. Yellow slimy tongue fur [舌苔黄腻 *shé tāi huáng nì*]. Soggy slippery or slippery rapid pulse [脉濡滑或滑数 *mài rú huá huò huá shuò*].

12.2.3   Qì Stagnation and Blood Stasis [气滞血瘀 *qì zhì xuè yū*]

Causes and Pathomechanism of Qì Stagnation and Blood Stasis

After herpes zoster has endured for a long time, enduring liver depression [肝郁 *gān yù*] can result in qì stagnation and blood stasis. In short, this pattern is the development of another pattern.

Important Signs of Qì Stagnation and Blood Stasis

Often seen in old people. Severe pain persists even after the fluid-filled blisters heal. There may be oppression in the chest [胸闷 *xiōng mèn*] and frequent sighing. Dark purple tongue, thin fur [舌质紫, 苔薄 *shé zhì zǐ, tāi bó*]. Rough or stringlike pulse [脉涩或弦 *mài sè huò xián*].

12.2.4   Yīn Depletion Blood Stagnation [阴亏血滞 *yīn kuī xuè zhì*]

Causes and Pathomechanism of Yīn Depletion Blood Stagnation

After herpes zoster has endured for a long time, it may also progressively damage yīn. When yīn is depleted the liver channel is not properly nourished, which results in dull pain [隐痛 *yǐn tòng*].

Important Signs of Yīn Depletion Blood Stagnation

After the fluid-filled blisters heal there is dull or stabbing pain in the rib-side and chest. Dry mouth and throat. The tongue has peeling fur or scant liquid [苔花剥或少津 *tāi huā bō huò shǎo jīn*]. Stringlike and thin pulse [脉弦细 *mài xián xì*].

12.3   TREATMENT OF HERPES ZOSTER USING CHINESE MEDICINALS

12.3.1   Liver-Gallbladder Exuberant Heat [肝胆热盛 *gān dǎn rè shèng*]

Method of Treatment for Liver-Gallbladder Exuberant Heat

Drain liver-gallbladder repletion fire, disinhibit triple burner damp-heat [泻肝胆实火，利三焦湿热 *xiè gān dǎn shí huǒ, lì sān jiāo shī rè*].

Gentian Liver-Draining Decoction [龙胆泻肝汤 *lóng dǎn xiè gān tāng*]	
gentian [龙胆草 *lóng dǎn cǎo*, Gentianae Radix]	6g
bupleurum [柴胡 *chái hú*, Bupleuri Radix]	6g
alisma [泽泻 *zé xiè*, Alismatis Rhizoma]	12g
plantago seed [车前子 *chē qián zǐ*, Plantaginis Semen]	9g
trifoliate akebia [木通 *mù tōng*, Akebiae Trifoliatae Caulis]	9g
dried/fresh rehmannia [生地黄 *shēng dì huáng*, Rehmanniae Radix seu Recens]	9g
Chinese angelica [当归 *dāng guī*, Angelicae Sinensis Radix]	3g
gardenia [栀子 *zhī zǐ*, Gardeniae Fructus]	9g
scutellaria [黄芩 *huáng qín*, Scutellariae Radix]	9g
licorice [甘草 *gān cǎo*, Glycyrrhizae Radix]	6g

Directions: Take decocted with water [水煎服 *shuǐ jiān fú*].

Prescription Analysis

Chief Medicinal

Gentian, which is extremely bitter and cold, is used to clear and drain liver-gallbladder repletion fire and to clear and disinhibit lower burner damp-heat.

Support Medicinals

The bitter and cold properties of scutellaria and gardenia drain fire [泻火 *xiè huǒ*] and help the chief medicinal to clear and drain liver-gallbladder repletion heat.

Assistant Medicinals

Alisma, trifoliate akebia, and plantago seed clear heat and disinhibit dampness as well as conduct fire out through the urine [引火从小便而出 *yǐn huǒ cóng xiǎo biàn ér chū*].

The liver stores blood [肝藏血 *gān cáng xuè*]. Therefore, heat in the liver easily damages yīn-blood. This is why the prescription uses Chinese angelica to supplement and quicken blood and dried/fresh rehmannia to nourish blood and boost yīn [养血益阴 *yǎng xuè yì yīn*]. Bupleurum courses liver-gallbladder depression [疏肝胆郁滞 *shū gān dǎn yù zhì*].

Licorice [*gān cǎo*] harmonizes the actions of all the other medicinals.

Using this combination of medicinals effectively supplements within draining [泻中有补 *xiè zhōng yǒu bǔ*] and nourishes within clearing [清中有养 *qīng zhōng yǒu yǎng*]. When liver-gallbladder repletion fire is drained, liver channel damp-heat is cleared, blood is nourished, and yīn is boosted.

Variation According to Signs

If the patient shows signs of vigorous heat [壮热 *zhuàng rè*], add crude gypsum [生石膏 *shēng shí gāo*]. If the patient also suffers from constipation, add rhubarb [*dà huáng*]. For localized severe pain, add frankincense [*rǔ xiāng*] and myrrh [*mò yào*]. If the upper extremities are involved, add turmeric [*jiāng huáng*] and cinnamon twig [*guì zhī*]. If the face is involved, add arctium [*niú bàng zǐ*] and wild chrysanthemum flower [*yě jú huā*].

12.3.2   Damp-Heat in the Spleen Channel [脾经湿热 *pí jīng shī rè*]

Method of Treatment for Damp-Heat in the Spleen Channel

Fortify the spleen and disinhibit dampness [健脾利湿 *jiàn pí lì shī*].

Dampness-Eliminating Stomach-Calming Poria Five Decoction **[除湿胃苓汤 *chú shī wèi líng tāng*]**	
atractylodes [苍术 *cāng zhú*, Atractylodis Rhizoma]	10g
white atractylodes [白术 *bái zhú*, Atractylodis Macrocephalae Rhizoma]	10g
official magnolia bark [厚朴 *hòu pò*, Magnoliae Officinalis Cortex]	9g
tangerine peel [陈皮 *chén pí*, Citri Reticulatae Pericarpium]	9g
poria [茯苓 *fú líng*, Poria]	12g
polyporus [猪苓 *zhū líng*, Polyporus]	15g
talcum [滑石 *huá shí*, Talcum]	15g
trifoliate akebia [木通 *mù tōng*, Akebiae Trifoliatae Caulis]	6g
licorice [甘草 *gān cǎo*, Glycyrrhizae Radix]	3g

Directions: Take decocted with water [水煎服 *shuǐ jiān fú*].

Prescription Analysis

Chief Medicinals

Atractylodes and white atractylodes dry dampness and fortify the spleen [燥湿健脾 *zào shī jiàn pí*], thus treating the root [治本 *zhì běn*].

Support Medicinals

Poria and polyporus disinhibit water and percolate dampness [利水渗湿 *lì shuǐ shèn shī*] to help the chief medicinals dispel dampness.

Assistant Medicinals

When qì moves then water also moves [气行则水行 *qì xíng zé shuǐ xíng*]; thus, the prescription uses tangerine peel and official magnolia bark to move qì and loosen the center [宽中 *kuān zhōng*].

Talcum and trifoliate akebia disinhibit the bladder to dispel dampness.

Licorice harmonizes the properties of all the medicinals [调和药性 *tiáo hé yào xìng*].

This combination of medicinals fortifies the spleen and disinhibits dampness. When damp evil is dispelled, all symptoms will disappear.

Variation According to Signs

If damp evil is severe and there are many vesicles, add agastache [*huò xiāng*], eupatorium [*pèi lán*], areca husk [*dà fù pí*], and plantago seed [*chē qián zǐ*] to reinforce the damp-dispelling action. If the heat toxin is extreme, add lonicera [*jīn yín huā*], gardenia [*zhī zǐ*], smooth greenbrier root [*tǔ fú líng*], and moutan [*mǔ dān pí*] to clear heat, cool blood, and resolve toxin.

12.3.3 Qì Stagnation and Blood Stasis [气滞血瘀 *qì zhì xuè yū*]

Method of Treatment for Qì Stagnation and Blood Stasis

Course the liver and rectify qì, quicken blood and check pain [疏肝理气, 活血止痛 *shū gān lǐ qì, huó xuè zhǐ tòng*].

Bupleurum Liver-Coursing Powder [柴胡疏肝散 *chái hú shū gān sǎn*]	
bupleurum [柴胡 *chái hú*, Bupleuri Radix]	6g
tangerine peel [陈皮 *chén pí*, Citri Reticulatae Pericarpium]	6g
white peony [白芍 *bái sháo*, Paeoniae Radix Alba]	5g
bitter orange [枳壳 *zhǐ ké*, Aurantii Fructus]	5g
chuanxiong [川芎 *chuān xiōng*, Chuanxiong Rhizoma]	5g
cyperus [香附 *xiāng fù*, Cyperi Rhizoma]	5g
honey-fried licorice [炙甘草 *zhì gān cǎo*, Glycyrrhizae Radix Preparata]	2g
Directions: Take decocted with water [水煎服 *shuǐ jiān fú*].	

Prescription Analysis

Chief Medicinals

Bupleurum courses the liver and resolves depression; chuanxiong quickens blood and checks pain. Both medicinals treat the root [治本 *zhì běn*].

Support Medicinals

Tangerine peel and bitter orange help the chief medicinals rectify qì and loosen the chest [宽胸 *kuān xiōng*], while white peony helps the chief medicinals regulate blood [调血 *tiáo xuè*].

Assistant Medicinals

Cyperus is one of the main medicinals for qì diseases and has an important function in gynecological diseases. It rectifies qì and regulates blood.

Honey-fried licorice and white peony make up Peony and Licorice Decoction [芍药甘草汤 *sháo yào gān cǎo tāng*], which relaxes tension and checks pain [缓急止痛 *huǎn jí zhǐ tòng*]. Honey-fried licorice also harmonizes the properties of all the medicinals [调和药性 *tiáo hé yào xìng*].

This combination of medicinals is effectively used to course the liver and rectify qì and to quicken blood and check pain.

Variation According to Signs

Bupleurum Liver-Coursing Powder is effective for moving qì and coursing the liver, but its power to quicken blood and check pain might be insufficient for this pattern. For such cases, add peach kernel [*táo rén*], carthamus [*hóng huā*], moutan [*mǔ dān pí*], red peony [*chì sháo*], and corydalis [*yán hú suǒ*] to improve the blood-quickening and pain-checking actions.

12.3.4   Yīn Depletion Blood Stagnation [阴亏血滞 *yīn kuī xuè zhì*]

Method of Treatment for Yīn Depletion Blood Stagnation

Enrich yīn and quicken blood [滋阴活血 *zī yīn huó xuè*].

All-the-Way-Through Brew [一贯煎 *yī guàn jiān*]	
glehnia [北沙参 *běi shā shēn*, Glehniae Radix]	10g
ophiopogon [麦冬 *mài dōng*, Ophiopogonis Radix]	10g
dried/fresh rehmannia [生地黄 *shēng dì huáng*, Rehmanniae Radix seu Recens]	30g
lycium berry [枸杞子 *gǒu qǐ zǐ*, Lycii Fructus]	12g
toosendan [川楝子 *chuān liàn zǐ*, Toosendan Fructus]	5g
Directions: Take decocted with water [水煎服 *shuǐ jiān fú*].	

Prescription Analysis

Chief Medicinal

Dried/fresh rehmannia strongly enriches and supplements liver and kidney yīn.

Support Medicinals

Glehnia, ophiopogon, and lycium berry help the chief medicinal enrich and supplement yīn.

Assistant Medicinal

Toosendan drains fire, courses the liver, and checks pain [泻火疏肝止痛 *xiè huǒ shū gān zhǐ tòng*].

This combination of medicinals enriches yīn and courses the liver.

Variation According to Signs

The strength of All-the-Way-Through Brew lies in enriching yīn and coursing the liver. Its power to quicken blood is comparatively lacking, so if there are strong signs of blood stagnation, add peach kernel [*táo rén*], carthamus [*hóng huā*], and chuanxiong [*chuān xiōng*]. If the blood stagnation is severe, further add pangolin scales [*chuān shān jiǎ*], vaccaria [*wáng bù liú xíng*], sparganium [*sān léng*], and curcuma rhizome [*é zhú*] to improve the ability to quicken blood, transform stasis, and check pain. If there is blood stagnation with heat, add red peony [*chì sháo*], moutan [*mǔ dān pí*], and puccoon [*zǐ cǎo*] to clear heat and to cool and quicken blood [清热凉血活血 *qīng rè liáng xuè huó xuè*].

12.4   ACUPUNCTURE TREATMENT FOR HERPES ZOSTER

12.4.1   Base Acupuncture Prescription for Herpes Zoster

This base prescription should be modified according to the identified patterns that are discussed below and according to the condition of the individual patient.

Treatment Method for Herpes Zoster

Dispel evil and check pain [祛邪止痛 *qū xié zhǐ tòng*].

Base Acupuncture Prescription for Herpes Zoster
Select points for local bloodletting (i.e., network vessel pricking [局部刺络放血 *jú bù cì luò fàng xuè*])

Prescription Analysis

Local bloodletting makes evil toxins [邪毒 *xié dú*] that are accumulated in the skin drain [泻 *xiè*] out of the body along with the blood. Thus, the procedure dispels evil toxins and checks pain [止痛 *zhǐ tòng*].

12.4.2   Points to Add to the Base Prescription

Points for Liver-Gallbladder Exuberant Heat [肝胆热盛 *gān dǎn rè shèng*]
TB-6 Branch Ditch [支沟 *zhī gōu*] GB-34 Yang Mound Spring [阳陵泉 *yáng líng quán*]

TB-6 and GB-34 are used to course the liver and gallbladder and to clear heat and disinhibit dampness [疏泄肝胆, 清热利湿 *shū xiè gān dǎn, qīng rè lì shī*].

Points for Damp-Heat in the Spleen Channel [脾经湿热 *pí jīng shī rè*]
SP-9 Yīn Mound Spring [阴陵泉 *yīn líng quán*]
LR-5 Woodworm Canal [蠡沟 *lǐ gōu*

These two points disinhibit dampness and resolve toxins [利湿解毒 *lì shī jiě dú*].

Points for Qì Stagnation and Blood Stasis [气滞血瘀 *qì zhì xuè yū*]
LR-3 Supreme Surge [太冲 *tài chōng*]
PC-6 Inner Pass [内关 *nèi guān*]
BL-40 Bend Center [委中 *wěi zhōng*]
SP-10 Sea of Blood [血海 *xuè hǎi*]

LR-3 and PC-6 are used to course the liver and resolve depression [疏肝解郁 *shū gān jiě yù*] and to regulate qì dynamic [调畅气机 *tiáo chàng qì jī*].

BL-40 and SP-10 quicken blood and transform stasis [活血化瘀 *huó xuè huà yū*]. SP-10 is indicated for all skin diseases related to the blood aspect [血分 *xuè fēn*] or damp qì [湿气 *shī qì*].

Points for Yīn Depletion Blood Stagnation [阴亏血滞 *yīn kuī xuè zhì*]
LR-2 Moving Between [行间 *xíng jiān*]
KI-7 Recover Flow [复溜 *fù liū*]
KI-6 Shining Sea [照海 *zhào hǎi*]

LR-2 is the spring point [荥穴 *yíng xué*] of the liver channel and has a heat-clearing function. When heat is gone, yīn can be preserved. KI-7 and KI-6 increase yīn humor [阴液 *yīn yè*]. When yīn is supplemented, blood stagnation can be freed.

CHAPTER 13
Chronic Gastritis

Chronic gastritis is the result of chronic inflammation of the stomach lining. Its main symptoms are discomfort and pain in the upper abdomen, indigestion, and nausea or heartburn. There may be bleeding or ulcers.

There are seven main forms of chronic gastritis:

- cold evil visiting the stomach [寒邪客胃 *hán xié kè wèi*]
- food collecting and stagnating [饮食停滞 *yǐn shí tíng zhì*]
- liver qì invading the stomach [肝气犯胃 *gān qì fàn wèi*]
- depressed heat of the liver-stomach [肝胃郁热 *gān wèi yù rè*]
- blood stasis collecting and stagnating [瘀血停滞 *yū xuè tíng zhì*]
- stomach yīn depletion [胃阴亏虚 *wèi yīn kuī xū*]
- spleen-stomach vacuity cold [脾胃虚寒 *pí wèi xū hán*]

13.1 POINTS OF ATTENTION FOR CHRONIC GASTRITIS

Chronic gastritis is often caused by emotional factors, such as anxiety [忧 *yōu*], excessive thought [思 *sī*], or anger [怒 *nù*], or by dietary irregularities [饮食不节 *yǐn shí bù jié*], such as eating too many spicy or raw foods, drinking too much alcohol, or excessive eating and drinking. The disease can also be due to enduring illness or to constitutional spleen and stomach vacuity.

13.1.1 Treatment

Chronic gastritis tends to be connected to liver depression and qì stagnation that cause spleen-stomach disharmony. Thus, methods that rectify qì and harmonize the stomach [理气和胃 *lǐ qì hé wèi*] are the basis of most treatments.

When treating liver-stomach depressed heat [肝胃郁热 *gān wèi yù rè*] or stomach yīn depletion [胃阴亏虚 *wèi yīn kuī xū*], be careful with the use of medicinals that rectify qì, as they have acrid-drying [辛燥 *xīn zào*] properties that can damage yīn.

In addition to the medicinal or acupuncture treatment, the patient has to avoid certain factors that could worsen his condition or prevent recovery. The patient should avoid stress, taxation fatigue, emotional disharmony, and skipping meals; he should also carefully schedule sufficient time for rest and meals. The patient should abstain from foods that irritate the stomach lining, alcohol, and smoking. He should eat in moderation, neither too little nor too much.

13.1.2   Differentiating the Nature of Pain

Vacuity Pattern or Repletion Pattern

Pain that is worse after eating indicates repletion pattern; pain that is exacerbated by an empty stomach indicates a vacuity pattern.

Distending stomach pain indicates repletion pattern; stomach pain without distention indicates vacuity pattern.

Pain that refuses pressure [拒按 *jù àn*] indicates a repletion pattern; pain that is relieved by pressure indicates a vacuity pattern.

Severe pain in a fixed area indicates repletion pattern; moderate pain indicates a vacuity pattern.

Cold Pattern or Heat Pattern

Pain relieved by warmth indicates a cold pattern. Scorching pain [灼痛 *zhuó tòng*] in the stomach duct indicates a heat pattern.

Qì Stagnation or Blood Stagnation

Qì stagnation occurs more in the beginning stage of the disease, whereas enduring pain tends to enter the network vessels and cause blood stasis.

Distending pain [胀痛 *zhàng tòng*] with belching indicates qì stagnation. Stabbing pain [刺痛 *cì tòng*] indicates blood stasis.

Pain that moves from one location to another [窜痛 *cuàn tòng*] indicates qì stagnation. Pain of fixed location indicates blood stasis.

13.2 CAUSES AND PATHOMECHANISM OF CHRONIC GASTRITIS; IDENTIFYING PATTERNS

13.2.1 Cold Evil Visiting the Stomach [寒邪客胃 *hán xié kè wèi*]

Causes and *Pathomechanism* of Cold Evil Visiting the Stomach

Wind-cold assails the exterior [风寒外袭 *fēng hán wài xí*] and passes into the interior where it assails the stomach [内侵胃腑 *nèi qīn wèi fǔ*]. This impairs the harmonious downbearing of the stomach [胃失和降 *wèi shī hé jiàng*] and results in stoppage in the network vessels, causing stomach pain.

Important Signs of Cold Evil Visiting the Stomach

Sudden appearance of stomach pain. Aversion to cold and liking for warmth. Pain is relieved by warmth and exacerbated by cold. Liking for warm drinks, no thirst. The tongue has a thin white coating [苔薄白 *tāi bó bái*]. Stringlike and tight pulse [脉弦紧 *mài xián jǐn*].

13.2.2 Food Collecting and Stagnating [饮食停滞 *yǐn shí tíng zhì*]

Causes and Pathomechanism of Food Collecting and Stagnating

Food collecting and stagnating causes obstruction of the qì dynamic in the middle burner [中焦气机阻塞 *zhōng jiāo qì jī zǔ sāi*].

Important Signs of Food Collecting and Stagnating

Stomach pain, distention and fullness in the stomach duct and abdomen [脘腹胀满 *wǎn fù zhàng mǎn*], and putrid belching and acid regurgitation [嗳腐吞酸 *ài fǔ tūn suān*]. Vomiting of undigested food. Pain is relieved by vomiting or flatus. Ungratifying defecation [大便不爽 *dà biàn bú shuǎng*]. The tongue has a thick and slimy fur [苔厚腻 *tāi hòu nì*]. Slippery pulse [脉滑 *mài huá*].

13.2.3 Liver Qì Invading the Stomach [肝气犯胃 *gān qì fàn wèi*]

Causes and Pathomechanism of Liver Qì Invading the Stomach

Binding depression of liver qì [肝气郁结 *gān qì yù jié*] invades the stomach [犯胃 *fàn wèi*] and causes the qì dynamic to stagnate. The result is stoppage in the network vessels, impaired harmonious downbearing of the stomach [胃失和降 *wèi shī hé jiàng*], and upward counterflow of the qì dynamic [气机上逆 *qì jī shàng nì*].

Important Signs of Liver Qì Invading the Stomach

Oppression and distention in the stomach duct and abdomen [胃脘胀闷 *wèi wǎn zhàng mèn*], with distention being more prominent. Pain in the stomach that spreads to the ribs. Belching and acid upflow [泛酸 *fàn suān*]. Nausea. Vexation and irascibility [心烦易怒 *xīn fán yì nù*]. Pain is set off or exacerbated by emotional discomfort. Frequent sighing. The tongue has thin white fur [苔薄白 *tāi bó bái*]. Deep and stringlike pulse [脉沉弦 *mài chén xián*].

13.2.4   Depressed Heat of the Liver-Stomach [肝胃郁热 *gān wèi yù rè*]

Causes and Pathomechanism of Depressed Heat of the Liver-Stomach

Liver depression transforms into fire, and fire evil invades the stomach; the result is impaired harmonious downbearing of the stomach [胃失和降 *wèi shī hé jiàng*].

Important Signs of Depressed Heat of the Liver-Stomach

Scorching pain in the stomach duct and abdomen [胃脘灼痛 *wèi wǎn zhuó tòng*]. Vexation and irascibility [心烦易怒 *xīn fán yì nù*]. Feeling of emptiness and burning in the stomach duct. Acid vomiting [吐酸 *tù suān*]. Bitter taste in the mouth [口苦 *kǒu kǔ*], dry mouth. Constipation, reddish urine. Red tongue with yellow fur [舌红苔黄 *shé hóng tāi huáng*]. Stringlike and rapid pulse [脉弦数 *mài xián shuò*].

13.2.5   Blood Stasis Collecting and Stagnating [瘀血停滞 *yū xuè tíng zhì*]

Causes and Pathomechanism of Blood Stasis Collecting and Stagnating

Enduring qì stagnation impedes the smooth flow of blood, and blood stasis collects internally, obstructing the stomach duct.

Important Signs of Blood Stasis Collecting and Stagnating

Enduring stomach pain. Stabbing pain [刺痛 *cì tòng*] in a fixed location that refuses pressure [拒按 *jù àn*]. Pain is worse after eating. Ejection of blood and black stools [吐血黑便 *tù xuè hēi biàn*]. Dark purple tongue, or stasis macules [舌质紫黯或有瘀斑 *shé zhì zǐ àn huò yǒu yū bān*]. Rough pulse [涩脉 *sè mài*].

13.2.6   Stomach Yīn Depletion [胃阴亏虚 *wèi yīn kuī xū*]

Causes and Pathomechanism of Stomach Yīn Depletion

Stomach yīn depletion can result when stomach yīn is scorched by: any of the following:

- enduring stomach pain
- cold evil transforming into heat
- qì depression transforming into fire
- stomach heat
- improper treatment using warm drying medicinals for too long
- liver yīn vacuity with ascendant liver yáng [肝阳上亢 *gān yáng shàng kàng*]
- Insufficiency of stomach yīn results in failure to moisten and downbear

Important Signs of Stomach Yīn Depletion

Dull scorching pain in the stomach duct [胃脘隐隐灼痛 *wèi wǎn yǐn yǐn zhuó tòng*]. Dry mouth and throat. Scant intake. Dry bound stool [大便干结 *dà biàn gān jié*]. Red tongue with scant fur [舌红少苔 *shé hóng shǎo tāi*]. Fine rapid pulse [脉细数 *mài xì shuò*].

13.2.7   Spleen-Stomach Vacuity Cold [脾胃虚寒 *pí wèi xū hán*]

Causes and Pathomechanism of Spleen-Stomach Vacuity Cold

Enduring stomach pain causes spleen-stomach yáng vacuity, impeded food intake and movement, and loss of warmth in the stomach. Thus, cold is engendered in the middle burner.

Important Signs of Spleen-Stomach Vacuity Cold

Slow onset and long duration of the disease. Discomfort in the stomach duct. Dull pain [隐痛 *yǐn tòng*] that is relieved by warmth and pressure. Preference for warm drinks. No appetite. Occasional vomiting of clear water [吐清水 *tù qīng shuǐ*]. Pain is stronger when stomach is empty and is relieved after eating. Fatigue and cold limbs. Cold hands and feet. Clear urine, sloppy stool [便溏 *biàn táng*]. Pale tender tongue, thin white fur [舌淡嫩，薄白苔 *shé dàn nèn, bò bái tāi*]. Fine weak pulse [脉细弱 *mài xì ruò*].

13.3   TREATMENT OF CHRONIC GASTRITIS USING CHINESE MEDICINALS

13.3.1   Cold Evil Visiting the Stomach [寒邪客胃 *hán xié kè wèi*]

Method of Treatment for Cold Evil Visiting the Stomach

Warm the center and dissipate cold, supplement and boost spleen and stomach [温中散寒，补益脾胃 *wēn zhōng sàn hán, bǔ yì pí wèi*].

Center-Rectifying Pill [理中丸 *lǐ zhōng wán*]	
ginseng [人参 *rén shēn*, Ginseng Radix]	90g
dried ginger [干姜 *gān jiāng*, Zingiberis Rhizoma]	90g
white atractylodes [白术 *bái zhú*, Atractylodis Macrocephalae Rhizoma]	90g
licorice [甘草 *gān cǎo*, Glycyrrhizae Radix]	90g

The original prescription is taken in pill form (the medicinals are ground into powder and formed into pills the size of egg yolks). In modern times, it is also taken as a decoction with the quantities of the medicinals proportionately decreased according to the proportion of the original prescription.

Prescription Analysis

Chief Medicinal

Dried ginger warms the center and dissipates cold, treating the root [治本 *zhì běn*].

Support Medicinals

Ginseng and white atractylodes supplement the center and boost qì [补中益气 *bǔ zhōng yì qì*].

Assistant and Conductor Medicinal

Licorice is used both to supplement the center and boost qì [补中益气 *bǔ zhōng yì qì*] and to harmonize the properties of all medicinals [调和药性 *tiáo hé yào xìng*].

This combination of medicinals warms the center and dissipates cold.

Variation According to Signs

Center-Rectifying Pill is often used to warm the center and dissipate cold. If there is severe cold pain in the stomach duct [胃脘冷痛剧烈 *wèi wǎn lěng tòng jù liè*], add aconite [*fù zǐ*] to warm yáng, dissipate cold and check pain, such as in Aconite Center-Rectifying Pill [附子理中丸 *fù zǐ lǐ zhōng wán*]. If there is distention and fullness in the stomach duct [胃脘胀满 *wèi wǎn zhàng mǎn*] with cold congealing and qì stagnating [寒凝气滞 *hán níng qì zhì*], add cyperus [*xiāng fù*], costusroot [*mù xiāng*], and lindera [*wū yào*] to move qì and eliminate fullness. If there is stomach cold ascending counterflow [胃寒上逆 *wèi hán shàng nì*] with vomiting and nausea [呕吐恶心 *ǒu tù ě xīn*], add fresh ginger [*shēng jiāng*] and pinellia [*bàn xià*] to downbear counterflow and check vomiting.

13.3.2 Food Collecting and Stagnating [饮食停滞 *yǐn shí tíng zhì*]

Method of Treatment for Food Collecting and Stagnating

Disperse food and harmonize the stomach [消食和胃 *xiāo shí hé wèi*].

Harmony-Preserving Pill [保和丸 *bǎo hé wán*]	
crataegus [山楂 *shān zhā*, Crataegi Fructus]	180g
medicated leaven [神曲 *shén qū*, Massa Medicata Fermentata]	60g
pinellia [半夏 *bàn xià*, Pinelliae Rhizoma]	90g
poria [茯苓 *fú líng*, Poria]	90g
tangerine peel [陈皮 *chén pí*, Citri Reticulatae Pericarpium]	30g
forsythia [连翘 *lián qiào*, Forsythiae Fructus]	30g
radish seed [莱菔子 *lái fú zǐ*, Raphani Semen]	30g

The original prescription is taken by grinding all of the above medicinals into fine powder, which is formed into pills and taken 6–9g each time, twice a day. The prescription can also be taken as a decoction with the quantities of the medicinals proportionally decreased according to the original prescription.

Prescription Analysis

Chief Medicinal

Crataegus disperses food stagnation, especially meat accumulation and stagnation [肉食积滞 *ròu shí jī zhì*].

Support Medicinals

Medicated leaven disperses food stagnation and fortifies the spleen [消食健脾 *xiāo shí jiàn pí*]; it also transforms alcohol and accumulations of putrid food [化酒陈腐之积 *huà jiǔ chén fǔ zhī jī*]. Radish seed disperses food stagnation and downbears qì; it is especially strong in dispersing wheat products and transforming phlegm. Both medicinals help the chief medicinal disperse food and transform accumulation [消食化积 *xiāo shí huà jī*].

Assistant Medicinals

Tangerine peel and pinellia move qì and loosen the center [行气宽中 *xíng qì kuān zhōng*] as well as dry dampness and transform phlegm [燥湿化痰 *zào shí huà tán*]. Poria fortifies the spleen, percolates dampness, and checks diarrhea [健脾渗湿而止泄 *jiàn pí shèn shī ér zhǐ xiè*]. Forsythia dissipates binds [散结 *sàn jié*] and clears the heat effusion caused by food accumulation [清食积之发热 *qīng shí jī zhī fā rè*].

This combination of medicinals is used to disperse food and abduct stagnation and to harmonize the stomach and check pain [消食导滞，和胃止痛 *xiāo shí dǎo zhì, hé wèi zhǐ tòng*].

Variation According to Signs

Harmony-Preserving Pill is often used to disperse food and harmonize the stomach. If there is severe pain in the stomach duct, add costusroot [*mù xiāng*] and corydalis [*yán hú suǒ*] to check pain. If there is distention and fullness in the stomach duct and abdomen [脘腹胀满 *wǎn fù zhàng mǎn*], add unripe bitter orange [*zhǐ shí*] and officinal magnolia bark [*hòu pò*] to move qì and eliminate fullness. If the patient is constipated, add rhubarb [*dà huáng*] and areca [*bīng láng*].

13.3.3   Liver Qì Invading the Stomach [肝气犯胃 *gān qì fàn wèi*]

Method of Treatment for Liver Qì Invading the Stomach

Course the liver and rectify qì, harmonize the stomach and check pain [疏肝理气，和胃止痛 *shū gān lǐ qì, hé wèi zhǐ tòng*].

Bupleurum Liver-Coursing Powder [柴胡疏肝散 *chái hú shū gān sǎn*]	
bupleurum [柴胡 *chái hú*, Bupleuri Radix]	6g
tangerine peel [陈皮 *chén pí*, Citri Reticulatae Pericarpium]	6g
bitter orange [枳壳 *zhǐ ké*, Aurantii Fructus]	5g
white peony [白芍 *bái sháo*, Paeoniae Radix Alba]	5g
chuanxiong [川芎 *chuān xiōng*, Chuanxiong Rhizoma]	5g
cyperus [香附 *xiāng fù*, Cyperi Rhizoma]	5g
licorice [甘草 *gān cǎo*, Glycyrrhizae Radix]	3g
Directions: Take decocted with water [水煎服 *shuǐ jiān fú*].	

Prescription Analysis

Chief Medicinal

Bupleurum courses the liver and resolves depression [疏肝解郁 *shū gān jiě yù*] to treat stagnant depression of liver qì [肝气郁滞 *gān qì yù zhì*].

Support Medicinals

Tangerine peel and bitter orange move qì and loosen the center [行气宽中 *xíng qì kuān zhōng*] to treat spleen-stomach qì stagnation and to eliminate distention and fullness in the stomach duct and abdomen.

Assistant Medicinals

White peony is used to supplement and emolliate the liver [补肝柔肝 *bǔ gān róu gān*] and to relax liver tension and check pain [缓肝之急而止痛 *huǎn gān zhī jí ér zhǐ tòng*]. Chuanxiong quickens blood and moves qì to check pain. Cyperus moves qì and soothes the liver to check pain [行气舒肝而止痛 *xíng qì shū gān ér zhǐ tòng*].

Licorice harmonizes the properties of all the medicinals [调和药性 *tiáo hé yào xìng*].

This combination of medicinals is used to course the liver and rectify qì and to harmonize the stomach and check pain.

Variation According to Signs

For severe pain, add toosendan [*chuān liàn zǐ*], corydalis [*yán hú suǒ*], and curcuma [*yù jīn*] to check pain. If there is belching [嗳气 *ài qì*] or vomiting, add fresh ginger [*shēng jiāng*] and pinellia [*bàn xià*] to harmonize the stomach, downbear counterflow, and check vomiting [和胃降逆止呕 *hé wèi jiàng nì zhǐ ǒu*]. If the patient has a bitter or sour taste in the mouth, add moutan [*mǔ dān pí*], gardenia [*zhī zǐ*], coptis [*huáng lián*], and evodia [*wú zhū yú*] to dissipate depression and clear heat [散郁清热 *sàn yù qīng rè*].

13.3.4 Depressed Heat of the Liver-Stomach [肝胃郁热 *gān wèi yù rè*]

Method of Treatment for Depressed Heat of the Liver-Stomach

Course the liver and harmonize the stomach, dissipate depression and clear heat [疏肝和胃，散郁清热 *shū gān hé wèi, sàn yù qīng rè*].

Liver-Transforming Brew [化肝煎 *huà gān jiān*]	
unripe tangerine peel [青皮 *qīng pí*, Citri Reticulatae Pericarpium Viride]	6g
tangerine peel [陈皮 *chén pí*, Citri Reticulatae Pericarpium]	6g
white peony [白芍 *bái sháo*, Paeoniae Radix Alba]	6g
moutan [牡丹皮 *mǔ dān pí*, Moutan Cortex]	5g
gardenia [栀子 *zhī zǐ*, Gardeniae Fructus]	5g
alisma [泽泻 *zé xiè*, Alismatis Rhizoma]	5g
bolbosteema [土贝母 *tǔ bèi mǔ*, Bolbostemmatis Rhizoma]	9g
Directions: Take decocted with water [水煎服 *shuǐ jiān fú*].	

Prescription Analysis

Chief Medicinal

Unripe tangerine peel treats the root [治本 *zhì běn*] by coursing the liver and breaking qì [疏肝破气 *shū gān pò qì*] and by clearing heat and draining fire.

Support Medicinals

Tangerine peel moves stagnant spleen and stomach qì to eliminate distention and fullness in the stomach duct and abdomen. White peony nourishes blood and emolliates the liver. Both medicinals help the chief medicinal course the liver and treat the root.

Assistant Medicinals

Moutan clears heat and cools blood. Gardenia drains fire-heat of the triple warmer. Alisma drains fire of the urinary bladder and disinhibits urine. Bolbosteema dissipates depression bind [散郁结 *sàn yù jié*] and disperses swelling of welling-abscess [消痈肿 *xiāo yōng zhǒng*].

This combination of medicinals is used to course the liver and harmonize the stomach and to dissipate depression and clear heat.

Variation According to Signs

For severe liver depression, add bupleurum [*chái hú*], curcuma [*yù jīn*], and corydalis [*yán hú suǒ*] to increase the liver-coursing, depression-resolving, and pain-checking effects. For acid upflow [泛酸 *fàn suān*], add coptis [*huáng lián*] and evodia [*wú zhū yú*] to clear heat and downbear counterflow. For constipation, add rhubarb [*dà huáng*], unripe bitter orange [*zhǐ shí*], and areca [*bīng láng*] to abduct stagnation.

13.3.5   Blood Stasis Collecting and Stagnating [瘀血停滞 *yū xuè tíng zhì*]

Method of Treatment for Blood Stasis Collecting and Stagnating

Quicken the blood and transform stasis, move qì and check pain [活血化瘀，行气止痛 *huó xuè huà yū, xíng qì zhǐ tòng*].

Infradiaphragmatic Stasis-Expelling Decoction **[膈下逐瘀汤 *gé xià zhú yū tāng*]**	
peach kernel [桃仁 *táo rén*, Persicae Semen]	10g
carthamus [红花 *hóng huā*, Carthami Flos]	10g
Chinese angelica [当归 *dāng guī*, Angelicae Sinensis Radix]	10g

chuanxiong [川芎 *chuān xiōng*, Chuanxiong Rhizoma]	10g
moutan [牡丹皮 *mǔ dān pí*, Moutan Cortex]	6g
red peony [赤芍 *chì sháo*, Paeoniae Radix Rubra]	6g
flying squirrel's droppings [五灵脂 *wǔ líng zhī*, Trogopteri Faeces]	6g
corydalis [延胡索 *yán hú suǒ*, Corydalis Rhizoma]	6g
lindera [乌药 *wū yào*, Linderae Radix]	6g
cyperus [香附 *xiāng fù*, Cyperi Rhizoma]	6g
bitter orange [枳壳 *zhǐ ké*, Aurantii Fructus]	6g
licorice [甘草 *gān cǎo*, Glycyrrhizae Radix]	3g

Directions: Take decocted with water [水煎服 *shuǐ jiān fú*].

Prescription Analysis

Chief Medicinals

Peach kernel and carthamus treat the root [治本 *zhì běn*] by quickening blood and transforming stasis.

Support Medicinals

Chinese angelica, chuanxiong, moutan, red peony, flying squirrel's droppings, and corydalis help the chief medicinals quicken blood, transform stasis, and check pain.

Assistant Medicinals

When qì moves, then blood also moves [气行则血行 *qì xíng zé xuè xíng*]; thus, lindera, cyperus, and bitter orange are used to move qì in order to help move blood.

Licorice harmonizes the properties of all the medicinals [调和药性 *tiáo hé yào xìng*].

This combination of medicinals is used to quicken blood and transform stasis and to move qì and check pain.

Variation According to Signs

For severe pain, add frankincense [*rǔ xiāng*] and myrrh [*mò yào*] to quicken blood and check pain. For congealed cold qì stagnation [寒凝气滞 *hán níng qì zhì*] with distention and fullness in the stomach duct and abdomen, add dried ginger [*gān jiāng*], cinnamon twig [*guì zhī*], or even aconite [*fù zǐ*] to warm the center and dissipate cold.

13.3.6   Stomach Yīn Depletion [胃阴亏虚 *wèi yīn kuī xū*]

Method of Treatment for Stomach Yīn Depletion

Boost the stomach and engender liquid [益胃生津 *yì wèi shēng jīn*].

Stomach-Boosting Decoction [益胃汤 *yì wèi tāng*]	
adenophora/glehnia [沙参 *shā shēn*, Adenophorae Radix]	10g
ophiopogon [麦冬 *mài dōng*, Ophiopogonis Radix]	15g
dried/fresh rehmannia [生地黄 *shēng dì huáng*, Rhmanniae Radix seu Recens]	15g
Solomon's seal [玉竹 *yù zhú*, Polygonati Odorati Rhizoma]	6g
rock sugar [冰糖 *bīng táng*, Saccharon Crystallinum]	10g
Directions: Take decocted with water [水煎服 *shuǐ jiān fú*].	

Prescription Analysis

Chief Medicinals

Adenophora/glehnia, ophiopogon, dried/fresh rehmannia, Solomon's seal, and rock sugar are all sweet and cold [甘寒 *gān hán*] and nourish yīn. They strongly supplement stomach yīn.

The above prescription is excellent for supplementing stomach yīn, yet, because all medicinals in the prescription have similar characteristics, modifying its ingredients according to signs is particularly important.

Variations According to Signs

For hunger but no desire to eat [饥不欲食 *è bú yù shí*], add medicated leaven [*shén qū*], barley sprout [*mài yá*], gizzard lining [*jī nèi jīn*], and radish seed [*lái fú zǐ*] to open the stomach [开胃 *kāi wèi*]. For acid upflow [泛酸 *fàn suān*], add ark shell [*wǎ léng zǐ*]. For dry stool [大便干燥 *dà biàn gān zào*], add hemp seed [*má zǐ rén*], bush cherry kernel [*yù lǐ rén*], and trichosanthes seed [*guā lóu rén*] to moisten the intestines and free the stool [润肠通便 *rùn cháng tōng biàn*].

13.3.7   Spleen-Stomach Vacuity Cold [脾胃虚寒 *pí wèi xū hán*]

Method of Treatment for Spleen-Stomach Vacuity Cold

Warm the center and supplement vacuity, dissipate cold and check pain [温中补虚, 散寒止痛 *wēn zhōng bǔ xū, sàn hán zhǐ tòng*].

Minor Center-Fortifying Decoction [小建中汤 *xiǎo jiàn zhōng tāng*]	
malt sugar [饴糖 *yí táng*, Maltosum]	30g
white peony [白芍 *bái sháo*, Paeoniae Radix Alba]	20g
cinnamon twig [桂枝 *guì zhī*, Cinnamomi Ramulus]	10g
honey-fried licorice [炙甘草 *zhì gān cǎo*, Glycyrrhizae Radix Preparata]	6g
fresh ginger [生姜 *shēng jiāng*, Zingiberis Rhizoma Recens]	3 slices
jujube [大枣 *dà zǎo*, Jujubae Fructus]	6 pieces

Directions: Take decocted with water [水煎服 *shuǐ jiān fú*].

Prescription Analysis

Chief Medicinal

Malt sugar, which is sweet and warm [甘温 *gān wēn*], enters the spleen, warms the center and supplements vacuity, harmonizes the interior [和里 *hé lǐ*], and relaxes tension and checks pain [缓急止痛 *huǎn jí zhǐ tòng*].

Support Medicinals

Cinnamon twig warms the center and dissipates cold, warms and frees the channels, and checks pain. White peony nourishes yīn and supplements blood, harmonizes the interior [和里 *hé lǐ*], and relaxes tension and checks pain [缓急止痛 *huǎn jí zhǐ tòng*].

Assistant Medicinals

Fresh ginger and jujube promote the source of qì and blood formation [资气血生化之源 *zī qì xuè shēng huà zhī yuán*].

Licorice harmonizes the properties of all the medicinals [调和药性 *tiáo hé yào xìng*].

This combination of medicinals is used to warm the center and supplement vacuity and to dissipate cold and check pain.

Variation According to Signs

Minor Center-Fortifying Decoction both warms and supplements; it strongly warms the center and fortifies the spleen and also dissipates cold and checks pain. If the patient vomits clear water, add dried ginger [*gān jiāng*] to warm the center and dissipate cold. If the patient vomits and suffers from acid upflow [泛酸 *fàn suān*], add coptis [*huáng lián*] and evodia [*wú zhū yú*]. Use Minor Center-Fortifying Decoction together with Saussurea and Amomum Stomach-Nourishing Pill [香砂养胃丸 *xiāng shā yǎng wèi wán*] for increased effectiveness.

13.4   ACUPUNCTURE TREATMENT FOR CHRONIC GASTRITIS

13.4.1   Base Acupuncture Prescription for Chronic Gastritis

This base prescription should be modified according to the identified patterns that are discussed below and according to the condition of the individual patient.

Treatment Method for Chronic Gastritis

Harmonize the stomach and check pain [和胃止痛 *hé wèi zhǐ tòng*].

Base Acupuncture Prescription for Chronic Gastritis
CV-12 Center Stomach Duct [中脘 *zhōng wǎn*]
ST-36 Leg Three Lǐ [足三里 *zú sān lǐ*]
ST-34 Beam Hill [梁丘 *liáng qiū*]
PC-6 Inner Pass [内关 *nèi guān*]

Prescription Analysis

CV-12 is the alarm point [募穴 *mù xué*] of the stomach and a meeting point [会穴 *huì xué*] for the bowels. ST-36 is the lower uniting point [下合穴 *xià hé xué*] of the stomach. Lower uniting points treat the diseases of the six bowels [合治内府 *hé zhì nèi fǔ*]. ST-36 fortifies the spleen and stomach and supplements center qì [中气 *zhōng qì*]. Together, CV-12 and ST-36 harmonize the stomach.

PC-6, the network point [络穴 *luò xué*] of the pericardium channel, regulates the qì dynamic [调气机 *tiáo qì jī*]. Network points are often used to treat the network vessels themselves rather than internal diseases; in this case, PC-6 is used to quicken the network vessels and settle pain [活络镇痛 *huó luò zhèn tòng*]. ST-34, the cleft point [郄穴 *xī xué*] of the foot yáng brightness channel, has an exceptionally strong capacity to check pain. Qì and blood accumulate at the cleft points, and they are mostly used in acute patterns, especially in the treatment of pain. Together, PC-6 and ST-34 move qì and check pain [行气止痛 *xíng qì zhǐ tòng*].

13.4.2   Points to Add to the Base Prescription

Points for Cold Evil Visiting the Stomach [寒邪客胃 *hán xié kè wèi*]
CV-12 Center Stomach Duct [中脘 *zhōng wǎn*] (moxa)
ST-25 Celestial Pivot [天枢 *tiān shū*]

This pair of points is used to dissipate cold evil [散寒邪 *sàn hán xié*].

Points for Food Collecting and Stagnating [饮食停滞 *yǐn shí tíng zhì*]
ST-44 Inner Court [内庭 *nèi tíng*] ST-21 Beam Gate [梁门 *liáng mén*]

In this pattern, food is collecting and stagnating and there is an accumulation of heat [积热 *jī rè*]. As ST-44 is a spring point, it has a strong ability to clear heat.

ST-21 Beam Gate [梁门 *liáng mén*] fortifies the spleen and stomach and assists transformation and movement [健脾胃，助运化 *jiàn pí wèi, zhù yùn huà*]. Here it is used to disperse food and transform stagnation [消食化滞 *xiāo shí huà zhì*].

Points for Liver Qì Invading the Stomach [肝气犯胃 *gān qì fàn wèi*]
LR-3 Supreme Surge [太冲 *tài chōng*]

LR-3 courses the liver [疏肝 *shū gān*].

Points for Depressed Heat of the Liver-Stomach [肝胃郁热 *gān wèi yù rè*]
ST-44 Inner Court [内庭 *nèi tíng*] LR-2 Moving Between [行间 *xíng jiān*]

Both points are spring points [荥穴 *yíng xué*] and thus have a strong ability to clear the heat evil of their respective channels.

Points for Blood Stasis Collecting and Stagnating [瘀血停滞 *yū xuè tíng zhì*]
LR-13 Camphorwood Gate [章门 *zhāng mén*] LR-14 Cycle Gate [期门 *qī mén*]

This pair of points quickens blood and transforms phlegm. LR-13 is the alarm point [募穴 *mù xué*] of the spleen; LR-14 is the alarm point [募穴 *mù xué*] of the liver. The spleen manages blood [脾统血 *pí tǒng xuè*] and the liver stores the blood [肝藏血 *gān cáng xuè*]. Needling both alarm points quickens blood and transforms stasis.

Points for Stomach Yīn Depletion [胃阴亏虚 *wèi yīn kuī xū*]
KI-7 Recover Flow [复溜 *fù liū*] KI-6 Shining Sea [照海 *zhào hǎi*]

Both points enrich and nourish kidney yīn [滋养肾阴 *zī yǎng shèn yīn*]. Because kidney yīn is the basis of yīn of the entire body, nourishing kidney yīn nourishes the yīn of all the other organs. When kidney yīn is ample, stomach yīn will recover.

Points for Spleen-Stomach Vacuity Cold [脾胃虚寒 *pí wèi xū hán*]
CV-12 Center Stomach Duct [中腕 *zhōng wǎn*] (moxa)
CV-11 Interior Strengthening [建里 *jiàn lǐ*] (moxa)
BL-20 Spleen Transport [脾俞 *pí shū*]
BL-21 Stomach Transport [胃俞 *wèi shū*]

These points fortify the spleen, nourish the stomach, and warm center yáng.

CHAPTER 14

Gallstones

Gallstones refers to a calculus or calculi in the gallbladder or the bile ducts. Gallstones may lie dormant and not cause any symptoms for some time, but when the stones shift and obstruct the gallbladder or bile duct, they may cause severe pain in the upper abdomen. This can be set off by eating, especially eating fatty foods. The pain is typically sharp, and it comes and goes (colic).

There are four main patterns associated with gallstones:

- Liver-gallbladder qì stagnation [肝胆气滞 *gān dǎn qì zhì*]
- Damp-heat brewing internally [湿热内蕴 *shī rè nèi yùn*]
- Exuberant heat toxin [热毒炽盛 *rè dú chì shèng*]
- Liver yīn insufficiency [肝阴不足 *gān yīn bù zú*]

14.1   POINTS OF ATTENTION FOR GALLSTONES

14.1.1   Physiology

The gallbladder is called the bowel of center clearness [胆为中清之腑 *dǎn wéi zhōng qīng zhī fǔ*] because it secretes gall, which is a clear fluid, and because it does not pass and transform food or waste. Normally, the direction of its function is descending.

The gallbladder and liver stand in exterior-interior realtionship [肝胆相表里 *gān dǎn xiāng biǎo lǐ*]. The liver is the source of bile; bile is formed by the liver's replete qì, which spills into the gallbladder and accumulates into bile.

Thus, gallstones may be caused by a variety of of factors that disturb the liver's capacity to govern free coursing [肝主疏泄 *gān zhǔ shū xiè*] or the gallbladder's function of descending and secreting bile.

14.1.2   Pathomechanism

Pathological changes primarily affect the liver, gallbladder, spleen, and stomach.

Liver and gallbladder qì stagnation and damp-heat congestion cause bile to accumulate and bind into stones. Qì stagnation and damp-heat influence each other; when there is qì stagnation, damp-heat cannot be transformed. When there is damp-heat, the qì dynamic cannot flow smoothly. Due to impaired free coursing of the liver and disturbed descending function of the gallbladder, the qì dynamic is obstructed, giving rise to pain.

14.1.3   Treatment

In the dormant stage of the disease, the main patterns are liver-gallbladder qì stagnation [肝胆气滞 *gān dǎn qì zhì*] and liver yīn insufficiency [肝阴不足 *gān yīn bù zú*].

In the stage of attack, depending on the level of heat transformation, the main patterns are damp-heat brewing internally [湿热内蕴 *shī rè nèi yùn*] and exuberant heat toxin [热毒炽盛 *rè dú chì shèng*].

Based on the close relationship between the gallbladder and liver, the main treatment principles are to course the liver and rectify qì [疏肝理气 *shū gān lǐ qì*], clear heat and resolve toxins [清热解毒 *qīng rè jiě dú*], and free the interior with offensive precipitation [通里攻下 *tōng lǐ gōng xià*], according to the respective pattern and stage of the illness.

14.2   CAUSES AND PATHOMECHANISM OF GALLSTONES; IDENTIFYING PATTERNS

14.2.1   Liver-Gallbladder Qì Stagnation [肝胆气滞 *gān dǎn qì zhì*]

Causes and Pathomechanism of Liver-Gallbladder Qì Stagnation

This pattern appears in the beginning or resting stage of the disease. Affect-mind binding depression [情志郁结 *qíng zhì yù jié*] or sudden bursts of anger damage the liver and disturb the liver's function of governing free coursing [肝主疏泄 *gān zhǔ shū xiè*]. Bile gets depressed and over time binds to form stones that obstruct qì and create stoppage and pain.

Important Signs of Liver-Gallbladder Qì Stagnation

Oppression, distention, and pain in the middle or right upper abdomen. Sometimes gripping pain [绞痛 *jiǎo tòng*]. Pain is set off or exacerbated by emotional instability. Pain is sustained but varies in intensity. Right upper abdomen is painful to the touch. Nausea, vomiting, belching, bitter taste in the mouth [口苦 *kǒu kǔ*]. No pleasure in eating and abdominal distention after eating. Mouth is not dry, no heat effusion, no jaundice. Constipation or dry stool. Thin white or yellow tongue coating [苔薄白或薄黄 *tāi bó bái huò bó huáng*]. Stringlike pulse or stringlike tight pulse [脉弦或弦紧 *mài xián huò xián jǐn*].

14.2.2 Damp-Heat Brewing Internally [湿热内蕴 *shī rè nèi yùn*]

Causes and Pathomechanism of Damp-Heat Brewing Internally

This pattern results from external contraction of damp-heat invading the liver, gallbladder, spleen, and stomach. Another cause may be dietary irregularities, e.g., eating too many foods that generate heat such as fatty, sweet foods and alcohol, which impede movement and transformation in the middle burner and cause dampness obstruction and brewing heat. Another possible cause of this pattern is liver-gallbladder qì stagnation that transforms into heat after enduring depression and combines with spleen damp. Damp-heat binds with bile and, over time, forms stones.

Important Signs of Damp-Heat Brewing Internally

Severe gripping [绞痛 *jiǎo tòng*] or distending [胀痛 *zhàng tòng*] pain in the upper right or middle abdomen. Pain spreads to the chest and right shoulder blade. The upper abdomen is painful or hard to the touch. Alternating heat effusion and aversion to cold [往来寒热 *wǎng lái hán rè*]. Bitter taste in the mouth [口苦 *kǒu kǔ*], torpid intake [纳呆 *nà dāi*]. Fullness and distention in the stomach duct and abdomen. Constipation. Short voidings of yellow urine. There may be jaundice. Red tongue with yellow slimy fur [舌红，苔黄腻 *shé hóng, tāi huáng nì*]. Stringlike slippery rapid pulse [脉弦滑数 *mài xián huá shuò*].

14.2.3 Exuberant Heat-Toxin [热毒炽盛 *rè dú chì shèng*]

Causes and Pathomechanism of Exuberant Heat-Toxin

This pattern can be caused by enduring damp-heat depression or liver depression that transforms into heat. It may also result from external contraction or internal damage that causes liver-gallbladder damp-heat to intensify. Damp-heat and gallstones combine and obstruct the biliary tract, channels and network vessels, thus causing pain in the right upper abdomen.

Important Signs of Exuberant Heat-Toxin

Continuous gripping [绞痛 *jiǎo tòng*] or distending [胀痛 *zhàng tòng*] pain in the upper right or middle abdomen that is sometimes severe. Pain is exacerbated by pressing on the upper abdomen. Pain spreads to the chest and right shoulder blade. Abdominal muscles are hard and refuse pressure [拒按 *jù àn*]. Oppression and distention in the chest and abdomen. Strong heat effusion and shivering. Nausea, vomiting. Dry mouth and tongue. Constipation. Short voidings of red urine.

When the pattern gets worse, there may be clouded spirit and delirious speech [神昏谵语 *shén hūn zhān yǔ*] that can transform into indifference and apathy. Heat reversal in the extremities. Crimson tongue with rough yellow fur [舌红绛苔黄糙 *shé hóng jiàng tāi huáng cāo*]. Stringlike slippery rapid pulse or, in a later stage, fine rapid forceless [脉弦滑数或细数无力 *mài xián huá shuò huò xì shuò wú lì*].

14.2.4　Liver Yīn Insufficiency [肝阴不足 *gān yīn bù zú*]

Causes and Pathomechanism of Liver Yīn Insufficiency

Insufficient liver yīn may be due to the disease enduring for a long time. Other reasons are taxation, or yīn essence depletion due to old age in combination with gallstones. This causes failure to nourish the liver, the network vessels are not moistened, and liver-gallbladder qì does not spread freely.

Important Signs of Liver Yīn Insufficiency

Dull pain [隐痛 *yǐn tòng*] or fullness and distention in the right rib-side. The patient is thin. Decreased food intake. Distention is exacerbated by eating. Dry mouth and throat, thirst. Vexation and irascibility [心烦易怒 *xīn fán yì nù*], dizziness, unclear vision. Red and cracked tongue, with scant or no fur [舌红有裂纹, 少苔或无苔 *shé hóng yǒu liè wén, shǎo tāi huò wú tāi*]. Stringlike and fine pulse [脉弦细 *mài xián xì*].

14.3　TREATMENT OF GALLSTONES USING CHINESE MEDICINALS

14.3.1　Liver-Gallbladder Qì Stagnation [肝胆气滞 *gān dǎn qì zhì*]

Method of Treatment for Liver-Gallbladder Qì Stagnation

Course the liver and rectify qì, disinhibit the gallbladder and expel stones [疏肝理气，利胆排石 *shū gān lǐ qì, lì dǎn pái shí*].

Major Bupleurum Decoction [大柴胡汤 *dà chái hú tāng*]	
bupleurum [柴胡 *chái hú*, Bupleuri Radix]	9g
scutellaria [黄芩 *huáng qín*, Scutellariae Radix]	9g
white peony [白芍 *bái sháo*, Paeoniae Radix Alba]	9g
pinellia [半夏 *bàn xià*, Pinelliae Rhizoma]	9g
unripe bitter orange [枳实 *zhǐ shí*, Aurantii Fructus Immaturus]	9g
rhubarb [大黄 *dà huáng*, Rhei Rhizoma et Radix]	6g
fresh ginger [生姜 *shēng jiāng*, Zingiberis Rhizoma Recens]	12g
jujube [大枣 *dà zǎo*, Jujubae Fructus]	4 pieces
Directions: Take decocted with water [水煎服 *shuǐ jiān fú*].	

Prescription Analysis

Chief Medicinals

Bupleurum and scutellaria harmonize the lesser yáng [和解少阳 *hé jiě shào yáng*]. Bupleurum also courses and discharges liver-gallbladder depression and stagnation [疏泄肝胆郁滞 *shū xiè gān dǎn yù zhì*], thus treating the root [治本 *zhì běn*].

Support Medicinals

Rhubarb and unripe bitter orange drain yáng brightness bowel repletion [泻阳明之腑实 *xiè yáng míng zhī fǔ shí*]. They free and abduct the large intestine [通导大肠 *tōng dǎo dà cháng*] in order to disinhibit and expel the stones.

Assistant Medicinals

White peony is used to help bupleurum course the liver and move qì-blood depression and stagnation. Pinellia downbears stomach qì [降胃气 *jiàng wèi qì*] to help its downward movement [助下行 *zhù xià xíng*].

Fresh ginger downbears stomach qì and resolves the toxicity of pinellia. The combination of fresh ginger and jujube harmonizes construction and defense [调和营卫 *tiáo hé yíng wèi*].

This combination of medicinals is used to course the liver and rectify qì and to disinhibit the gallbladder and expel stones.

Variation According to Signs

Major Bupleurum Decoction was originally designed to treat lesser yáng and yáng brightness combination disease [少阳阳明合病 *shào yáng yáng míng hé bìng*]. Its scope of application was expanded with clinical use.

For constipation, add mirabilite [*máng xiāo*] to free and abduct the large intestine. If the left rib-side is painful and if it is hard to turn when lying, add corydalis [*yán hú suǒ*], trichosanthes [*guā lóu*], and unripe tangerine peel [*qīng pí*] to move qì and check pain. If the stones are hard to expel, add corydalis [*yán hú suǒ*], gizzard lining [*jī nèi jīn*], lygodium spore [*hǎi jīn shā*], and moneywort [*jīn qián cǎo*] to disinhibit and expel the stones. If there are signs of jaundice, add capillaris [*yīn chén hāo*], gardenia [*zhī zǐ*], phellodendron [*huáng bǎi*], and moneywort to disinhibit the gallbladder and abate jaundice [退黄 *tuì huáng*].

14.3.2 Damp-Heat Brewing Internally [湿热内蕴 *shī rè nèi yùn*]

Method of Treatment for Damp-Heat Brewing Internally

Clear heat and disinhibit dampness [清热利湿 *qīng rè lì shī*].

Capillaris Decoction [茵陈蒿汤 *yīn chén hāo tāng*]	
capillaris [茵陈蒿 *yīn chén hāo*, Artemisiae Capillaris Herba]	30g
gardenia [栀子 *zhī zǐ*, Gardeniae Fructus]	15g
rhubarb [大黄 *dà huáng*, Rhei Rhizoma et Radix]	10g
Directions: Take decocted with water [水煎服 *shuǐ jiān fú*].	

Prescription Analysis

Chief Medicinal

Capillaris clears heat and disinhibits dampness [清热利湿 *qīng rè lì shī*].

Support Medicinals

Gardenia clears and drains triple burner fire [清泻三焦火 *qīng xiè sān jiāo huǒ*] and disinhibits urine [利小便 *lì xiǎo biàn*], thereby dispelling damp-heat.

Assistant Medicinal

Rhubarb drains heat to free and abduct the stool [泻热而通导大便 *xiè rè ér tōng dǎo dà biàn*] and also dispels damp-heat and gallstones through the large intestine.

This combination of medicinals clears heat, disinhibits dampness, expels stones and abates jaundice.

Variation According to Signs

Capillaris Decoction is the chief prescription used for treating damp-heat jaundice. It is therefore also highly suitable to treat the root [治本 *zhì běn*] of gallstones that are caused by damp-heat brewing internally. To enhance the stone-expelling strength, add bupleurum [*chái hú*], curcuma [*yù jīn*], corydalis [*yán hú suǒ*], and talcum [*huá shí*], to disinhibit and expel the stones by coursing and disinhibiting the liver and gallbladder.

If there are signs of jaundice, increase the amount of capillaris and add phellodendron [*huáng bǎi*], moneywort [*jīn qián cǎo*], lygodium spore [*hǎi jīn shā*], plantago seed [*chē qián zǐ*], and dandelion [*pú gōng yīng*] to disinhibit the gallbladder and abate jaundice. If there are strong signs of damp evil, add agastache [*huò xiāng*], eupatorium [*pèi lán*], atractylodes [*cāng zhú*], and officinal magnolia bark [*hòu pò*] to transform dampness with aroma [芳香化湿 *fāng xiāng huà shī*].

14.3.3 Exuberant Heat-Toxin [热毒炽盛 *rè dú chì shèng*]

Method of Treatment for Exuberant Heat-Toxin

Clear and drain liver-gallbladder repletion heat [清泻肝胆实热 *qīng xiè gān dǎn shí rè*].

Gentian Liver-Draining Decoction [龙胆泻肝汤 *lóng dǎn xiè gān tāng*]	
gentian [龙胆草 *lóng dǎn cǎo*, Gentianae Radix]	6g
bupleurum [柴胡 *chái hú*, Bupleuri Radix]	6g
alisma [泽泻 *zé xiè*, Alismatis Rhizoma]	12g
plantago seed [车前子 *chē qián zǐ*, Plantaginis Semen]	9g
trifoliate akebia [木通 *mù tōng*, Akebiae Trifoliatae Caulis]	9g
dried/fresh rehmannia [生地黄 *shēng dì huáng*, Rehmanniae Radix seu Recens]	9g
Chinese angelica [当归 *dāng guī*, Angelicae Sinensis Radix]	3g
gardenia [栀子 *zhī zǐ*, Gardeniae Fructus]	9g
scutellaria [黄芩 *huáng qín*, Scutellariae Radix]	9g
licorice [甘草 *gān cǎo*, Glycyrrhizae Radix]	6g
Directions: Take decocted with water [水煎服 *shuǐ jiān fú*].	

Prescription Analysis

Chief Medicinal

Gentian, which is extremely cold and bitter, clears and drains liver-gallbladder heat toxin.

Support Medicinals

The bitter and cold properties of gardenia and scutellaria drain fire and help the chief medicinal treat the root [治本 *zhì běn*]. Alisma, trifoliate akebia, and plantago seed clear heat and disinhibit urine, which helps the chief medicinal clear heat and drain fire.

Assistant Medicinals

Chinese angelica quickens blood.

Dried/fresh rehmannia cools blood and nourishes yīn [凉血养阴 *liáng xuè yǎng yīn*].

Bupleurum courses and discharges liver-gallbladder depressed heat [疏泄肝胆郁热 *shū xiè gān dǎn yù rè*].

Licorice harmonizes the actions of the other medicinals.

This combination of medicinals clears and drains liver-gallbladder heat toxin.

Variation According to Signs

Gentian Liver-Draining Decoction [龙胆泻肝汤 *lóng dǎn xiè gān tāng*] clears and drains liver-gallbladder repletion fire and also clears and disinhibits damp-heat in the lower burner. It is an excellent prescription to treat the root [治本 *zhì běn*] of gallstones that are caused by liver-gallbladder repletion heat. To increase the stone-expelling strength, add gizzard lining [*jī nèi jīn*] to transform the stones [化石 *huà shí*], or add talcum [*huá shí*] and/or moneywort [*jīn qián cǎo]* to expel the stones. To check pain, loosen the bile duct, and disinhibit and expel the stones, add corydalis [*yán hú suǒ*] and scorpion [*quán xiē*].

14.3.4   Liver Yīn Insufficiency [肝阴不足 *gān yīn bù zú*]

Method of Treatment for Liver Yīn Insufficiency

Nourish blood and emolliate the liver, clear heat and disinhibit the gallbladder [养血柔肝，清热利胆 *yǎng xuè róu gān, qīng rè lì dǎn*].

All-the-Way-Through Brew [一贯煎 *yī guàn jiān*]	
dried/fresh rehmannia [生地黄 *shēng dì huáng*, Rehmanniae Radix seu Recens] 30g	
lycium berry [枸杞子 *gǒu qǐ zǐ*, Lycii Fructus]	12g
Chinese angelica [当归 *dāng guī*, Angelicae Sinensis Radix]	10g
glehnia [北沙参 *běi shā shēn*, Glehniae Radix]	10g
ophiopogon [麦冬 *mài dōng*, Ophiopogonis Radix]	10g
toosendan [川楝子 *chuān liàn zǐ*, Toosendan Fructus]	5g
Directions: Take decocted with water [水煎服 *shuǐ jiān fú*].	

Prescription Analysis

Chief Medicinal

Dried/fresh rehmannia strongly supplements liver and kidney yīn.

Support Medicinals

Glehnia, ophiopogon, Chinese angelica, and lycium berry enrich yīn and emolliate the liver [滋阴柔肝 *zī yīn róu gān*]. They help the chief medicinal enrich yīn.

Assistant Medicinal

A small quantity of toosendan courses the liver and qì [疏肝泄气 *shū gān xiè qì*].

This combination of medicinals nourishes blood and emolliates the liver.

Variation According to Signs

All-the-Way-Through Brew treats liver-kidney yīn vacuity, constrained liver qì [肝气不舒 *gān qì bù shū*], and pain in the rib-side. If it is necessary to enhance its stone-expelling strength, add talcum [*huá shí*], gizzard lining [*jī nèi jīn*], corydalis [*yán hú suǒ*], and bupleurum [*chái hú*] to course the liver, disinhibit the gallbladder, and expel the stones.

14.4 ACUPUNCTURE TREATMENT FOR GALLSTONES

14.4.1 Base Acupuncture Prescription for Gallstones

This base prescription should be modified according to the identified patterns that are discussed below and according to the condition of the individual patient.

Treatment Method

Course the liver and disinhibit the gallbladder [疏肝利胆 *shū gān lì dǎn*].

Base Acupuncture Prescription for Gallstones
LR-3 Supreme Surge [太冲 *tài chōng*]
GB-40 Hill Ruins [丘墟 *qiū xū*]
GB-24 Sun and Moon [日月 *rì yuè*]

Prescription Analysis

LR-3, the source point [原穴 *yuán xué*] of the liver channel, courses the liver. The source points of the yīn organs have a direct effect on the associated organs.

GB-40 is the source point [原穴 *yuán xué*] of the gallbladder channel; it disinhibits the gallbladder.

GB-24, the alarm point [募穴 *mù xué*] of the gallbladder, downbears counterflow and disinhibits the gallbladder, opens depression and checks pain [降逆利胆，开郁止痛 *jiàng nì lì dǎn, kāi yù zhǐ tòng*]. It regulates channel qì and expels stones [排石 *pái shí*].

14.4.2 Points to Add to the Base Prescription

Points for Liver-Gallbladder Qì Stagnation [肝胆气滞 *gān dǎn qì zhì*]

PC-6 Inner Pass [内关 *nèi guān*]

PC-6 regulates the qì dynamic [调畅气机 *tiáo chàng qì jī*] and courses and frees the channels [疏通经脉 *shū tōng jīng mài*].

Points for Damp-Heat Brewing Internally [湿热内蕴 *shī rè nèi yùn*]

GB-34 Yáng Mound Spring [阳陵泉 *yáng líng quán*]

GB-34 is the lower uniting point [下合穴 *xià hé xué*] of the gallbladder channel. Because lower uniting points treat diseases of the six bowels [合治内府 *hé zhì nèi fǔ*], GB-34 clears the liver and disinhibits the gallbladder, and clears and disinhibits damp-heat [清肝利胆，清利湿热 *qīng gān lì dǎn, qīng lì shī rè*].

Points for Exuberant Heat-toxin [热毒炽盛 *rè dú chì shèng*]

Apply needling and/or bloodletting [放血 *fàng xuè*] to
GB-44 Foot Orifice Yīn [足窍阴 *zú qiào yīn*]

GB-44 is the well point [井穴 *jǐng xué*] of the gallbladder channel. The *Classic of Difficult Issues, the 82nd Difficulty* [《难经六十八难》 *nán jīng liù shí bā nán*], says: "Well points are indicated in cases of fullness below the heart" [井主心下满 *jǐng zhǔ xīn xià mǎn*]. Bloodletting [放血 *fàng xuè*] at point GB-44 expels the heat toxin.

Points for Liver yīn insufficiency [肝阴不足 *gān yīn bù zú*]

KI-3 Great Ravine [太溪 *tài xī*]
LR-8 Spring at the Bend [曲泉 *qū quán*]

KI-3 enriches kidney yīn [滋肾阴 *zī shèn yīn*]. LR-8, the uniting (water) point [合 (水) 穴 *hé (shuǐ) xué*] of the liver channel, supplements liver yīn.

CHAPTER 15

Cholecystitis

Cholecystitis refers to inflammation of the gallbladder. Main symptoms of acute cholecystitis are severe pain in the right upper part of the abdomen (corresponding to the anatomical position of the gallbladder), fever, nausea, and vomiting. The main symptom of chronic cholecystitis is intermittent severe pain in the upper abdomen. Cholecystitis is often caused by gallstones.

There are four main forms of cholecystitis:

- liver-gallbladder qì stagnation [肝胆气滞 *gān dǎn qì zhì*]
- liver-gallbladder damp-heat [肝胆湿热 *gān dǎn shī rè*]
- blood stasis obstruction [瘀血阻滞 *yū xuè zǔ zhì*]
- liver-gallbladder fire toxin [肝胆火毒 *gān dǎn huǒ dú*]

15.1 POINTS OF ATTENTION FOR CHOLECYSTITIS

15.1.1 Pathomechanism of Cholecystitis

The four main forms of cholecystitis can appear separately or can influence and cause each other. In particular, several factors, such as affect-mind binding depression [情志郁结 *qíng zhì yù jié*], dietary irregularities (mainly greasy and/or sweet foods), or external contraction, can disturb free coursing of the liver-gallbladder [肝胆疏泄 *gān dǎn shū xiè*]. This results in obstructed qì dynamic, which in turn affects the upbearing and downbearing of the spleen and stomach [升降 *shēng jiàng*]. Damp-heat obstructing the middle burner further obstructs the qì dynamic. Qì is the commander of blood [气为血之帅 *qì wéi xuè zhī shuài*]; therefore, when qì is obstructed, blood also stagnates. When qì depression, blood stasis, and damp-heat combine, they form liver-gallbladder fire toxin.

15.1.2   Differentiating the Nature of Pain

Distending [胀痛 *zhàng tòng*], continuous, and scurrying (moving) [窜痛 *cuàn tòng*] pain in the right upper abdomen with intermittent periods of severe pain indicates qì stagnation and tends to appear in the beginning stage of the illness.

Blood stasis is indicated by stabbing pain [刺痛 *cì tòng*] in the right upper abdomen that is of fixed location and that refuses pressure.

Fire toxin is indicated by severe gripping pain [绞痛 *jiǎo tòng*] in the right upper abdomen with jaundice and strong heat effusion.

15.2   Causes and Pathomechanism of Cholecystitis; Identifying Patterns

15.2.1   Liver-Gallbladder Qì Stagnation [肝胆气滞 *gān dǎn qì zhì*]

Causes and Pathomechanism of Liver-Gallbladder Qì Stagnation

This pattern is the result of affect-mind binding depression [情志郁结 *qíng zhì yù jié*] or sudden bursts of anger that damage the liver. Depressed liver qì also influences the gallbladder and can cause liver-gallbladder qì stagnation; when qì obstructs the network vessels, it leads to fullness and distending pain in the right upper abdomen.

Important Signs of Liver-Gallbladder Qì Stagnation

Chronic Cholecystitis

Fullness and pain in the upper right abdomen that is distending [胀痛 *zhàng tòng*] and scurrying [窜痛 *cuàn tòng*]. Pain sometimes spreads to the right shoulder blade. Oppression in the chest. Frequent sighing. Rashness, impatience, and irascibility [急躁易怒 *jí zào yì nù*]. Pain is set off or exacerbated by emotional swings. Fullness in the stomach duct, torpid intake [纳呆 *nà dāi*]. Abdominal distention.

Acute Cholecystitis

Pain in the upper right abdomen that is gripping [绞痛 *jiǎo tòng*] and scurrying [窜痛 *cuàn tòng*]. Nausea, vomiting, dizziness, bitter taste in the mouth. Dry throat, no appetite. Dry stool, slight heat effusion. The tongue has a thin white coating [薄白苔 *bò bái tāi*]. Stringlike pulse [脉弦 *mài xián*].

15.2.2   Liver-Gallbladder Damp-Heat [肝胆湿热 *gān dǎn shī rè*]

Causes and Pathomechanism of Liver-Gallbladder Damp-Heat

This pattern is caused by dietary irregularities, such as eating too many fatty, spicy, or sweet foods, or by habitually drinking too much alcohol, which damage the spleen and stomach. Another possible cause is damp-heat evil assailing the body. When the spleen is impaired in its function of movement and transformation, water-dampness collects [停 *tíng*] and is not properly transformed. After some time, dampness transforms into heat, and damp-heat impairs the liver and gallbladder; this obstructs the qì dynamic and free coursing [气机疏泄不畅 *qì jī shū xiè bú chàng*].

Important Signs

Continuous distending pain [胀痛 *zhàng tòng*] and fullness in the right upper abdomen that is intermittently severe. Fullness and oppression in the chest and stomach duct. Heat effusion [发热 *fā rè*]. Bitter taste in the mouth. Dry throat. Nausea and vomiting. No thought of food. Yellowing of eyes and body. Yellow vaginal discharge. Short voidings of yellow or reddish urine. Constipation. The tongue has a yellow slimy coating [舌苔黄腻 *shé tāi huáng nì*]. Stringlike rapid pulse, or slippery rapid pulse [脉弦数或滑数 *mài xián shuò huò huá shuò*].

15.2.3   Blood Stasis Obstruction [瘀血阻滞 *yū xuè zǔ zhì*]

Causes and Pathomechanism of Blood Stasis Obstruction

When qì is obstructed, blood also stagnates; thus, depressed liver qì stagnation can lead to blood stasis.

Important Signs of Blood Stasis Obstruction

Stabbing pain in the right upper abdomen that has a fixed location. The pain refuses pressure [拒按 *jù àn*]. Rashness, impatience, and irascibility [急躁易怒 *jí zào yì nù*]. Glomus lump [痞块 *pǐ kuài*] below the right rib-side. The tongue is purple or has stasis macules [舌紫或有瘀斑 *shé zǐ huò yǒu yū bān*]. Rough pulse [脉涩 *mài sè*].

15.2.4   Liver-Gallbladder Fire Toxin [肝胆火毒 *gān dǎn huǒ dú*]

Causes and Pathomechanism of Liver-Gallbladder Fire Toxin

Enduring liver-gallbladder damp-heat depression combines with toxin and transforms into fire toxin. Fire toxin presses bile out and into the muscle and skin.

When fire toxin sinks into heart construction [心营 *xīn yíng*] there is clouded spirit and delirious speech [神昏谵语 *shén hūn zhān yǔ*]. When fire toxin distresses [迫 *pò*] blood, there are stasis macules [瘀斑 *yū bān*] on the skin.

Important Signs of Liver-Gallbladder Fire Toxin

Sudden gripping pain [绞痛 *jiǎo tòng*] in the upper abdomen that refuses pressure. Abdominal fullness and distention. Rigid abdominal muscles, painful to the touch. Continuous strong heat effusion. Shivering. Dry lips and mouth. Deep yellowing of the body and eyes. Dry stool. Short voidings of reddish urine [小便短赤 *xiǎo biàn duǎn chì*] that feel scorching hot. In cases of extreme heat there may be clouded spirit and delirious speech [神昏谵语 *shén hūn zhān yǔ*], stasis macules on the skin, and reversal cold of the limbs. Crimson tongue with dry yellow fur [舌红绛, 苔黄干 *shé hóng jiàng, tāi huáng gān*]. Stringlike slippery rapid pulse or fine rapid pulse [脉弦滑数或细数 *mài xián huá shuò huò xì shuò*].

15.3   TREATMENT OF CHOLECYSTITIS USING CHINESE MEDICINALS

15.3.1   Liver-Gallbladder Qì Stagnation [肝胆气滞 *gān dǎn qì zhì*]

Method of Treatment for Liver-Gallbladder Qì Stagnation

Course the liver and rectify qì, disinhibit the gallbladder and clear heat [疏肝理气，利胆清热 *shū gān lǐ qì, lì dǎn qīng rè*].

Major Bupleurum Decoction [大柴胡汤 *dà chái hú tāng*]	
bupleurum [柴胡 *chái hú*, Bupleuri Radix]	9g
scutellaria [黄芩 *huáng qín*, Scutellariae Radix]	9g
white peony [白芍 *bái sháo*, Paeoniae Radix Alba]	9g
pinellia [半夏 *bàn xià*, Pinelliae Rhizoma]	9g
unripe bitter orange [枳实 *zhǐ shí*, Aurantii Fructus Immaturus]	9g
rhubarb [大黄 *dà huáng*, Rhei Rhizoma et Radix]	6g
fresh ginger [生姜 *shēng jiāng*, Zingiberis Rhizoma Recens]	12g
jujube [大枣 *dà zǎo*, Jujubae Fructus]	4 pieces
Directions: Take decocted with water [水煎服 *shuǐ jiān fú*].	

Prescription Analysis

Chief Medicinals

Bupleurum and scutellaria harmonize the lesser yáng [和解少阳 *hé jiě shào yáng*].

Support Medicinals

Rhubarb and unripe bitter orange drain yáng brightness repletion heat [泻阳明实热 *xiè yáng míng shí rè*].

Assistant Medicinals

Because of heat transformation [化热 *huà rè*] in the lesser yáng and wood overwhelming earth [木乘土 *mù chéng tǔ*], white peony [*bái sháo*] is used to help bupleurum and scutellaria clear liver and gallbladder heat [清肝胆之热 *qīng gān dǎn zhī rè*].

Pinellia harmonizes the stomach, downbears counterflow, and checks vomiting [和胃降逆止呕 *hé wèi jiàng nì zhǐ ǒu*].

Fresh ginger and jujube harmonize construction and defense [调和营卫 *tiáo hé yíng wèi*].

This combination of medicinals courses the liver and rectifies qì, disinhibits the gallbladder and clears heat.

Variation According to Signs

For phlegm and heat binding together [痰热互结 *tán rè hù jié*], which is marked by glomus and oppression in the chest and stomach [胸脘痞闷 *xiōng wǎn pǐ mèn*] that is painful to the touch and by yellow and slimy tongue fur [舌苔黄腻 *shé tāi huáng nì*], add trichosanthes [瓜蒌 *guā lóu*] and coptis [*huáng lián*] to clear heat and transform phlegm.

For qì stagnation and damp obstruction [气滞湿阻 *qì zhì shī zǔ*], which is marked by: distention and fullness in the stomach duct and abdomen [脘腹胀满 *wǎn fù zhàng mǎn*]; belching and sour regurgitation [嗳气反酸 *ài qì fǎn suān*]; and aversion to greasy, oily food [厌油腻 *yàn yóu nì*], add bitter orange [*zhǐ ké*], officinal magnolia bark [*hòu pò*], agastache [*huò xiāng*], eupatorium [*pèi lán*], and Buddha's hand [*fó shǒu*] to eliminate dampness and move qì.

If there are stones as well, add moneywort [*jīn qián cǎo*], lygodium spore [*hǎi jīn shā*], capillaris [*yīn chén hāo*], and gizzard lining [*jī nèi jīn*] to expel stones and disinhibit the gallbladder [排石利胆 *pái shí lì dǎn*].

15.3.2　Liver-Gallbladder Damp-Heat [肝胆湿热 *gān dǎn shī rè*]

Method of Treatment for Liver-Gallbladder Damp-Heat

Clear heat and disinhibit dampness [清热利湿 *qīng rè lì shī*].

Capillaris Decoction [茵陈蒿汤 *yīn chén hāo tāng*]	
capillaris [茵陈蒿 *yīn chén hāo*, Artemisiae Capillaris Herba]	30g
gardenia [栀子 *zhī zǐ*, Gardeniae Fructus]	10g
rhubarb [大黃 *dà huáng*, Rhei Rhizoma et Radix]	10g
Directions: Take decocted with water [水煎服 *shuǐ jiān fú*].	

Prescription Analysis

Chief Medicinal

Capillaris clears and disinhibits liver-gallbladder damp-heat.

Support Medicinal

Gardenia clears heat and disinhibits dampness [清热利湿 *qīng rè lì shī*] and drains triple burner damp-heat [泻三焦湿热 *xiè sān jiāo shī rè*].

Assistant Medicinal

Rhubarb drains heat to free the large intestine [泻热而通大肠 *xiè rè ér tōng dà cháng*] and dispels damp-heat through the large intestine.

Capillaris in combination with gardenia dispels damp-heat through the small intestine; capillaris in combination with rhubarb dispels damp-heat through the large intestine. Together, these three medicinals clear heat and disinhibit dampness.

Variation According to Signs

The above prescription very strongly clears heat and disinhibits dampness. For severe pain, add bupleurum [*chái hú*], scutellaria [*huáng qín*], corydalis [*yán hú suǒ*], curcuma [*yù jīn*], and costusroot [*mù xiāng*] to course the liver and check pain [疏肝止痛 *shū gān zhǐ tòng*].

15.3.3　Blood Stasis Obstruction [瘀血阻滞 *yū xuè zǔ zhì*]

Method of Treatment

Quicken blood and transform stasis, course the liver and free the network vessels [活血化瘀，疏肝通络 *huó xuè huà yū, shū gān tōng luò*].

Infradiaphragmatic Stasis-Expelling Decoction **[膈下逐瘀汤 *gé xià zhú yū tāng*]**	
Chinese angelica [当归 *dāng guī*, Angelicae Sinensis Radix]	10g
peach kernel [桃仁 *táo rén*, Persicae Semen]	10g

carthamus [红花 *hóng huā*, Carthami Flos]	10g
chuanxiong [川芎 *chuān xiōng*, Chuanxiong Rhizoma]	6g
red peony [赤芍 *chì sháo*, Paeoniae Radix Rubra]	6g
flying squirrel's droppings [五灵脂 *wǔ líng zhī*, Trogopteri Faeces]	6g
moutan [牡丹皮 *mǔ dān pí*, Moutan Cortex]	6g
lindera [乌药 *wū yào*, Linderae Radix]	6g
corydalis [延胡索 *yán hú suǒ*, Corydalis Rhizoma	4g
cyperus [香附 *xiāng fù*, Cyperi Rhizoma]	4g
bitter orange [枳壳 *zhǐ ké*, Aurantii Fructus]	4g
licorice [甘草 *gān cǎo*, Glycyrrhizae Radix]	3g

Directions: Take decocted with water [水煎服 *shuǐ jiān fú*].

Prescription Analysis

Chief Medicinals

Chinese angelica, peach kernel, and carthamus [*hóng huā*] quicken blood, transform stasis, and check pain.

Support Medicinals

Chuanxiong, red peony, moutan, and flying squirrel's droppings help the chief medicinals quicken blood and transform stasis.

Assistant Medicinals

Lindera, cyperus, bitter orange, and corydalis move qì in order to help move blood.

Licorice harmonizes the properties of all the medicinals [调和药性 *tiáo hé yào xìng*].

This combination of medicinals is used to quicken blood and transform stasis and to course the liver and check pain.

Variation According to Signs

For strong stabbing pain [刺痛 *cì tòng*], add frankincense [*rǔ xiāng*] and myrrh [*mò yào*] to stop pain. For signs of heat, remove Chinese angelica and cyperus and add isatis root [*bǎn lán gēn*] and scutellaria [*huáng qín*]. For jaundice [黄疸 *huáng dǎn*], add capillaris [*yīn chén hāo*], gardenia [*zhī zǐ*], and rhubarb [*dà huáng*] to disinhibit the gallbladder and abate jaundice [退黄 *tuì huáng*].

15.3.4 Liver-Gallbladder Fire Toxin [肝胆火毒 *gān dǎn huǒ dú*]

Method of Treatment for Liver-Gallbladder Fire Toxin

Drain fire and resolve toxins [泻火解毒 *xiè huǒ jiě dú*].

Coptis Toxin-Resolving Decoction [黄连解毒汤 *huáng lián jiě dú tāng*]	
coptis [黄连 *huáng lián*, Coptidis Rhizoma]	9g
scutellaria [黄芩 *huáng qín*, Scutellariae Radix]	6g
phellodendron [黄柏 *huáng bǎi*, Phellodendri Cortex]	6g
gardenia [栀子 *zhī zǐ*, Gardeniae Fructus]	9g
Directions: Take decocted with water [水煎服 *shuǐ jiān fú*].	

Prescription Analysis

Chief Medicinal

Coptis, which is cold and bitter, powerfully drains heart fire.

Support Medicinals

Scutellaria drains lung and upper burner fire. Phellodendron drains lower burner fire. Gardenia drains triple burner fire and abducts the heat downwards [导热下行 *dǎo rè xià xíng*]. All support medicinals help the chief medicinal drain fire.

All four medicinals together free and drain exuberant triple burner fire [三焦火盛 *sān jiāo huǒ shèng*].

Variation According to Signs

Coptis Toxin-Resolving Decoction drains fire toxin with great strength. If the specific draining action on the liver and gallbladder is insufficient, add bupleurum [*chái hú*], curcuma [*yù jīn*], and gentian [*lóng dǎn cǎo*] to drain liver-gallbladder fire toxin.

If heat evil intensifies and becomes so exuberant that it leads to symptoms such as clouded spirit or delirious spirit [神昏谵神 *shén hūn zhān shén*], prescribe Peaceful Palace Bovine Bezoar Pill [安宫牛黄丸 *ān gōng niú huáng wán*] in addition to the above prescription in order to open the orifices and arouse the spirit [开窍醒神 *kāi qiào xǐng shén*].

15.4 ACUPUNCTURE TREATMENT FOR CHOLECYSTITIS

15.4.1 Base Acupuncture Prescription for Cholecystitis

This base prescription should be modified according to the identified patterns that are discussed below and according to the condition of the individual patient.

Treatment Method for Cholecystitis

Course the liver and disinhibit the gallbladder [疏肝利胆 *shū gān lì dǎn*].

Base Acupuncture Prescription for Cholecystitis

LR-3 Supreme Surge [太冲 *tài chōng*]
GB-40 Hill Ruins [丘墟 *qiū xū*]

Prescription Analysis

LR-3, the source point [原穴 *yuán xué*] of the liver channel, courses the liver; GB-40, the source point [原穴 *yuán xué*] of the gallbladder channel, disinhibits the gallbladder. The combination of the source points of these interior-exterior channels strongly stimulates the channel qì and expels evil from the body.

15.4.2   Points to Add to the Base Prescription

Points for Liver-Gallbladder Qì Stagnation [肝胆气滞 *gān dǎn qì zhì*]

PC-6 Inner Pass [内关 *nèi guān*]
GB-37 Bright Light [光明 *guāng míng*]

PC-6 regulates the qì dynamic [调畅气机 *tiáo chàng qì jī*]. GB-37 courses and frees the channels.

Points for Liver-Gallbladder Damp-Heat [肝胆湿热 *gān dǎn shī rè*]

GB-34 Yáng Mound Spring [阳陵泉 *yáng líng quán*]

GB-34 is the lower uniting point of the gallbladder channel. Because lower uniting points treat the diseases of the six bowels [合治内府 *hé zhì nèi fǔ*], GB-24 is used to treat diseases of the gallbladder; it also clears and disinhibits damp-heat.

Points for Blood Stasis Obstruction [瘀血阻滞 *yū xuè zǔ zhì*]

LR-14 Cycle Gate [期门 *qī mén*]
GB-24 Sun and Moon [日月 *rì yuè*]
GB-36 Outer Hill [外丘 *wài qiū*]

LR-14 and GB-24, the alarm points [募穴 *mù xué*] of the liver and gallbladder, clear heat and quicken blood. GB-36 is the cleft point [郄穴 *xī xué*] of the gallbladder channel. Qì and blood accumulate at the cleft points, and they are mostly used in acute patterns, especially in the treatment of pain. GB-36 frees the channels and quickens the network vessels [通经活络 *tōng jīng huó luò*].

Liver-Gallbladder Fire Toxin [肝胆火毒 *gān dǎn huǒ dú*]

LR-2 Moving Between [行间 *xíng jiān*]
GB-43 Pinched Ravine [侠溪 *xiá xī*]

LR-2 clears liver heat. GB-43 clears gallbladder heat. Both points are spring points [荥穴 *yíng xué*] and have heat-clearing and toxin-resolving properties.

CHAPTER 16
Ulcerative Colitis

Ulcerative colitis is a chronic inflammatory and ulcerative disease of the colon. Main symptoms are diarrhea with blood and mucus, lower abdominal cramps, and pain. There is also inflammation and ulceration of the mucous membrane of the colon and periods of diarrhea of varying intensity and duration that alternate with symptom-free periods. Ulcerative colitis appears in all age groups.

Before beginning treatment, check that the colitis is not due to infection, e.g., by *Entamoeba histolytica*, or by bacteria such as salmonella or *Shigella dysenteriae*.

There are five main forms of ulcerative colitis:

- damp-heat stagnating in the intestines [湿热滞肠 *shī rè zhì cháng*]
- disharmony of the liver and spleen [肝脾不和 *gān pí bù hé*]
- spleen vacuity qì fall [脾虚气陷 *pí xū qì xiàn*]
- spleen-kidney yáng vacuity [脾肾阳虚 *pí shèn yáng xū*]
- blood stasis in the intestine network vessels [血瘀肠络 *xuè yū cháng luò*]

16.1 POINTS OF ATTENTION FOR ULCERATIVE COLITIS

16.1.1 Different Stages of Ulcerative Colitis

Early Stage

In many cases, ulcerative colitis begins with dietary irregularities that damage the spleen and stomach, or the patient already has damp-heat brewing internally and eats too many fatty, sweet, and/or unclean foods.

In other cases, affect-mind internal damage [情志内伤 *qíng zhì nèi shāng*] causes the liver to lose its function of coursing and discharging [肝失疏泄 *gān shī shū xiè*]. Liver qì then overwhelms the spleen and invades the stomach, which disturbs the moving and transforming function of the spleen and stomach.

Damage to the spleen and stomach influences the intestines, which impairs the intestine's ability to separate the clear and the turbid and to discharge waste from the body. This leads to the internal engendering of water-damp; when the water-damp is depressed, it transforms into fire. Damp-heat toxin binds in the intestines, scorching the network vessels, and causing blood to spill outside of the channel, or qì-blood congeals and stagnates and transforms into pus. Spilt blood and pus are discharged together with the stool.

Advanced Stage

Frequent relapses of ulcerative colitis weaken spleen qì. Spleen vacuity impairs the production of qì and blood and results in qì-blood vacuity. When the spleen is vacuous, clear yáng fails to bear upwards [清阳不升 *qīng yáng bù shēng*] and center qì falls [中气下陷 *zhōng qì xià xiàn*], which makes recovery even more difficult. The spleen disease affects the kidney, resulting in both spleen and kidney vacuity and weak yáng qì.

In most cases, this disease either starts out with a vacuous root (spleen and kidney vacuity) or it develops towards a vacuous root, while the tip is a repletion (damp-heat toxin brewing in the intestines). In the acute stage, the tip/repletion is prominent. In the chronic stage, the root/vacuity is prominent.

16.1.2 Treatment for Ulcerative Colitis

In the acute stage of ulcerative colitis the repletion pattern [实证 *shí zhèng*] is prominent, and dispelling evil [祛邪 *qū xié*] is the main treatment principle. If the illness persists, the vacuity pattern [虚证 *xū zhèng*] becomes prominent, and supplementation is the main treatment principle, such as supplementing the spleen and kidney, securing and astricting [固涩 *gù sè*], and checking diarrhea.

16.2   CAUSES AND PATHOMECHANISM OF ULCERATIVE COLITIS; IDENTIFYING PATTERNS

16.2.1   Damp-Heat Stagnating in the Intestines [湿热滞肠 *shī rè zhì cháng*]

Causes and Pathomechanism of Damp-Heat Stagnating in the Intestines

This pattern is the result of external contraction of damp-heat or of dietary irregularities, such as consumption of unclean foods, or excessive consumption of greasy, sweet, or raw foods that engender damp-heat. Damp-heat brews internally, causes qì to stagnate and qì-blood to coagulate, and transforms into blood mixed with pus.

Important Signs of Damp-Heat Stagnating in the Intestines

Abdominal pain and distention, diarrhea. Abdominal urgency and rectal heaviness (tenesmus) [里急后重 *lǐ jí hòu zhòng*]. Malodorous stool mixed with blood or with pus and blood. Scorching heat sensation in the rectum, yellow turbid urine, heat effusion. Bitter taste in the mouth, or sticky feeling in the mouth. The tongue has a yellow slimy coating [舌苔黄腻 *shé tāi huáng nì*]. Slippery rapid pulse [脉滑数 *mài huá shuò*].

16.2.2 Disharmony of the Liver and Spleen [肝脾不和 *gān pí bù hé*]

Causes and Pathomechanism of Disharmony of the Liver and Spleen

Affect-mind internal damage [情志内伤 *qíng zhì nèi shāng*] causes the liver to lose its function of coursing and discharging [肝失疏泄 *gān shī shū xiè*]. Liver qì overwhelms the spleen [肝气乘脾 *gān qì chéng pí*] and invades the stomach, which disturbs the moving and transforming function of the spleen and stomach. This gives rise to inhibited upbearing and downbearing of the qì dynamic [气机升降不利 *qì jī shēng jiàng bú lì*], qì stagnation, and blood stasis in the stomach and intestines.

Important Signs of Disharmony of the Liver and Spleen

Abdominal pain and diarrhea. Pain is relieved after an attack of diarrhea. Stool is watery and yellow or sticky. Rumbling intestines, flatus [失气 *shī qì*]. Feeling of fullness and blockage in the stomach duct and abdomen. Reduced food intake. The condition is influenced by emotional swings. Pale tongue with thin white coating [舌淡苔薄白 *shé dàn tāi bó bái*]. Stringlike fine pulse [脉弦细 *mài xián xì*].

16.2.3 Spleen Vacuity Qì Fall [脾虚气陷 *pí xū qì xiàn*]

Causes and Pathomechanism of Spleen Vacuity Qì Fall

When the spleen is vacuous, clear yáng fails to bear upwards [清阳不升 *qīng yáng bù shēng*] and center qì falls [中气下陷 *zhōng qì xià xiàn*], resulting in diarrhea and dysentery [下利 *xià lì*].

Important Signs of Spleen Vacuity Qì Fall

When people suffer from this pattern and are not cautious with food, they easily develop watery stools. The stool is mixed with sticky fluid, undigested food, or vanquished blood [败血 *bài xuè*]. There may be incontinence and sagging distention in the abdomen [腹部坠胀 *fù bù zhuì zhàng*]. Continuous abdominal pain, weak limbs, loss of appetite, and torpid intake [纳呆 *nà dāi*]. Lusterless facial complexion [面色不华 *miàn sè bù huá*]. Pale tongue with white coating [舌淡苔白 *shé dàn tāi bái*]. Deep pulse or fine weak pulse [脉沉或细弱 *mài chén huò xì ruò*].

16.2.4   Spleen-Kidney Yáng Vacuity [脾肾阳虚 *pí shèn yáng xū*]

Causes and Pathomechanism of Spleen-Kidney Yáng Vacuity

Long-standing diarrhea causes vacuity of spleen qì that in turn affects the kidney, resulting in both spleen-kidney vacuity and weak yáng qì. Or, weak kidney qì due to insufficiency of the inherited constitution can bring about spleen vacuity. Insufficiency of spleen-kidney yáng qì causes impaired movement and transformation and results in enduring diarrhea.

Important Signs of Spleen-Kidney Yáng Vacuity

Lower abdominal cold pain [少腹冷痛 *shào fù lěng tòng*]. Fifth-watch diarrhea,[11] or clear-food diarrhea [下利清谷 *xià lì qīng gǔ*]. The pain is relieved after defecation and with warmth. Stool may be mixed with vanquished blood [败血 *bài xuè*]. Aching, weak lumbus. Aversion to cold, cold limbs. Pale and enlarged tongue with white fur [舌淡胖，苔白 *shé dàn pàng, tāi bái*]. Deep forceless pulse [脉沉无力 *mài chén wú lì*].

16.2.5   Blood Stasis in the Intestine Network Vessels
             [血瘀肠络 *xuè yū cháng luò*]

Causes and Pathomechanism of Blood Stasis in the Intestine Network Vessels

This pattern results from qì-blood stagnating in and congesting the intestines and from blood stasis obstructing the intestinal network vessels. This causes the blood to spill out of the channels.

Important Signs of Blood Stasis in the Intestine Network Vessels

Severe abdominal pain that refuses pressure [拒按 *jù àn*]. Pain location is fixed. Stool is mixed with purple-black blood clots. Dark purple tongue or the tongue has stasis macules [舌质紫暗或有瘀斑 *shé zhì zǐ àn huò yǒu yū bān*]. Deep rough pulse [脉沉涩 *mài chén sè*].

---

[11] Fifth-watch diarrhea refers to diarrhea before daybreak. (Ed.)

16.3 **TREATMENT OF ULCERATIVE COLITIS USING CHINESE MEDICINALS**

16.3.1 **Damp-Heat Stagnating in the Intestines [湿热滞肠 *shī rè zhì cháng*]**

Method of Treatment for Damp-Heat Stagnating in the Intestines

Clear heat and dry dampness, upbear yáng and check dysentery [清热燥湿，升阳止痢 *qīng rè zào shī, shēng yáng zhǐ lì*].

Pueraria, Scutellaria, and Coptis Decoction [葛根芩连汤 *gé gēn qín lián tāng*]	
pueraria [葛根 *gé gēn*, Puerariae Radix]	15g
scutellaria [黄芩 *huáng qín*, Scutellariae Radix]	9g
coptis [黄连 *huáng lián*, Coptidis Rhizoma]	9g
licorice [甘草 *gān cǎo*, Glycyrrhizae Radix]	3g
Directions: Take decocted with water [水煎服 *shuǐ jiān fú*].	

Prescription Analysis

Chief Medicinal

Pueraria clears heat, upbears and effuses spleen-stomach clear yáng qì [升发脾胃清阳之气 *shēng fā pí wèi qīng yáng zhī qì*], and treats diarrhea and dysentery [治下利 *zhì xià lì*].

Support Medicinals

The cold quality of scutellaria and coptis clears heat in the stomach and intestines. Their bitter [苦 *kǔ*] flavor dries dampness in the stomach and intestines.

Licorice harmonizes the center and harmonizes the actions of all the other medicinals.

This combination of medicinals is used to clear heat and dry dampness and to upbear yáng and check dysentery.

Variation According to Signs

The primary indication for Pueraria, Scutellaria, and Coptis Decoction is damp-heat dysentery. For heat-toxin blood dysentery [热毒血痢 *rè dú xuè lì*], if the stool contains pus and blood with copious blood and little pus [赤多白少 *chì duō bái shǎo*], add pulsatilla [*bái tóu wēng*] and ash [*qín pí*] to cool blood and check dysentery. For severe abdominal pain, add white peony [*bái sháo*] and more licorice to harmonize the interior, relax tension, and check pain [和里，缓急，止痛 *hé lǐ, huǎn jí, zhǐ tòng*]. If the stool has copious pus, add moutan [*mǔ dān pí*], red peony [*chì sháo*], and lonicera [*jīn yín huā*] to cool blood and resolve toxin [凉血解毒 *liáng xuè jiě dú*]. If there is severe tenesmus [里急后重 *lǐ jí hòu zhòng*], add costusroot [*mù xiāng*], areca husk [*dà fù pí*], and Chinese chive [*xiè bái*] to move qì and abduct stagnation [行气导滞 *xíng qì dǎo zhì*].

16.3.2   Disharmony of the Liver and Spleen [肝脾不和 *gān pí bù hé*]

Method of Treatment for Disharmony of the Liver and Spleen

Course the liver and supplement the spleen [疏肝补脾 *shū gān bǔ pí*].

Pain and Diarrhea Formula [痛泻要方 *tòng xiè yào fāng*]	
white peony [白芍 *bái sháo*, Paeoniae Radix Alba]	60g
white atractylodes [白术 *bái zhú*, Atractylodis Macrocephalae Rhizoma]	90g
tangerine peel [陈皮 *chén pí*, Citri Reticulatae Pericarpium]	45g
saposhnikovia [防风 *fáng fēng*, Saposhnikoviae Radix]	60g

Directions: The original prescription was taken as a powder [散 *sàn*] or pill [丸 *wán*]. Nowadays, it is taken as a decoction [水煎服 *shuǐ jiān fú*] with the quantities of medicinals proportionately decreased according to the original ratio.

Prescription Analysis

Chief Medicinals

White atractylodes dries dampness and fortifies the spleen [燥湿健脾 *zào shī jiàn pí*]. White peony relaxes tension and checks pain [缓急止痛 *huǎn jí zhǐ tòng*].

Support Medicinals

Tangerine peel, which rectifies qì and regulates the middle [理气调中 *lǐ qì tiáo zhōng*] and also transforms dampness and harmonizes the stomach, helps white atractylodes fortify the spleen and dispel dampness. The acrid flavor and warm characteristic of saposhnikovia enter the liver and spleen channels, helping the chief medicinals course the liver and rectify the spleen.

This combination of medicinals drains the liver, supplements the spleen, and regulates the qì dynamic.

Variation According to Signs

The indication for Pain and Diarrhea Formula is diarrhea with abdominal pain that is caused by depressed wood restraining earth [木郁克土 *mù yù kè tǔ*].

For spleen qì vacuity (distention and fullness in the stomach duct and abdomen [脘腹胀满 *wǎn fù zhàng mǎn*], no thought of food and drink [不思饮食 *bù sī yǐn shí*], sloppy diarrhea [大便溏泻 *dà biàn táng xiè*], and enlarged tongue [舌体胖大 *shé tǐ pàng dà*] with dental impressions), add mix-fried astragalus [*zhì huáng qí*], codonopsis [*dǎng shēn*], dioscorea [*shān yào*], and poria [*fú líng*] to supplement and boost center qì. For severe stagnant depression of liver qì [肝气郁滞 *gān qì yù zhì*] (distention and fullness in the ribs, vexation, agitation and irascibility [烦躁易怒 *fán zào yì nù*]), add bupleurum [*chái hú*] and curcuma [*yù jīn*] to course the liver. For cold pain in the stomach duct and abdomen [脘腹冷痛 *wǎn fù lěng tòng*], add dried ginger [*gān jiāng*] to warm the center, dissipate cold, and check pain.

16.3.3   Spleen Vacuity Qì Fall [脾虚气陷 *pí xū qì xiàn*]

Method of Treatment for Spleen Vacuity Qì Fall

Supplement qì and upbear yáng [补气升阳 *bǔ qì shēng yáng*].

Center-Supplementing Qì-Boosting Decoction [补中益气汤 *bǔ zhōng yì qì tāng*]	
astragalus [黄芪 *huáng qí*, Astragali Radix]	15g
ginseng [人参 *rén shēn*, Ginseng Radix] or	
(codonopsis [党参 *dǎng shēn*, Codonopsis Radix])	10g
Chinese angelica [当归 *dāng guī*, Angelicae Sinensis Radix]	10g
tangerine peel [橘皮 *jú pí*, Citri Reticulatae Pericarpium]	6g
licorice [甘草 *gān cǎo*, Glycyrrhizae Radix]	5g
cimicifuga [升麻 *shēng má*, Cimicifugae Rhizoma]	3g
bupleurum [柴胡 *chái hú*, Bupleuri Radix]	3g
white atractylodes [白术 *bái zhú*, Atractylodis Macrocephalae Rhizoma]	10g
Directions: Take decocted with water [水煎服 *shuǐ jiān fú*].	

Prescription Analysis

Chief Medicinal

Astragalus supplements the center and boosts qì, upbears yáng and secures the exterior [升阳固表 *shēng yáng gù biǎo*].

Support Medicinals

Codonopsis, white atractylodes, and licorice support the chief medicinal in supplementing the center and boosting qì.

Assistant Medicinals

Tangerine peel rectifies qì and harmonizes the center [理气和中 *lǐ qì hé zhōng*]. Chinese angelica supplements and harmonizes blood. Cimicifuga and bupleurum uplift falling yáng qì [升提下陷之阳气 *shēng tí xià xiàn zhī yáng qì*].

This combination of medicinals supplements qì and upbears yang.

Variation According to Signs

The primary indication for Center-Supplementing Qì-Boosting Decoction is spleen-stomach qì vacuity and center qì fall [中气下陷 *zhōng qì xià xiàn*]. For severe sloppy diarrhea [大便溏泻 *dà biàn táng xiè*], add dioscorea [*shān yào*] and remove Chinese angelica. If the patient has no thought of food and drink [不思饮食 *bù sī yǐn shí*], add gizzard lining [*jī nèi jīn*], medicated leaven [*shén qū*], barley sprout [*mài yá*], and radish seed [*lái fú zǐ*] for abductive dispersion [消导 *xiāo dǎo*].

16.3.4   Spleen-Kidney Yáng Vacuity [脾肾阳虚 *pí shèn yáng xū*]

Method of Treatment for Spleen-Kidney Yáng Vacuity

Warm and supplement spleen and kidney, astringe the intestines and check diarrhea [温补脾肾，涩肠止泻 *wēn bǔ pí shèn, sè cháng zhǐ xiè*].

Four Spirits Pill [四神丸 *sì shén wán*]	
psoralea [补骨脂 *bǔ gǔ zhī*, Psoraleae Fructus]	15g
nutmeg [肉豆蔻 *ròu dòu kòu*, Myristicae Semen]	10g
schisandra [五味子 *wǔ wèi zǐ*, Schisandrae Fructus	10g
evodia [吴茱萸 *wú zhū yú*, Evodiae Fructus]	5g

Directions: Decoct in water with six slices of fresh ginger [生姜 *shēng jiāng*, Zingiberis Rhizoma Recens] and ten pieces of jujube [大枣 *dà zǎo*, Jujubae Fructus].

Prescription Analysis

Chief Medicinal

Psorealea strongly supplements the life gate fire [大补命门之火 *dà bǔ mìng mén zhī huǒ*] to warm and nourish spleen yáng.

Support Medicinals

Evodia warms the center and dissipates cold. Nutmeg is used to warm the kidney and spleen and to astringe the intestines and check diarrhea [涩肠止泻 *sè cháng zhǐ xiè*]. Both medicinals help the chief medicinal treat the root [治本 *zhì běn*].

Assistant Medicinals

Schisandra, which is sour [酸 *suān*], constrains [敛 *liǎn*], secures [固 *gù*], and astringes [涩 *sè*] to check diarrhea. Fresh ginger helps evodia warm the center and dissipate cold. Jujube supplements the spleen and nourishes the stomach.

This combination of medicinals is used to warm and supplement the spleen and kidney and to astringe the intestines and check diarrhea.

16.3.5   Blood Stasis in the Intestine Network Vessels
[血瘀肠络 *xuè yū cháng luò*]

Method of Treatment for Blood Stasis in the Intestine Network Vessels

Quicken blood and dissipate stasis, free the channels and check pain [活血散瘀，通经止痛 *huó xuè sàn yū, tōng jīng zhǐ tòng*].

Lesser Abdomen Stasis-Expelling Decoction [少腹逐瘀汤 *shào fù zhú yū tāng*]	
fennel [小茴香 *xiǎo huí xiāng*, Foeniculi Fructus]	7 grains
dried ginger [干姜 *gān jiāng*, Zingiberis Rhizoma]	2g
corydalis [延胡索 *yán hú suǒ*, Corydalis Rhizoma]	3g
myrrh [没药 *mò yào*, Myrrha]	3g
Chinese angelica [当归 *dāng guī*, Angelicae Sinensis Radix]	9g
chuanxiong [川芎 *chuān xiōng*, Chuanxiong Rhizoma]	3g
cinnamon bark [肉桂 *ròu guì*, Cinnamomi Cortex]	3g
red peony [赤芍 *chì sháo*, Paeoniae Radix Rubra]	6g
typha pollen [蒲黄 *pú huáng*, Typhae Pollen]	5g
flying squirrel's droppings [五灵脂 *wǔ líng zhī*, Trogopteri Faeces]	6g
Directions: Take decocted with water [水煎服 *shuǐ jiān fú*].	

Prescription Analysis

Chief Medicinals

Chinese angelica and chuanxiong quicken blood and transform stasis to treat the root [治本 *zhì běn*].

Support Medicinals

Red peony, myrrh, typha pollen, flying squirrel's droppings, and corydalis help the chief medicinals quicken blood and check pain.

Assistant Medicinals

Fennel, dried ginger, and cinnamon bark warm the channels and dispel cold, and quicken blood and free the channels to help move blood and transform stasis.

This combination of medicinals is used to quicken blood and transform stasis and to free the channels and check pain.

Variation According to Signs

For copious pus and blood in the stool, add sanguisorba [*dì yú*] and notoginseng [*sān qī*] to transform stasis and stanch bleeding [化瘀止血 *huà yū zhǐ xuè*]. For tenesmus [里急后重 *lǐ jí hòu zhòng*], add costusroot [*mù xiāng*] and Chinese chive [*xiè bái*] to move qì and abduct stasis [行气导滞 *xíng qì dǎo zhì*]. For fatigue [身体倦怠 *shēn tǐ juàn dài*], add astragalus [*huáng qí*] and ginseng [*rén shēn*] to supplement qì.

16.4   ACUPUNCTURE TREATMENT FOR ULCERATIVE COLITIS

16.4.1   Base Acupuncture Prescription for Ulcerative Colitis

This base prescription should be modified according to the identified patterns that are discussed below and according to the condition of the individual patient.

Treatment Method for Ulcerative Colitis

Move qì and abduct stagnation [行气导滞 *xíng qì dǎo zhì*].

Base Acupuncture Prescription for Ulcerative Colitis
PC-6 Inner Pass [内关 *nèi guān*]
ST-36 Leg Three Lǐ [足三里 *zú sān lǐ*]
ST-37 Upper Great Hollow [上巨虚 *shàng jù xū*]
ST-39 Lower Great Hollow [下巨虚 *xià jù xū*]

Prescription Analysis

PC-6 moves qì. ST-36, ST-37, and ST-39 are the lower uniting points [下合穴 *xià hé xué*] of the stomach, large intestine, and small intestine, respectively. Lower uniting points treat the diseases of the six bowels [合治内府 *hé zhì nèi fǔ*]; they abduct stagnation and move it downwards. The inflammation [炎症 *yán zhèng*] in ulcerative colitis is caused by stagnation. When the stagnation is abducted, the inflammation will disappear.

16.4.2 Points to Add to the Base Prescription

Points for Damp-Heat Stagnating in the Intestines [湿热滞肠 *shī rè zhì cháng*]
GB-34 Yáng Mound Spring [阳陵泉 *yáng líng quán*]   LR-5 Woodworm Canal [蠡沟 *lǐ gōu*]

GB-34 clears heat and disinhibits dampness [清热利湿 *qīng rè lì shī*]. LR-5, the network point [络穴 *luò xué*] of the liver channel, also clears heat and disinhibits dampness.

Points for Disharmony of the Liver and Spleen [肝脾不和 *gān pí bù hé*]
LR-3 Supreme Surge [太冲 *tài chōng*]   SP-3 Supreme White [太白 *tài bái*]   SP-6 Three Yīn Intersections [三阴交 *sān yīn jiāo*]

LR-3 courses the liver [疏肝 *shū gān*]. SP-3 and SP-6 fortify the spleen [健脾 *jiàn pí*].

Points for Spleen Vacuity Qì Fall [脾虚气陷 *pí xū qì xiàn*]
CV-6 Sea of Qì [气海 *qì hǎi*]   GV-20 Hundred Convergences [百会 *bǎi huì*]

This pair of points is used to boost qì and fortify the spleen and to upbear yáng and raise the fall [益气健脾，升阳举陷 *yì qì jiàn pí, shēng yáng jǔ xiàn*].

Points for Spleen-Kidney Yáng Vacuity [脾肾阳虚 *pí shèn yáng xū*]
CV-4 Pass Head [关元 *guān yuán*] (moxa)   SP-2 Great Metropolis [大都 *dà dū*]

CV-4 boosts qì and assists yáng [益气助阳 *yì qì zhù yáng*]. SP-2 is a spring/fire point [荥火穴 *yíng huǒ xué*]; because fire engenders earth [火生土 *huǒ shēng tǔ*], SP-2 assists spleen yáng.

Points for Blood Stasis in the Intestine Network Vessels [血瘀肠络 *xuè yū cháng luò*]
ST-25 Celestial Pivot [天枢 *tiān shū*]

ST-25 is the alarm point [募穴 *mù xué*] of the large intestine; it stimulates intestinal peristalsis and disperses stagnation in the intestine.

CHAPTER 17

Urethritis and Cystitis (Strangury)

Inflammation of the urethra and the urinary bladder are called urethritis and cystitis, respectively, in Western medicine. In traditional Chinese medicine, these symptoms are both ascribed to strangury [淋证 *lín zhèng*]. The main symptoms are painful urination; frequent urination; and short, scant, and rough voidings of urine [尿痛，小便频数，小便短少而涩 *niào tòng, xiǎo biàn pín shuò, xiǎo biàn duǎn shǎo ér sè*].

There are five main forms of strangury:

- damp-heat in the urinary bladder [膀胱湿热 *páng guāng shī rè*]
- repletion heat in the small intestine [小肠实热 *xiǎo cháng shí rè*]
- depressed liver channel heat [肝经郁热 *gān jīng yù rè*]
- liver-kidney yīn vacuity [肝肾阴虚 *gān shèn yīn xū*]
- spleen-kidney yáng vacuity [脾肾阳虚 *pí shèn yáng xū*]

17.1 Points of Attention for Strangury

In the beginning stage, this symptom tends to be associated with kidney vacuity and brewing heat in the urinary bladder [膀胱蕴热 *páng guāng yùn rè*]. It often occurs after eating greasy sweet foods, which cause internal damp-heat to become abundant. Damp-heat then pours down into the bladder [湿热下注膀胱 *shī rè xià zhù páng guāng*] where it disturbs qì transformation [气化 *qì huà*] and produces the above signs.

17.1.1 Differentiate Between False and Real Signs of External Contraction

In some cases of strangury, there are symptoms such as aversion to cold and heat effusion [畏寒发热 *wèi hán fā rè*]. If there are no further signs of external contraction, these are not signs of external evil assailing the exterior [外邪袭表 *wài xié xí biǎo*] but signs of damp-heat sweltering [熏蒸 *xūn zhēng*] and evil and right fighting each other [邪正相搏 *xié zhèng xiāng bó*]. Thus, in such cases, it is wrong to promote sweating and resolve the exterior [发汗解表 *fā hàn jiě biǎo*], as this not only fails to abate heat [退热 *tuì rè*] but also damages yīn [伤阴 *shāng yīn*].

If the patient contracts external evil [感外邪 *gǎn wài xié*], then in addition to aversion to cold and heat effusion there will be symptoms such as blocked nose with nasal discharge, coughing, sore throat, and other symptoms of external contraction. In the event of external contraction, add acrid-cool [辛凉 *xīn liáng*] medicinals to a prescription to promote sweat and resolve the exterior. As strangury involves heat in the urinary bladder and insufficiency of yīn and humor [液液 *yè*], contracted cold evil in a strangury patient quickly transforms into heat [化热 *huà rè*]; thus, it is advisable to avoid acrid-warm [辛温 *xīn wēn*] medicinals for treating strangury.

17.2 CAUSES AND PATHOMECHANISM OF STRANGURY; IDENTIFYING PATTERNS

17.2.1 Damp-Heat in the Urinary Bladder [膀胱湿热 *páng guāng shī rè*]

Causes and Pathomechanism of Damp-Heat in the Urinary Bladder

Damp-heat pours down into the bladder [湿热下注膀胱 *shī rè xià zhù páng guāng*], or foul turbidity [秽浊 *huì zhuó*] assails upwards [上侵 *shàng qīn*] into the bladder, where it inhibits qì transformation [气化 *qì huà*].

Important Signs of Damp-Heat in the Urinary Bladder

Feeling of scorching heat and rough pain during urination [小便灼热涩痛 *xiǎo biàn zhuó rè sè tòng*], urinary urgency and frequent urination [尿急尿频 *niào jí niào pín*], dribbling urination. Dark-colored turbid urine. Distending pain and tense fullness in the smaller abdomen [小腹拒急胀痛 *xiǎo fù jù jí zhàng tòng*]. Bitter taste in the mouth [口苦 *kǒu kǔ*] and vexation [心烦 *xīn fán*]. Oppression in the stomach duct [脘闷 *wǎn mèn*], ungratifying defecation [大便不爽 *dà biàn bú shuǎng*]. Red tongue with yellow slimy coating [舌红苔黄腻 *shé hóng tāi huáng nì*]. Soggy rapid pulse or slippery rapid pulse [脉濡数或滑数 *mài rú shuò huò huá shuò*].

17.2.2 Repletion Heat in the Small Intestine [小肠实热 *xiǎo cháng shí rè*]

Causes and Pathomechanism of Repletion Heat in the Small Intestine

This pattern is the result of heart fire spreading heat to the small intestine [心火移热于小肠 *xīn huǒ yí rè yú xiǎo cháng*], which leads to heat settling in the bladder. The heat damages the blood network vessels [热伤血络 *rè shāng xuè luò*] and blood fails to stay in the channels [血不循经 *xuè bù xún jīng*].

Important Signs of Repletion Heat in the Small Intestine

Stabbing pain [刺痛 *cì tòng*] and a feeling of heat and roughness during urination, urinary urgency, and frequent urination [尿急尿频 *niào jí niào pín*]. Short voidings of scant urine [小便短少 *xiǎo biàn duǎn shǎo*]. Dark-colored urine, or bloody urine [尿血 *niào xuè*]. Vexation [心烦 *xīn fán*]. Mouth sores [口疮 *kǒu chuāng*]. Thirst and constipation. Red tip on the tongue, yellow coating [舌尖红苔 黄 *shé jiān hóng tāi huáng*]. Slippery rapid pulse [脉滑数 *mài huá shuò*].

17.2.3   Depressed Liver Channel Heat [肝经郁热 *gān jīng yù rè*]

Causes and Pathomechanism of Depressed Liver Channel Heat

Liver depression transforms into fire [肝郁化火 *gān yù huà huǒ*]. Fire gets depressed in the lower burner and obstructs the qì transformation [气化 *qì huà*] of the bladder.

Important Signs of Depressed Liver Channel Heat

Short and rough voidings of urine. Dribbling urination that is hard to pass. Distending pain in the smaller abdomen [小腹胀痛 *xiǎo fù zhàng tòng*]. Red face and eyes [面红目赤 *miàn hóng mù chì*]. Rashness, impatience, and irascibility [急躁易怒 *jí zào yì nù*]. Chest and rib-side distention and fullness [胸胁胀满 *xiōng xié zhàng mǎn*]. Bitter taste in the mouth, dry mouth. Red tongue, thin yellow coating [舌红苔薄黄 *shé hóng tāi bó huáng*]. Stringlike rapid pulse [脉弦 数 *mài xián shuò*].

17.2.4   Liver-Kidney Yīn Vacuity [肝肾阴虚 *gān shèn yīn xū*]

Causes and Pathomechanism of Liver-Kidney Yīn Vacuity

The damaged yīn essence in this pattern can be caused by persistent damp-heat damaging yīn, by constitutional yīn-depletion, or by the five minds (joy, anger, anxiety, thought, fear) forming fire [五志化火 *wǔ zhì huà huǒ*]. This causes internal development of vacuity heat and inhibits qì transformation. Effulgent yīn vacuity fire [阴虚火旺 *yīn xū huǒ wàng*] damages the network vessels and causes the symptoms explained below.

Important Signs of Liver-Kidney Yīn Vacuity

Short, rough voidings of urine. Stabbing pain [刺痛 *cì tòng*] and feeling of scorching heat during urination. Dribbling urination [小便淋沥 *xiǎo biàn lín lì*]. Ungratifying urination [小便不爽 *xiǎo biàn bú shuǎng*]. Yellow and turbid urine that may be bloody. Sometimes light and sometimes strong signs, frequent relapses. Dry mouth and throat. Heat vexation [烦热 *fán rè*]. Dizziness, tinnitus, sleeplessness.

Aching lumbus and limp knees [腰酸膝软 *yāo suān xī ruǎn*]. Red tongue with scant fur [舌红少苔 *shé hóng shǎo tāi*]. Thin rapid pulse [脉细数 *mài xì shuò*].

17.2.5 Spleen-Kidney Yáng Vacuity [脾肾阳虚 *pí shèn yáng xū*]

Causes and Pathomechanism of Spleen-Kidney Yáng Vacuity

This pattern is the result of long-standing illness with vacuity of right [正虚 *zhèng xū*]. Vacuous spleen qì causes clear qì to fall [清气下陷 *qīng qì xià xiàn*]. Kidney vacuity causes insecurity of the lower origin [下元不固 *xià yuán bú gù*], which affects the ability to discharge urine. Because right qì is vacuous and cannot remove evil, there is no true recovery and the illness relapses again and again.

Important Signs of Spleen-Kidney Yáng Vacuity

Frequent urination [小便频数 *xiǎo biàn pín shuò*], dribbling urinary incontinence [小便淋沥不禁 *xiǎo biàn lín lì bú jìn*], turbid urine [小便混浊 *xiǎo biàn hún zhuó*]. Distention in the smaller abdomen, limp aching lumbus and legs [腰腿酸软 *yāo tuǐ suān ruǎn*], shortness of breath and fatigued spirit [气短神疲 *qì duǎn shén pí*]. Aversion to cold and cold limbs, reduced intake, sloppy stool [便溏 *biàn táng*]. Even small exertion worsens the symptoms. Pale enlarged tongue with teeth-marks, white moist coating [舌淡胖有齿痕, 苔白润 *shé dàn pàng yǒu chǐ hén, tāi bái rùn*]. Fine weak pulse [脉细弱 *mài xì ruò*].

17.3 TREATMENT OF STRANGURY USING CHINESE MEDICINALS

17.3.1 Damp-Heat in the Urinary Bladder [膀胱湿热 *páng guāng shī rè*]

Method of Treatment for Damp-Heat in the Urinary Bladder

Clear heat and disinhibit dampness, free strangury and check pain [清热利湿, 通淋止痛 *qīng rè lì shī, tōng lín zhǐ tòng*].

Eight Corrections Powder [八正散 *bā zhèng sǎn*]	
trifoliate akebia [木通 *mù tōng*, Akebiae Trifoliatae Caulis]	6g
dianthus [瞿麦 *qū mài*, Dianthi Herba]	15g
plantago seed [车前子 *chē qián zǐ*, Plantaginis Semen]	15g
knotgrass [萹蓄 *biǎn xù*, Polygoni Avicularis Herba]	15g
talcum [滑石 *huá shí*, Talcum]	30g
honey-fried licorice [炙甘草 *zhì gān cǎo*, Glycyrrhizae Radix Preparata]	6g
rhubarb [大黃 *dà huáng*, Rhei Rhizoma et Radix]	9g
gardenia [山栀子 *shān zhī zǐ*, Gardeniae Fructus]	9g
juncus [灯心草 *dēng xīn cǎo*, Junci Medulla]	2g
Directions: Take decocted with water [水煎服 *shuǐ jiān fú*].	

Prescription Analysis

Chief Medicinals

Trifoliate akebia, dianthus, plantago seed, knotgrass, and talcum are all used to disinhibit water and free strangury and to clear heat and disinhibit dampness, treating the root [治本 *zhì běn*].

Support Medicinals

Gardenia clears and disinhibits triple burner exuberant heat [清利三焦热盛 *qīng lì sān jiāo rè shèng*]. Rhubarb drains heat and cools blood [泻热凉血 *xiè rè liáng xuè*]. Juncus conducts heat downwards [导热下行 *dǎo rè xià xíng*].

Assistant Medicinal

Licorice harmonizes the actions of all the other medicinals. It also prevents damage to the stomach by the mostly bitter-cold [苦寒 *kǔ hán*] medicinals in the prescription.

This combination of medicinals is used to clear heat and drain fire and to disinhibit water and free strangury. When damp-heat is dispelled, heat strangury [热淋 *rè lín*] stops.

Variation According to Signs

If heat evil is strong and the patient shows signs like a dry mouth, vexation and agitation [烦躁 *fán zào*], and constipation, add lonicera [*jīn yín huā*], forsythia [*lián qiào*], and scutellaria [*huáng qín*]. For roughness and pain in the urethra, add imperata [*bái máo gēn*] to free strangury and check pain. For blood in the urine, add lotus root node [*ǒu jié*], typha pollen [*pú huáng*], and notoginseng [*sān qī*] to cool blood and stanch bleeding [凉血止血 *liáng xuè zhǐ xuè*]. For exuberant heat damaging yīn [热盛伤阴 *rè shèng shāng yīn*], with signs such as dry mouth and red tongue, add ophiopogon [*mài dōng*], dried/fresh rehmannia [*shēng dì huáng*], and adenophora/glehnia [*shā shēn*] to nourish yīn and engender liquid [养阴生津 *yǎng yīn shēng jīn*].

17.3.2 Repletion Heat in the Small Intestine [小肠实热 *xiǎo cháng shí rè*]

Method of Treatment for Repletion Heat in the Small Intestine

Clear heat and disinhibit water [清热利水 *qīng rè lì shuǐ*].

Red-Abducting Powder [导赤散 *dǎo chì sǎn*]
dried/fresh rehmannia [生地黄 *shēng dì huáng*, Rehmanniae Radix seu Recens] trifoliate akebia [木通 *mù tōng*, Akebiae Trifoliatae Caulis]

bamboo leaf [竹叶 *zhú yè*, Lophatheri Folium]
licorice [甘草 *gān cǎo*, Glycyrrhizae Radix]

Directions: Use equal parts of all the ingredients. The original prescription was ground into a powder and 9g taken at a time, cooked in water. In modern times, the prescription is taken as a decoction [水煎服 *shuǐ jiān fú*].

Prescription Analysis

Chief Medicinals

Dried/fresh rehmannia clears heat, cools blood, and nourishes yīn [清热，凉血，养阴 *qīng rè, liáng xuè, yǎng yīn*]. Bitter-cold [苦寒 *kǔ hán*] trifoliate akebia clears heart fire and disinhibits urine and also abducts heart fire downwards [导心火下行 *dǎo xīn huǒ xià xíng*].

Support Medicinal

Bamboo leaf helps trifoliate akebia clear heart fire, disinhibit urine, and conduct heat out through the urine [从小便排出 *cóng xiǎo biàn pái chū*].

Assistant Medicinal

Licorice clears heat and resolves toxin [清热解毒 *qīng rè jiě dú*] as well as checks pain and harmonizes the actions of all the other medicinals.

This combination of medicinals is used to clear the heart and nourish yīn and to abduct heart fire downwards [清心养阴，导心火下行 *qīng xīn yǎng yīn, dǎo xīn huǒ xià xíng*]. Thus, the prescription is called "Red-Abducting Powder" [导赤散 *dǎo chì sǎn*].

Variation According to Signs

For exuberant heart fire, add coptis [*huáng lián*] and gardenia [*zhī zǐ*] to clear and drain exuberant heart channel fire [清泻心经火盛 *qīng xiè xīn jīng huǒ shèng*].

17.3.3 Depressed Liver Channel Heat [肝经郁热 *gān jīng yù rè*]

Method of Treatment for Depressed Liver Channel Heat

Course the liver and resolve depression, disinhibit urine and free strangury [疏肝解郁，利尿通淋 *shū gān jiě yù, lì niào tōng lín*].

Aquilaria Powder [沉香散 *chén xiāng sǎn*]	
aquilaria [沉香 *chén xiāng*, Aquilariae Lignum Resinatum]	15g
pyrrosia [石韦 *shí wéi*, Pyrrosiae Folium]	15g
talcum [滑石 *huá shí*, Talcum]	15g
Chinese angelica [当归 *dāng guī*, Angelicae Sinensis Radix]	15g
vaccaria [王不留行 *wáng bù liú xíng*, Vaccariae Semen]	15g
dianthus [瞿麦 *qū mài*, Dianthi Herba]	15g
mallow seed [冬葵子 *dōng kuí zǐ*, Malvae Semen]	20g
red peony [赤芍 *chì sháo*, Paeoniae Radix Rubra]	20g
white atractylodes [白术 *bái zhú*, Atractylodis Macrocephalae Rhizoma]	20g
honey-fried licorice [炙甘草 *zhì gān cǎo*, Glycyrrhizae Radix Preparata]	10g

Directions: The original prescription was ground into a powder and taken 6g at a time, cooked in water. In modern times, the prescription is taken decocted with water [水煎服 *shuǐ jiān fú*], with the quantities of the medicinals proportionally reduced.

Prescription Analysis

Chief Medicinal

Aquilaria courses the liver and downbears qì, treating the root [治本 *zhì běn*].

Support Medicinals

Pyrrosia, talcum, dianthus, and mallow seed disinhibit water and free strangury, treating the tip [治标 *zhì biāo*].

Assistant Medicinals

Chinese angelica, vaccaria, and red peony quicken blood and check pain. White atractylodes fortifies the spleen and disinhibits water.

Licorice harmonizes the actions of all the other medicinals.

This combination of medicinals is used to course the liver and resolve depression and to disinhibit urine and free strangury.

Variation According to Signs

For severe distending pain in the smaller abdomen [小腹胀痛 *xiǎo fù zhàng tòng*], add curcuma [*yù jīn*] and areca [*bīng láng*] to rectify qì and dissipate binds [理气散结 *lǐ qì sàn jié*]. If there are signs of exuberant heat damaging yīn [热盛伤阴 *rè shèng shāng yīn*], add dried/fresh rehmannia [*shēng dì huáng*], chaenomeles [*mù guā*], and lycium berry [*gǒu qǐ zǐ*] to nourish blood and emolliate the liver [养血柔肝 *yǎng xuè róu gān*]. For stabbing pain in the smaller abdomen [小腹刺痛

xiǎo fù cì tòng], add leonurus [*yì mǔ cǎo*], salvia [*dān shēn*], and cyathula [*chuān niú xī*] to quicken blood and transform stasis and thereby check pain.

17.3.4 Liver-Kidney Yīn Vacuity [肝肾阴虚 *gān shèn yīn xū*]

Method of Treatment for Liver-Kidney Yīn Vacuity

Enrich yīn and downbear fire [滋阴降火 *zī yīn jiàng huǒ*].

Anemarrhena, Phellodendron, and Rehmannia Pill **[知柏地黄丸 *zhī bǎi dì huáng wán*]**	
cooked rehmannia [熟地黄 *shú dì huáng*, Rehmanniae Radix Conquita]	20g
cornus [山茱萸 *shān zhū yú*, Corni Fructus]	12g
dioscorea [山药 *shān yào*, Dioscoreae Rhizoma]	20g
anemarrhena [知母 *zhī mǔ*, Anemarrhenae Rhizoma]	9g
phellodendron [黄柏 *huáng bǎi*, Phellodendri Cortex]	9g
alisma [泽泻 *zé xiè*, Alismatis Rhizoma]	9g
poria [茯苓 *fú líng*, Poria]	12g
moutan [牡丹皮 *mǔ dān pí*, Moutan Cortex]	9g

Directions: The original prescription was made into pills and taken 6g at a time, two times a day. In modern times, the prescription is taken decocted with water [水煎服 *shuǐ jiān fú*].

Prescription Analysis

Chief Medicinals

Cooked rehmannia and cornus enrich and supplement liver and kidney yīn.

Support Medicinals

Anemarrhena and phellodendron enrich yīn and downbear fire.

Assistant Medicinals

Dioscorea and poria fortify the spleen and percolate dampness [健脾渗湿 *jiàn pí shèn shī*], to promote the source of engendering transformation of later heaven [资后天生化之源 *zī hòu tiān shēng huà zhī yuán*]. Alisma and moutan disinhibit dampness and downbear ministerial fire [降相火 *jiàng xiàng huǒ*].

This combination of medicinals enriches yīn and downbears fire.

Variation According to Signs

Anemarrhena, Phellodendron, and Rehmannia Pill is a famous prescription for enriching yīn and downbearing fire. If vacuity fire is strong, and dizziness and tinnitus, tidal heat and night sweat [潮热盗汗 *cháo rè dào hàn*] are intense, add baiwei [*bái wēi*], lycium root bark [*dì gǔ pí*], and sweet wormwood [*qīng hāo*] to constrain yīn [敛阴 *liǎn yīn*] and check perspiration [止汗 *zhǐ hàn*]. If vacuity fire scorches the network vessels [虚火灼络 *xū huǒ zhuó luò*], producing signs such as coughing of blood [咳血 *ké xuè*], add biota leaf [*cè bǎi yè*] and notoginseng [*sān qī*] to stanch bleeding [止血 *zhǐ xuè*]. For strong signs of damp-heat, such as urine that is sometimes clear and sometimes turbid and severe rough pain [涩痛 *sè tòng*], add smooth greenbrier root [*tǔ fú líng*], mallow seed [*dōng kuí zǐ*], gardenia [*zhī zǐ*], and trifoliate akebia [*mù tōng*] to clear heat and disinhibit dampness.

17.3.5 Spleen-Kidney Yáng Vacuity [脾肾阳虚 *pí shèn yáng xū*]

Method of Treatment for Spleen-Kidney Yáng Vacuity

Warm yáng and disinhibit dampness, separate the clear and turbid [温阳利湿，分清别浊 *wēn yáng lì shī, fēn qīng bié zhuó*].

Fish Poison Yam Clear-Turbid Separation Beverage [萆薢分清饮 *bì xiè fēn qīng yǐn*]	
fish poison yam [萆薢 *bì xiè*, Dioscoreae Hypoglaucae Rhizoma]	12g
alpinia [益智仁 *yì zhì rén*, Alpiniae Oxyphyllae Fructus]	9g
acorus [石菖蒲 *shí chāng pú*, Acori Tatarinowii Rhizoma]	9g
lindera [乌药 *wū yào*, Linderae Radix]	9g
Directions: Take decocted with water [水煎服 *shuǐ jiān fú*].	

Prescription Analysis

Chief Medicinals

Fish poison yam warms yáng and disinhibits dampness and also separates the clear and the turbid.

Support Medicinals

Alpinia warms and supplements spleen and kidney yáng and reduces urine [缩尿 *suō niào*].

Assistant Medicinals

Lindera warms and supplements spleen and kidney yáng and also dissipates cold and moves qì [散寒行气 *sàn hán xíng qì*]. Acorus transforms damp turbidity [化湿浊 *huà shī zhuó*].

This prescription uses only a few medicinals, but its function is powerful and focused. It warms yáng and disinhibits dampness to separate the clear and turbid.

Variation According to Signs

If spleen yáng vacuity is more pronounced (turbid urine [小便浑浊 *xiǎo biàn hún zhuó*] that is congealed like fat [凝如膏脂 *níng rú gāo zhī*], oppression in the stomach duct, and loss of appetite), add atractylodes [*cāng zhú*], white atractylodes [*bái zhú*], dioscorea [*shān yào*], and amomum [*shā rén*] to strengthen movement and transformation [运化 *yùn huà*] of the spleen. If kidney yáng vacuity is more pronounced (dribbling urinary incontinence [小便淋沥不禁 *xiǎo biàn lín lì bú jìn*], turbid urine resembling animal fat [浑浊如膏 *hún zhuó rú gāo*], aversion to cold, and cold limbs), add mantis egg-case [*sāng piāo xiāo*] and rubus [*fù pén zǐ*] to secure essence and reduce urine [固精缩尿 *gù jīng suō niào*]. If there is sloppy stool [便溏 *biàn táng*] or fifth-watch diarrhea [五更泄 *wǔ gēng xiè*], add psoralea [*bǔ gǔ zhī*], nutmeg [*ròu dòu kòu*], and evodia [*wú zhū yú*] to warm yáng and check diarrhea.

17.4   ACUPUNCTURE TREATMENT FOR STRANGURY

17.4.1   Base Acupuncture Prescription for Strangury

This base prescription should be modified according to the identified patterns that are discussed below and according to the condition of the individual patient.

Treatment Method for Strangury

Clear heat and disinhibit dampness, free strangury and check pain [清热利湿，通淋止痛 *qīng rè lì shī, tōng lín zhǐ tòng*].

Base Acupuncture Prescription for Strangury
CV-3 Central Pole [中极 *zhōng jí*]
GB-34 Yáng Mound Spring [阳陵泉 *yáng líng quán*]
LR-2 Moving Between [行间 *xíng jiān*]
KI-7 Recover Flow [复溜 *fù liū*]
SP-9 Yīn Mound Spring [阴陵泉 *yīn líng quán*]

Prescription Analysis

The combination of GB-34, LR-2, KI-7, and SP-9 has been validated in clinical practice for the treatment of urethritis and cystitis. It clears heat and disinhibits dampness.

CV-3 is the alarm point of the urinary bladder and is commonly used in cases of urinary disease. Here CV-3 frees strangury and checks pain.

17.4.2 Points to Add to the Base Prescription

For damp-heat in the urinary bladder [膀胱湿热 *páng guāng shī rè*], repletion heat in the small intestine [小肠实热 *xiǎo cháng shí rè*], and depressed liver channel heat [肝经郁热 *gān jīng yù rè*], the base prescription is satisfactory.

Points for Liver-Kidney Yīn Vacuity [肝肾阴虚 *gān shèn yīn xū*]
LR-8 Spring at the Bend [曲泉 *qū quán*]
KI-10 Yīn Valley [阴谷 *yīn gǔ*]

This pair of points supplements liver and kidney yīn.

LR-8 is mainly indicated for disinhibiting dampness [利湿 *lì shī*], especially cases of damp-heat in the lower burner that cause urinary or gynecological diseases. Also, LR-8 is the uniting point [合穴 *hé xué*] of the liver channel, and as such it supplements the liver, nourishes yīn, and moistens the liver [养阴濡肝 *yǎng yīn rú gān*]. This is true because the uniting points of the yīn channels correspond to water, and according to the "supplement the mother, drain the child" method [补母泻子法 *bǔ mǔ xiè zǐ fǎ*], the liver corresponds to wood and LR-8 corresponds to water. Wood is engendered by water, because water is the mother of wood [水为木之母 *shuǐ wéi mù zhī mǔ*].

KI-10 is the uniting point [合穴 *hé xué*] of the kidney channel and corresponds to water. Although KI-10 does not nourish kidney yīn as well as KI-6 [*zhào hǎi*], it is chosen here for its ability to both nourish kidney yīn and disinhibit dampness [利湿 *lì shī*] in the lower burner.

Points for Spleen-Kidney Yáng Vacuity [脾肾阳虚 *pí shèn yáng xū*]
BL-20 Spleen Transport [脾俞 *pí shū*]
BL-23 Kidney Transport [肾俞 *shèn shū*]

This pair of points fortifies the spleen and boosts the kidney [健脾益肾 *jiàn pí yì shèn*]. Both points are back transport points [背俞 *bèi shū*], which are specifically indicated for yīn patterns, e.g., interior patterns, cold patterns, vacuity patterns, and chronic diseases; back transport points above the diaphragm are also used to treat yáng patterns like external contraction.

CHAPTER 18
Menstrual Pain

Pain that occurs shortly before, during, or after menstruation and that is located in the smaller abdomen, sometimes involving the lumbus, is called menstrual pain.

There are five main forms of menstrual pain:

- qì stagnation and blood stasis [气滞血瘀 *qì zhì xuè yū*]
- cold congealing in the uterus [寒凝胞中 *hán níng bāo zhōng*], which can be divided into:

     1) yáng vacuity internal cold [阳虚内寒 *yáng xū nèi hán*], and

     2) congealing cold-damp [寒湿凝滞 *hán shī níng zhì*]
- damp-heat pouring downward [湿热下注 *shī rè xià zhù*]
- qì-blood vacuity [气血虚弱 *qì xuè xū ruò*]
- liver-kidney depletion [肝肾亏损 *gān shèn kuī sǔn*]

Menstrual pain can also be caused by an underdeveloped, malformed, or abnormally placed uterus.

18.1 POINTS OF ATTENTION FOR MENSTRUAL PAIN

18.1.1 Pain and Female Physiology

When treating gynecological pain, it is important to consider the distinguishing characteristics of female physiology in order to properly understand the causes of pain, pathomechanisms, and treatment methods.

The Governing Factor in Female Physiology is Blood **[妇人以血为主 *fù rén yǐ xuè wéi zhǔ*].**

Female physiological functions, such as menstruation and gestation, heavily depend on blood. Blood, the material basis of menstruation, is the mother of qì, and qì is the driving force that moves the blood in the vessels. Hence, disharmony of qì and blood [气血失调 *qì xuè shī tiáo*] causes menstrual problems.

In gynecology, morbid changes occurring due to disharmony of qì and blood mainly manifest as blood and qì depletion [血亏气虚 *xuè kuī qì xū*] or blood stasis with qì stagnation [血瘀气滞 *xuè yū qì zhì*].

A Woman's Earlier Heaven is Governed by the Liver [妇人以肝为先天 *fù rén yǐ gān wéi xiān tiān*].

This statement stresses the importance of the liver in gynecology. It imitates the statement: "the kidney is the root of earlier heaven" [肾为先天之本 *shèn wéi xiān tiān zhī běn*], which means that the kidney is the basis of our inherited constitution. Reproduction, part of the inherited constitution, therefore depends on the condition of the kidney, but in female physiology it also heavily depends on the healthy function of the liver. The liver stores the blood [肝藏血 *gān cáng xuè*], the material basis of menstruation, and governs the sea of blood [肝主血海 *gān zhǔ xuè hǎi*]. Failure to do so can lead to disturbed blood-flow into the penetrating [冲脉 *chōng mài*] and controlling vessels [任脉 *rèn mài*], resulting in menstrual disorders. The liver also governs free coursing [肝主疏泄 *gān zhǔ shū xiè*]. Binding depression of liver qì that causes stagnation of qì and blood can lead to qì and blood stagnation in the penetrating and controlling vessels, which inhibits the menstrual flow and—according to the principle "when there is stoppage, there is pain" [不通则痛 *bù tōng zé tòng*]—causes pain.

The Penetrating [冲脉 *chōng mài*] and Controlling Vessels [任脉 *rèn mài*] both originate from the kidney and regulate the uterus and menstruation.

Treatment principles for gynecological disorders are likely to involve coursing the liver and rectifying qì [疏肝理气 *shū gān lǐ qì*], nourishing the blood and emolliating the liver [养血柔肝 *yǎng xuè róu gān*], restoring blood flow and freeing the vessels [通利血脉 *tōng lì xuè mài*], and regulating the qì and blood of the penetrating and controlling vessels.

18.1.2 Disease Pattern Identification

Differentiating the Nature of Pain

When does the pain occur?

- Pain occurring before or during menstruation (and that refuses pressure) reflects a repletion [实 *shí*], such as qì stagnation or blood stasis.

- Pain occurring after menstruation (and relieved by pressure) reflects a vacuity [虚 *xū*]. For example, aching pain that occurs after menstruation and that is located in the lumbus and relieved by pressure is a sign of liver-kidney depletion [肝肾亏损 *gān shèn kuī sǔn*].

Where does it hurt?

- Pain in the lesser abdomen [少腹 *shào fù*], frequently accompanied by pain in the chest and rib-side [胸胁 *xiōng xié*], indicates qì stagnation.[12]
- Pain in the smaller abdomen [小腹 *xiǎo fù*] indicates blood stagnation.[13]
- Pain at both sides of the lesser abdomen indicates the liver.
- Pain involving the lumbus indicates the kidney.
- Pain in the whole abdomen [全腹 *quán fù*] often indicates a spleen-stomach disharmony [脾胃不和 *pí wèi bù hé*].

Menstruation

Menstrual Periodicity

- Advanced menstruation [月经先期 *yuè jīng xiān qī*] indicates either qì vacuity or blood heat.
- Delayed menstruation [月经后期 *yuè jīng hòu qī*] indicates cold congealing [寒凝 *hán níng*] or blood vacuity.
- Menstruation at irregular intervals [月经先后无定期 *yuè jīng xiān hòu wú dìng qī*] indicates kidney vacuity or liver depression.

Volume of Menstrual Flow

- Profuse menstruation [月经过多 *yuè jīng guò duō*] indicates blood heat or qì vacuity.
- Scant menstruation [月经过少 *yuè jīng guò shǎo*] indicates blood vacuity, blood stasis, or cold congealing.
- Menstruation that irregularly switches between profuse and scant indicates liver stagnation or kidney vacuity.

Color of Menstrual Flow

- Dark red menstrual flow is an indication of normal health.
- Purple or bright red menstrual flow indicates blood heat.
- Purple menstrual flow indicates blood stasis.
- Pale menstrual flow indicates qì and blood vacuity.

---

[12] "Lesser abdomen" refers to the lateral lower abdomen, i.e., the sides of the smaller abdomen (see following note). (Ed.)

[13] "Smaller abdomen" refers to the area of the abdomen below the umbilicus. (Ed.)

Quality of Menstrual Flow

- Thick flow indicates heat.
- Thin flow indicates vacuity cold.
- Clotted menstrual flow indicates blood stasis.

Vaginal Discharge [带下 *dài xià*]

- Profuse discharge with white color and no abnormal smell indicates spleen vacuity with dampness.
- Profuse discharge with yellow color that is thick like pus and has a foul smell [秽气 *huì qì*] indicates damp-heat pouring downward [湿热下注 *shī rè xià zhù*] or damp toxin [湿毒 *shī dú*].

Pulse

Because of the changes occurring within the body during menstruation, the normal pulse of a menstruating woman is different from a non-menstruating woman. A surging large [洪大 *hóng dà*] and slippery [滑 *huá*] pulse or a stringlike [弦 *xián*] pulse at both bar [关 *guān*] positions during menstruation indicates normal health.

18.1.3   Treatment

The basis of treating menstrual pain lies in regulating the qì and blood of the penetrating and controlling vessels by the following methods:

- moving qì [行气 *xíng qì*]
- quickening the blood [活血 *huó xuè*]
- dissipating cold [散寒 *sàn hán*]
- clearing heat [清热 *qīng rè*]
- supplementing vacuity [补虚 *bǔ xū*] or
- draining repletion [泻实 *xiè shí*].

These principles should govern treatments in accordance with the patient's signs [证侯 *zhèng hòu*] and patterns.

Caution

Do not indiscriminately "move qì" and "quicken the blood," but be sure to comprehend the underlying cause of qì stagnation and blood stasis and treat accordingly.

Example: When cold is congealing in the uterus, the underlying cause for blood stasis is cold. Warming the channels and dissipating cold [温经散寒 *wēn jīng sàn hán*] is essential to eliminating stasis, while transforming stasis [化瘀 *huà yū*] alone will be of little or no effect.

Treating the Tip [治标 *zhì biāo*] ***Versus Treating the* Root** [治本 *zhì běn*]

Treating pain patients, one should always consider including treating the tip, especially if the pain is severe. During menstruation, regulate the blood and check pain, which is considered treating the tip. Between menstrual periods, treat the root by identifying patterns and seeking the causes [辨证求因 *biàn zhèng qiú yīn*] according to the individual situation of each patient.

18.2 CAUSES AND PATHOMECHANISM OF MENSTRUAL PAIN; IDENTIFYING PATTERNS

18.2.1 Qì Stagnation and Blood Stasis [气滞血瘀 *qì zhì xuè yū*]

Causes and Pathomechanism of Qì Stagnation and Blood Stasis

In this pattern, the patient may have a depressed disposition or may have repeatedly suffered emotional damage [伤情志 *shāng qíng zhì*] that has resulted in liver depression [肝郁 *gān yù*]. The liver governs the sea of blood [肝主血海 *gān zhǔ xuè hǎi*]; it also governs free coursing [肝主疏泄 *gān zhǔ shū xiè*]. Depressed liver gives rise to qì stagnation, which in turn leads to blood stagnation. This inhibits the qì dynamic of the sea of blood, disturbs the menstrual blood flow, and results in menstrual pain.

Important Signs of Qì Stagnation and Blood Stasis

Distending pain in the smaller abdomen 1–2 days before menstruation and/or during menstruation; the patient refuses pressure on the pain. Distending pain in the chest, rib-side, and breasts. Scant menstruation. Deep purple menstrual flow with blood clots. Pain is relieved with the passing of blood clots. Pain diminishes when menstruation passes. Purple tongue that may show stasis macules [瘀点 *yū diǎn*]. Stringlike pulse [脉弦 *mài xián*], or stringlike slippery pulse [脉弦滑 *mài xián huá*].

18.2.2 Cold Congealing in the Uterus [寒凝胞中 *hán níng bāo zhōng*]

Causes and Pathomechanism of Cold Congealing in the Uterus

Yáng Vacuity Internal Cold [阳虚内寒 ***yáng xū nèi hán***]

A constitutional disposition for yáng vacuity can easily give rise to exuberant internal yīn cold [阴寒内盛 *yīn hán nèi shèng*] and vacuity cold in the penetrating and controlling vessels, which impairs menstrual blood flow. Both the penetrating and controlling vessels originate directly from the kidney—the kidney is called the root of the penetrating and controlling vessels [‘肾为冲任之

本 *shèn wéi chōng rèn zhī běn*]. Also, the uterine vessels that nourish the uterus are related to the kidney. Vacuous kidney yáng gives rise to vacuity cold and causes the penetrating, controlling, and uterine vessels to lose their source of warmth such that the vacuity cold will obstruct the blood flow, thus causing cold pain during or after menstruation.

Congealing Cold Damp [寒湿凝滞 *hán shī níng zhì*]

If cold-damp evil visits [客 *kè*] the penetrating and controlling vessels and the uterus, it can congeal menstrual blood and impede its downward movement, causing pain. The following factors may give rise to this pattern: Getting wet (especially getting wet feet during menstruation), swimming, external contraction of wind-cold or cold-damp, living in a damp environment, or eating too many raw or cold foods that produce internal cold damage. This last point is particularly common in Western countries where women diet or live a fast life-style that does not leave much time for cooking and/or eating warm meals.

Important Signs of Cold Congealing in the Uterus

Yáng Vacuity Internal Cold [阳虚内寒 *yáng xū nèi hán*]

Cold pain in the smaller abdomen during and after menstruation. Limp aching lumbus and legs [腰腿酸软 *yāo tuǐ suān ruǎn*], long voidings of clear urine [小便清长 *xiǎo biàn qīng cháng*]. Pain is relieved by pressure and rubbing. The tongue has a white moist tongue fur [苔白润 *tāi bái rùn*]. Sunken pulse [沉 *chén*].

Congealing Cold Damp [寒湿凝滞 *hán shī níng zhì*]

Cold pain in the smaller abdomen 1–2 days before menstruation, sometimes also during menstruation. The pain refuses pressure. Often accompanied by fear of cold [怕冷 *pà lěng*] and generalized pain [周身痛 *zhōu shēn tòng*]. The tongue has a white slimy fur [苔白腻 *tāi bái nì*]. Sunken and tight pulse [脉沉紧 *mài chén jǐn*].

In both of the above patterns, pain is relieved by the application of warmth, there is scant menstruation, and the menses is almost black and has blood clots.

18.2.3   Damp-Heat Pouring Downward [湿热下注 *shī rè xià zhù*]

Causes and Pathomechanism of Damp-Heat Pouring Downward

This pattern results from long-standing damp-heat brewing internally [湿热内蕴 *shī rè nèi yùn*] that pours into the penetrating and controlling vessels, obstructing qì and blood. Alternatively, damp-heat evil may be contracted during menstruation, shortly after giving birth, or after an abortion or miscarriage; it then settles in the penetrating and controlling vessels or brews [蕴结 *yùn jié*] in the uterus. When damp-heat mixes with menstrual blood and disturbs normal menstrual flow, the result is pain.

Important Signs of Damp-Heat Pouring Downward

Pain that refuses pressure in the smaller abdomen 1–2 days before and during menstruation, feeling of scorching heat [灼热 *zhuó rè*]. Often accompanied by distending pain in the lower back or frequent pain in the lesser abdomen that is aggravated by menstruation. Dark red, thick menstrual flow with blood clots. Yellow discharge, thick like pus, with a foul smell. Short voidings of yellow urine [小便短黄 *xiǎo biàn duǎn huáng*]. Red tongue with yellow slimy tongue fur [舌红苔黄腻 *shé hóng tāi huáng nì*]. Stringlike rapid pulse [脉弦数 *mài xián shuò*] or soggy rapid pulse [脉濡数 *mài rú shuò*].

18.2.4 Qì-Blood Vacuity [气血虚弱 *qì xuè xū ruò*]

Causes and Pathomechanism of Qì-Blood Vacuity

A predisposition to a weak spleen and stomach, or a severe or long-standing illness can lead to qì and blood vacuity, including qì and blood vacuity of the penetrating and controlling vessels. Such patterns lead to the sea of blood[14] being empty after menstruation [血海空虚 *xuè hǎi kōng xū*] and unable to nourish the uterine vessels. Because of qì vacuity, qì does not have enough driving force to move the blood in the vessels, which causes blood stasis.

Important Signs of Qì-Blood Vacuity

Dull pain in the smaller abdomen towards the end of menstruation and 1–2 days after menstruation that is relieved by pressure [喜按 *xǐ àn*] and rubbing. Scant, pale, and thin menstrual flow. These signs are accompanied by lassitude of spirit [神疲 *shén pí*] and lack of strength [乏力 *fá lì*], lusterless facial complexion [面色不华 *miàn sè bù huá*], reduced food intake [纳少 *nà shǎo*], and sloppy stool [便溏 *biàn táng*]. Pale tongue [舌淡 *shé dàn*]. Fine weak pulse [脉细弱 *mài xì ruò*].

18.2.5 Liver-Kidney Depletion [肝肾亏损 *gān shèn kuī sǔn*]

Causes and Pathomechanism of Liver-Kidney Depletion

Insufficiency of essence and blood can be caused by a weak constitution with long-standing liver-kidney depletion, numerous births, or sexual taxation [房劳 *fáng láo*] that harms the liver and kidney. This will result in insufficiency of the penetrating and controlling vessels and deprivation of nourishment of the uterine vessel. Menstruation will aggravate the insufficiency of essence and blood even more, resulting in painful menstruation.

---

[14] In this instance, "sea of blood" means the penetrating vessel.

Important Signs of Liver-Kidney Depletion

Continuous pain in the smaller abdomen towards the end of menstruation and 1–2 days after menstruation, accompanied by aching pain [酸痛 *suān tòng*] in the lumbus. Scant, pale, and thin menstrual flow. Tinnitus [耳鸣 *ěr míng*], dizzy head [头晕 *tóu yūn*], tidal heat [潮热 *cháo rè*]. The tongue has thin white or thin yellow fur [苔薄白或薄黄 *tāi bó bái huò bó huáng*]. Fine weak or sunken fine pulse [脉细弱或沉细 *mài xì ruò huò chén xì*].

18.3 TREATMENT OF MENSTRUAL PAIN USING CHINESE MEDICINALS[15]

18.3.1 Qì Stagnation and Blood Stasis [气滞血瘀 *qì zhì xuè yū*]

Method of Treatment for Qì Stagnation and Blood Stasis

Coursing the liver and rectifying qì [疏肝理气 *shū gān lǐ qì*], transforming stasis [化瘀 *huà yū*], checking pain [止痛 *zhǐ tòng*].

Dr. Zhū Shēng-Ān's Formula for Qì-Stagnation and Blood-Stasis Menstrual Pain	
raw typha pollen [生蒲黄 *shēng pú huáng*, Typhae Pollen Crudum]	10g
flying squirrel's droppings [五灵脂 *wǔ líng zhī*, Trogopteri Faeces]	10g
red peony [赤芍 *chì sháo*, Paeoniae Radix Rubra]	15g
bitter orange [枳壳 *zhǐ ké*, Aurantii Fructus]	10g
unripe tangerine peel [青皮 *qīng pí*, Citri Reticulatae Pericarpium Viride]	10g
Chinese angelica [当归 *dāng guī*, Angelicae Sinensis Radix]	15g
chuanxiong [川芎 *chuān xiōng*, Chuanxiong Rhizoma]	15g
moutan [牡丹皮 *mǔ dān pí*, Moutan Cortex]	10g
sparganium [三棱 *sān léng*, Rhizoma Sparganii]	10g
curcuma rhizome [莪术 *é zhú*, Curcumae Rhizoma]	10g
frankincense [乳香 *rǔ xiāng*, Olibanum]	10g
myrrh [没药 *mò yào*, Myrrha]	10g

Directions: One medicinal preparation per day. Split preparation in two equal parts and take in the morning and in the evening, one hour after meals. Stop taking this prescription before the anticipated start of menstruation.

---

[15] The medicinal and acupuncture prescriptions of this chapter are handed down from earlier generations of the family [家传 *jiā chuán*] of Dr. Zhū Shēng-Ān [朱生安大夫].

Prescription Analysis

Chinese angelica nourishes the blood [养血 *yǎng xuè*] and quickens the blood [活血 *huó xuè*].

Bitter orange, red peony, and unripe tangerine peel rectify qì [理气 *lǐ qì*] and resolve depression [解郁 *jiě yù*].

Chuanxiong, frankincense, and myrrh quicken the blood [活血 *huó xuè*] and check pain [止痛 *zhǐ tòng*].

Sparganium and curcuma rhizome break blood [破血 *pò xuè*] and transform stasis [化瘀 *huà yū*].

Raw typha pollen and flying squirrel's droppings transform stasis [化瘀 *huà yū*] and check pain [止痛 *zhǐ tòng*].

Moutan quickens the blood [活血 *huó xuè*] and transforms stasis [化瘀 *huà yū*].

Variation According to Signs

In some patients, liver depression might transform into heat [肝郁化热 *gān yù huà rè*]. Those patients may show profuse menstruation instead of the typical scant menstruation associated with this pattern. For profuse menstruation, use charred typha pollen[16] [蒲黄炭 *pú huáng tàn*], which stanches bleeding [止血 *zhǐ xuè*]. Remove sparganium and curcuma rhizome. Add charred cooked rhubarb [*shú jūn tàn*] and blast-fried charred ginger [*páo jiāng tàn*] to stanch bleeding [止血 *zhǐ xuè*].

If the patient's general constitution tends to be hot, move blood and clear heat [行血清热 *xíng xuè qīng rè*] by adding 10 grams of anomalous artemisia [*liú jì nú*] and 10 grams of earthworm [*dì lóng*].

18.3.2   Cold Congealing in the Uterus [寒凝胞中 *hán níng bāo zhōng*]

Method of Treatment for Cold Congealing in the Uterus

Yáng Vacuity Internal Cold [阳虚内寒 *yáng xū nèi hán*]

Warm the channels and dissipate cold [温经散寒 *wēn jīng sàn hán*] and check pain [止痛 *zhǐ tòng*].

---

[16] When a medicinal is charred [制炭 *zhì tàn*] it is heated until its outer part is charred and gains a blood-stanching property. Its inner part becomes yellowish-brown and retains the original properties of the drug. *Zhì tàn* is translated in English as "mix-fried." A more precise selection for "charred" is *chǎo tàn*.

<u>Congealing Cold Damp</u> [寒湿凝滞 *hán shī níng zhì*]

Warm the channels and dissipate cold [温经散寒 *wēn jīng sàn hán*], eliminate dampness [除湿 *chú shī*], transform stasis [化瘀 *huà yū*], and check pain [止痛 *zhǐ tòng*].

Dr. Zhū Shēng-Ān's Formula for Yáng Vacuity Internal Cold [阳虚内寒 *yáng xū nèi hán*]	
Chinese angelica [当归 *dāng guī*, Angelicae Sinensis Radix]	6g
chuanxiong [川芎 *chuān xiōng*, Chuanxiong Rhizoma]	0g
white peony [白芍 *bái sháo*, Paeoniae Radix Alba]	10g
bitter orange [枳壳 *zhǐ ké*, Aurantii Fructus]	10g
processed aconite [制附子 *zhì fù zǐ*, Aconiti Tuber Laterale Praeparata]	6g
ophiopogon [麦冬 *mài dōng*, Ophiopogonis Radix]	12g
moutan [牡丹皮 *mǔ dān pí*, Moutan Cortex]	10g
mugwort [艾叶 *ài yè*, Artemisiae Argyi Folium]	10g
fennel [小茴香 *xiǎo huí xiāng*, Foeniculi Fructus]	15g
licorice [甘草 *gān cǎo*, Glycyrrhizae Radix]	6g

Directions: One medicinal preparation per day. Split preparation in two equal parts and take in the morning and in the evening, one hour after a meal.

Prescription *Analysis*

Chinese angelica and chuanxiong nourish the blood [养血 *yǎng xuè*] and quicken the blood [活血 *huó xuè*].

White peony, bitter orange, and licorice relax tension [缓急 *huǎn jí*], harmonize the center (spleen and stomach) [和中 *hé zhōng*], and check pain.

Ophiopogon and moutan nourish yīn [养阴 *yǎng yīn*] and downbear fire [降火 *jiàng huǒ*].

Mugwort, fennel, and processed aconite tuber dissipate cold [散寒 *sàn hán*] and check pain [止痛 *zhǐ tòng*].

Dr. Zhū Shēng-Ān's Formula for Congealing Cold Damp [寒湿凝滞 *hán shī níng zhì*]	
atractylodes [苍术 *cāng zhú*, Atractylodis Rhizoma]	10g
white atractylodes [白术 *bái zhú*, Atractylodis Macrocephalae Rhizoma]	10g
poria [茯苓 *fú líng*, Poria]	10g
bitter orange [枳壳 *zhǐ ké*, Aurantii Fructus]	10g
plantago seed [车前子 *chē qián zǐ*, Plantaginis Semen]	15g

Chinese angelica [当归 *dāng guī*, Angelicae Sinensis Radix]	10g
chuanxiong [川芎 *chuān xiōng*, Chuanxiong Rhizoma]	10g
red peony [赤芍 *chì sháo*, Paeoniae Radix Rubra]	15g
corydalis [延胡索 *yán hú suǒ*, Corydalis Rhizoma]	10g
fennel [小茴香 *xiǎo huí xiāng*, Foeniculi Fructus]	10g
cyperus [香附 *xiāng fù*, Cyperi Rhizoma]	10g
processed aconite [制附子 *zhì fù zǐ*, Aconiti Tuber Laterale Praeparata]	6g

Directions: Start taking this formula one week before menstruation and continue taking it until menstruation begins. Take one medicinal preparation per day. Split preparation in two equal parts and take in the morning and in the evening, one hour after meals. Take for three consecutive months.

Prescription Analysis

Atractylodes and white atractylodes fortify the spleen and dry dampness [健脾燥湿 *jiàn pí zào shī*].

Poria and plantago seed disinhibit water and percolate dampness [利水渗湿 *lì shuǐ shèn shī*].

Chinese angelica, chuanxiong, red peony, and corydalis nourish the blood, quicken the blood, and check pain [养血活血止痛 *yǎng xuè huó xuè zhǐ tòng*].

Fennel, cyperus, and processed aconite are used to warm and invigorate kidney yáng [温壮肾阳 *wēn zhuàng shèn yáng*] and to warm the uterus and check pain [暖宫止痛 *nuǎn gōng zhǐ tòng*].

18.3.3   Damp-Heat Pouring Downward [湿热下注 *shī rè xià zhù*]

Treatment Method for Damp-Heat Pouring Downward

Clear heat and eliminate dampness [清热除湿 *qīng rè chú shī*], transform stasis and check pain [化瘀止痛 *huà yū zhǐ tòng*].

Dr. Zhū Shēng-Ān's Formula for Damp-Heat Pouring Downward Menstrual Pain	
coptis [黄连 *huáng lián*, Coptidis Rhizoma]	6g
phellodendron [黄柏 *huáng bǎi*, Phellodendri Cortex]	10g
dried/fresh rehmannia [生地黄 *shēng dì huáng*, Rehmanniae Radix seu Recens]	15g
chuanxiong [川芎 *chuān xiōng*, Chuanxiong Rhizoma]	10g
Chinese angelica [当归 *dāng guī*, Angelicae Sinensis Radix]	6g

peach kernel [桃仁 *táo rén*, Persicae Semen]	10g
carthamus [红花 *hóng huā*, Carthami Flos]	10g
coix [薏苡仁 *yì yǐ rén*, Semen Coicis]	20g
poria [茯苓 *fú líng*, Poria]	15g
patrinia [败酱草 *bài jiàng cǎo*, Patriniae Herba]	10g

Directions: One medicinal preparation per day. Split preparation in two equal parts and take in the morning and in the evening, one hour after a meal.

Prescription Analysis

Coptis, phellodendron, and dried/fresh rehmannia enrich yīn [滋阴 *zī yīn*], disperse inflammation [消炎 *xiāo yán*], and clear lower burner heat.

Chuanxiong, Chinese angelica, peach kernel, and carthamus quicken blood, transform stasis, and check pain.

Coix and poria clear heat, resolve toxin [解毒 *jiě dú*], and eliminate dampness.

Patrinia clears heat, resolves toxin [解毒 *jiě dú*], and transforms stasis and checks pain [化瘀止痛 *huà yū zhǐ tòng*].

18.3.4   Qì-Blood Vacuity [气血虚弱 *qì xuè xū ruò*]

Treatment Method for Qì-Blood Vacuity

Boost qì [益气 *yì qì*], supplement the blood [补血 *bǔ xuè*], and check pain [止痛 *zhǐ tòng*].

Dr. Zhū Shēng-Ān's Formula for Qì-Blood Vacuity Menstrual Pain	
cooked rehmannia [熟地黄 *shú dì huáng*, Rehmanniae Radix Conquita]	15g
white peony [白芍 *bái sháo*, Paeoniae Radix Alba]	10g
Chinese angelica [当归 *dāng guī*, Angelicae Sinensis Radix]	6g
chuanxiong [川芎 *chuān xiōng*, Chuanxiong Rhizoma]	10g
adenophora/glehnia [沙参 *shā shēn*, Adenophorae Radix]	10g
raw astragalus [生黄芪 *shēng huáng qí*, Astragali Radix Cruda]	20g
costusroot [木香 *mù xiāng*, Aucklandiae Radix]	10g
leonurus [益母草 *yì mǔ cǎo*, Leonuri Herba]	15g

Directions: One medicinal preparation per day. Split preparation in two equal parts and take in the morning and in the evening, one hour after a meal.

Prescription Analysis

The combination of adenophora/glehnia and astragalus supplements qì.

Four Agents Decoction [四物汤 *sì wù tāng*] (Chinese angelica, chuanxiong, white peony, and cooked rehmannia) supplements and regulates blood [调血 *tiáo xuè*].

Costusroot and leonurus regulate qì, and ease and smooth the blood vessels of the lower burner, thus checking pain.

Variation According to Signs

If there is blood vacuity with liver depression [血虚肝郁 *xuè xū gān yù*] and distending pain [胀痛 *zhàng tòng*] in the smaller abdomen, add fennel [*xiǎo huí xiāng*], lindera [*wū yào*], bupleurum [*chái hú*], and toosendan [*chuān liàn zǐ*].

For dizzy head and sleeplessness, add gastrodia [*tiān má*] and spiny jujube kernel [*suān zǎo rén*].

For aching lumbus and heavy legs [腰酸腿沉 *yāo suān tuǐ chén*], add dipsacus [*xù duàn*], mistletoe [*sāng jì shēng*], and achyranthes [*niú xī*].

18.3.5 Liver-Kidney Depletion [肝肾亏损 *gān shèn kuī sǔn*]

Treatment Method for Liver-Kidney Depletion

Boost the kidney [益肾 *yì shèn*], nourish the liver [养肝 *yǎng gān*], harmonize blood [和血 *hé xuè*], and check pain.

Dr. Zhū Shēng-Ān's Formula for Liver-Kidney Depletion Menstrual Pain	
Chinese angelica [当归 *dāng guī*, Angelicae Sinensis Radix]	6g
chuanxiong [川芎 *chuān xiōng*, Chuanxiong Rhizoma]	10g
evodia [吴茱萸 *wú zhū yú*, Evodiae Fructus]	6g
dioscorea [山药 *shān yào*, Dioscoreae Rhizoma]	15g
moutan [牡丹皮 *mǔ dān pí*, Moutan Cortex]	10g
white peony [白芍 *bái sháo*, Paeoniae Radix Alba]	6g
notoginseng [三七 *sān qī*, Notoginseng Radix]	10g
costusroot [木香 *mù xiāng*, Aucklandiae Radix]	10g
cyperus [香附 *xiāng fù*, Cyperi Rhizoma]	10g
corydalis [延胡索 *yán hú suǒ*, Corydalis Rhizoma]	10g
curcuma [郁金 *yù jīn*, Curcumae Radix]	10g
licorice [甘草 *gān cǎo*, Glycyrrhizae Radix]	6g

Directions: One medicinal preparation per day. Split preparation in two equal parts and take in the morning and in the evening, one hour after a meal.

Prescription Analysis

Chinese angelica and chuanxiong quicken and supplement blood.

Evodia and dioscorea enrich and supplement kidney essence and fortify the spleen [健脾 *jiàn pí*].

Chinese angelica and white peony emolliate the liver [柔肝 *róu gān*] and nourish the blood [养血 *yǎng xuè*].

Notoginseng and corydalis quicken the blood and check pain.

Costusroot and curcuma soothe and rectify the qì dynamic [气机 *qì jī*].

Licorice harmonizes the properties of all the medicinals [调和药性 *tiáo hé yào xìng*] and regulates the spleen and stomach.

Moutan and costusroot move qì and clear heat.

18.4   ACUPUNCTURE TREATMENTS FOR MENSTRUAL PAIN

Treatment Method for Menstrual Pain

Regulate penetrating and controlling vessels [调理冲任 *tiáo lǐ chōng rèn*], free the channels and check pain [通经止痛 *tōng jīng zhǐ tòng*].

18.4.1   Qì Stagnation and Blood Stasis [气滞血瘀 *qì zhì xuè yū*]

Base Acupuncture Prescription for Qì Stagnation and Blood Stasis Menstrual Pain
LR-2 Moving Between [行间 *xíng jiān*]
SP-6 Three Yīn Intersections [三阴交 *sān yīn jiāo*]
CV-6 Sea of Qì [气海 *qì hǎi*]
CV-3 Central Pole [中极 *zhōng jí*]
BL-32 Second Bone Hole [次髎 *cì liáo*]

Prescription Analysis

This type of menstrual pain is due to depressed liver that gives rise to qì stagnation, which in turn leads to blood stagnation. LR-2 and SP-6 course the liver and resolve depression [疏肝解郁 *shū gān jiě yù*].

LR-2 is the spring point [荥穴 *yíng xué*] of the liver channel and corresponds to fire, while the liver corresponds to wood in the five phases. Thus, LR-2 is the child point of the liver channel, and according to the principle "repletion is treated by draining the child" [实则泻其子 *shí zé xiè qí zǐ*], it can be used to treat liver repletion patterns such as liver depression.

SP-6 is the intersection point of the spleen, liver, and kidney channels and is therefore indicated for diseases of the reproductive system, blood patterns, and gynecological diseases. SP-6 courses the liver, quickens the blood, and transforms stasis.

Qì is the driving force that moves the blood in the vessels. If qì is moving, blood will be able to flow. As its name says, CV-6 (Sea of Qì [气海 *qì hǎi*]) is an extremely important point for qì diseases. It strongly supplements [大补 *dà bǔ*] original qì [元气 *yuán qì*], and it regulates the qì dynamic of the lower burner. This point treats all qì-related blood patterns, e.g., blood stasis caused by qì stagnation.

CV-3 is the intersection point of the controlling vessel [任脉 *rèn mài*] and the three yīn channels of the foot (liver, spleen, kidney), which are all strongly related to the reproductive functions. CV-3 is therefore indicated for reproductive system, gynecological, and smaller abdominal diseases. CV-3 frees the channels and quickens the blood.

Together CV-6 and CV-3 regulate the qì of the lower burner and thereby transform stasis.

BL-32 is a clinically proven point for menstrual pain. It frees the penetrating and controlling vessels, transforms stasis, and conducts menstrual blood downwards.

18.4.2   Cold Congealing in the Uterus [寒凝胞中 *hán níng bāo zhōng*]

Base Acupuncture Prescription for Yáng Vacuity Internal Cold Menstrual Pain
CV-4 Pass Head [关元 *guān yuán*] (moxa)
CV-6 Sea of Qì [气海 *qì hǎi*]
CV-3 Central Pole [中极 *zhōng jí*]
BL-23 Kidney Transport [肾俞 *shèn shū*]

Prescription Analysis

All four points boost and supplement kidney qì.

Cold causes qì to stagnate and congeals blood. Together CV-4, CV-6, and CV-3 regulate the qì of the lower burner and thereby transform stasis (when qì moves, blood flows). Using moxibustion on CV-4 warms lower burner yáng.

CV-4, located 3 body-inches below the umbilicus, is sometimes called "cinnabar field" [丹田 *dān tián*] or the "chamber of essence" in men and the "uterus" in women. It is also an intersection point of the controlling vessel [任脉

rèn mài] and the three yīn channels of the foot (liver, spleen, kidney). CV-4 strongly supplements [大补 *dà bǔ*] original yáng [元阳 *yuán yáng*] and is a principal point [要穴 *yào xué*] for invigorating yáng [壮阳 *zhuàng yáng*]. When this point is tender, it often indicates a gynecological or reproductive system disease. Using moxibustion for 10–30 minutes on this point warms the original qì of the lower burner and the uterus; it also dissipates cold evil.

The actions of CV-6 and CV-3 are discussed above on page 192.

BL-23 dissipates cold in the lower burner by supplementing kidney yáng.

Base Acupuncture Prescription for Congealing Cold Damp Menstrual Pain

M-BW-25 (Extra Point) Seventeenth Vertebra Point [十七椎穴 *shí qī zhuī xué*]
CV-4 Pass Head [关元 *guān yuán*]
ST-25 Celestial Pivot [天枢 *tiān shū*]
CV-8 Spirit Gate Tower [神阙 *shén què*]
SP-6 Three Yīn Intersections [三阴交 *sān yīn jiāo*]

Prescription Analysis

M-BW-25 is an extra point located below the spinous process of the 5th lumbar vertebra. It frees the channel and dissipates cold [通经散寒 *tōng jīng sàn hán*]. Apply draining method [泻法 *xiè fǎ*] to move qì and transform stasis.

CV-4, ST-25, and CV-8 warm and supplement the original qì of the lower burner [下元 *xià yuán*]. Applying moxibustion on CV-4, CV-8, and SP-6 dissipates cold and checks pain.

CV-4 with moxibustion is described in the preceding formula.

ST-25 has an alternate name that literally means "supplementing original qì" [补元 *bǔ yuán*]; it is used for yīn-cold congealing in the abdomen.

CV-8 is located between the middle and lower burner, in the umbilicus, which is said to be "the root of the five viscera and six bowels" [五脏六腑之本 *wǔ zàng liù fǔ zhī běn*]. At birth the umbilicus serves as the connective tissue to earlier heaven [先天 *xiān tiān*], and throughout life the umbilicus is circulated by the penetrating vessel. Thus, CV-8 is a principal point [要穴 *yào xué*] for warming yang. It treats vacuity of original qì and cold in the lower burner [下元 *xià yuán*], lack of vigor in center yáng (stomach and spleen), congealing cold with blood stasis, and so forth. This point should not be needled; use moxibustion.

For menstrual pain due to cold congealing blood, SP-6 is often used together with moxibustion on CV-4 to quicken blood, transform stasis, warm the channels, and check pain.

18.4.3 Damp-Heat Pouring Downward [湿热下注 *shī rè xià zhù*]

Base Acupuncture Prescription for Menstrual Pain due to Damp-Heat Pouring Downward
CV-3 Central Pole [中极 *zhōng jí*] SP-6 Three Yīn Intersection [三阴交 *sān yīn jiāo*] CV-4 Pass Head [关元 *guān yuán*] LI-4 Union Valley [合谷 *hé gǔ*]

Prescription Analysis

CV-3 and SP-6 conduct blood downwards [引血下行 *yǐn xuè xià xíng*] and dispel dampness [祛湿 *qū shī*].

CV-3, the alarm point [募穴 *mù xué*] of the urinary bladder, frees and disinhibits urine [通利小便 *tōng lì xiǎo biàn*] and promotes qì transformation and moves water [化气行水 *huà qì xíng shuǐ*]. It can thus be used for damp-heat pouring downward [湿热下注 *shī rè xià zhù*] and other dampness patterns that require dampness to be removed by freeing and disinhibiting urine. As discussed above, CV-3 is also indicated for reproductive system, gynecological, and smaller abdominal diseases, especially if they involve dampness patterns.

As discussed above, SP-6 is the intersection point of the spleen, liver, and kidney channels and is therefore indicated for diseases of the reproductive system, blood patterns, and gynecological diseases. Furthermore, as a point of the spleen channel, it fortifies the spleen and disinhibits dampness [健脾利湿 *jiàn pí lì shī*].

CV-4 and LI-4 free the channels [通经 *tōng jīng*], resolve heat [解热 *jiě rè*], and reinforce the actions of CV-3 and SP-6.

CV-4 strongly supplements [大补 *dà bǔ*] original yáng [元阳 *yuán yáng*], but it also clears heat and disinhibits dampness [清热利湿 *qīng rè lì shī*] and is used for damp-heat pouring downward.

Because LI-4 Union Valley [合谷 *hé gǔ*] frees the channels, rectifies qì, and quickens blood [理气活血 *lǐ qì huó xuè*], it is an important point for settling pain [镇痛 *zhèn tòng*]. The yáng brightness channel has abundant qì and blood [阳明经多气多血 *yáng míng jīng duō qì duō xuè*]; therefore, needling LI-4 rectifies qì and quickens blood, and it is indicated for gynecological diseases.

Every five minutes during needling, apply musk oil[麝香 *shè xiāng*] to the skin around the needles.[17]

---

[17] The advice to use musk oil is an example of the treatment experiences passed down within the family of Dr. Zhū Shēng-Ān.

18.4.4   Qì-Blood Vacuity [气血虚弱 *qì xuè xū ruò*]

Base Acupuncture Prescription for Qì-Blood Vacuity Menstrual Pain
BL-23 Kidney Transport [肾俞 *shèn shū*] GV-4 Life Gate [命门 *mìng mén*] CV-4 Pass Head [关元 *guān yuán*] ST-36 Leg Three Lǐ [足三里 *zú sān lǐ*] CV-12 Center Stomach Duct [中脘 *zhōng wǎn*] add moxibustion

Prescription Analysis

As discussed above, BL-23 supplements kidney yáng and dissipates cold in the lower burner.

GV-4 is a point on the governing vessel [督脉 *dū mài*], which governs the yáng of the whole body (regulates the yáng channels), homes to the brain, and nets the kidney. Thus, needling GV-4 supplements true yáng [真阳 *zhēn yáng*](kidney yáng).

The actions of CV-4 are discussed above on page 193.

ST-36, the uniting point [合穴 *hé xué*] of the stomach channel, belongs to earth and is the earth point of the earth channel. It is an important point for strengthening and invigorating because it supplements the spleen and kidney and boosts qì-blood [气血 *qì xuè*].

Applying moxibustion to CV-12 warms and supplements the qì of the middle burner.

The spleen and stomach are the root of later heaven [后天之本 *hòu tiān zhī běn*], the source of qì and blood formation [脾胃为生化气血之源 *pí wèi wéi shēng huà qì xuè zhī yuán*]. The combination of ST-36 and CV-12 is thus important for replenishing qì and blood.

18.4.5   Liver-Kidney Depletion [肝肾亏损 *gān shèn kuī sǔn*]

Base Acupuncture Prescription for Menstrual Pain due to Liver-Kidney Depletion
CV-4 Pass Head [关元 *guān yuán*] CV-3 Central Pole [中极 *zhōng jí*] SP-6 Three Yīn Intersections [三阴交 *sān yīn jiāo*] BL-23 Kidney Transport [肾俞 *shèn shū*] LR-3 Supreme Surge [太冲 *tài chōng*]

Prescription Analysis

When water (kidney) is abundant it nourishes wood (liver). If both are flourishing, the penetrating and controlling vessels will flourish and pain will be relieved.

CV-4 and CV-3 supplement earlier heaven original qì [先天之元气 *xiān tiān zhī yuán qì*]; they are discussed above on pages 193 and 192, respectively.

BL-23 is a principal point [要穴 *yào xué*] for treating kidney vacuity. It boosts the kidney and secures essence [益肾固精 *yì shèn gù jīng*], enriches and supplements kidney yīn [滋补肾阴 *zī bǔ shèn yīn*], and warms and invigorates kidney yáng [温壮肾阳 *wēn zhuàng shèn yáng*].

SP-6 is a principal point [要穴 *yào xué*] for treating blood patterns, as discussed on page 58.

LR-3 is the source point [原穴 *yuán xué*] of the liver channel (the point where the source qì of the liver collects). Because indications for source points are diseases of the internal organs related to the respective channel, this point is indicated for disorders of the liver itself.

CHAPTER 19
Chronic Lumbar Strain

Chronic lumbar strain refers to chronic ache of the lower back that is of varying severity and is usually due to strained muscles, fasciae, or ligaments of the lumbar region. There are two main forms of chronic lumbar strain.

- accumulation of taxation injury, qì-blood stagnation [积劳损伤，气血郁滞 *jī láo sǔn shāng, qì xuè yù zhì*]
- wind-cold-damp evil obstructing the channels and network vessels [风寒湿邪，痹阻经络 *fēng hán shī xié, bì zǔ jīng luò*]

19.1 POINTS OF ATTENTION FOR CHRONIC LUMBAR STRAIN

19.1.1 Physiology, Pathomechanism, and Treatment

***The lumbus is the house of the kidney** [腰为肾之府 **yāo wéi shèn zhī fǔ**].*

The lumbus is the house of the kidney [腰为肾之府 *yāo wéi shèn zhī fǔ*], and the kidney governs the bones [肾主骨 *shèn zhǔ gǔ*]. If there is no kidney vacuity, chronic low backache will not arise.

Kidney vacuity is the root of this disease [本 *běn*], and wind-cold-damp evil is the tip [标 *biāo*] because it exploits [乘 *chéng*] vacuity and enters the body. Another cause for lumbar strain is accumulation of taxation injury that repeatedly damages the sinew vessels and blocks the channels and network vessels.

Therefore, in addition to treating the immediate cause, such as qì-blood stagnation or wind-cold-damp evil, the kidney has to be supplemented. This is reflected in both the acupuncture treatment and the medicinal treatment.

The Kidney, Bladder Channel, Liver, and Spleen in Relation to Lumbar Strain

The lumbus is the house of the kidney [腰为肾之府 *yāo wéi shèn zhī fǔ*]. The kidney governs the bones [肾主骨 *shèn zhǔ gǔ*].

The foot greater yáng bladder channel [足太阳膀胱经 *zú tài yáng páng guāng jīng*] passes the lumbar area. The lumbus is the house of the kidney, and the kidney and bladder channels stand in interior-exterior relationship. When external evil is contracted, it first enters the foot greater yáng bladder channel.

If there is no kidney vacuity, chronic low backache will not arise. The liver and spleen can contribute to kidney vacuity due to their relation with the kidney: the liver promotes kidney qì [肝资肾气 *gān zī shèn qì*]and the source of the kidney's essential qì [精气 *jīng qì*] is the spleen. These dynamics merit consideration during diagnosis and treatment.

19.2 CAUSES AND PATHOMECHANISM OF CHRONIC LUMBAR STRAIN; IDENTIFYING PATTERNS

19.2.1 Accumulation of Taxation Injury; Qì-Blood Stagnation [积劳损伤，气血郁滞 *jī láo sǔn shāng, qì xuè yù zhì*]

Causes and Pathomechanism of Accumulation of Taxation Injury and Qì-Blood Stagnation

This pattern is the result of chronic overstrain damaging the sinews and gradually damaging kidney qì [耗伤肾气 *hào shāng shèn qì*], or it is the result of knocks and falls causing sprain and bruising [闪挫 *shǎn cuò*] which do not heal for a long time; in both circumstances there is obstruction of the network vessels that leads to qì stagnation and blood stasis [气滞血瘀 *qì zhì xuè yū*]. When there is stoppage, there is pain [不通则痛 *bù tōng zé tòng*]. As blood stasis is an evil that has a physical form and is thus considered yīn [属阴 *shǔ yīn*], the pain caused by blood stasis is lighter during daytime and worse during nighttime.

Important Signs of Accumulation of Taxation Injury and Qì-Blood Stagnation

Stabbing or distending pain [刺痛或胀痛 *cì tòng huò zhàng tòng*] in the lumbar region, as well as hypertonicity. The pain is in a fixed location and refuses pressure [拒按 *jù àn*]. The lumbus is hard as a board. Inhibited bending, stretching, and turning of the waist. Pain is lighter during daytime and worse during nighttime. Dark purple tongue, or tongue with stasis macules [舌暗紫或有瘀斑 *shé àn zǐ huò yǒu yū bān*]. Rough pulse [涩脉 *sè mài*].

19.2.2 Wind-Cold-Damp Evil Obstructing the Channels and Network Vessels [风寒湿邪，痹阻经络 *fēng hán shī xié, bì zǔ jīng luò*]

Causes and Pathomechanism of Wind-Cold-Damp Evil Obstructing the Channels and Network Vessels

This pattern is the result of wind, cold, and damp evils assailing [侵袭 *qīn xí*] the body and blocking the channels and network vessels [闭阻经络 *bì zǔ jīng luò*]. This inhibits the free flow of qì-blood [气血运行不畅 *qì xuè yùn xíng bú chàng*], causing pain.

Important Signs of Wind-Cold-Damp Evil Obstructing the Channels

Cold heavy pain [冷痛重痛 *lěng tòng zhòng tòng*] in the lumbar region that is relieved by warmth and by rubbing and pressing [揉按 *róu àn*]. Hypertonicity [拘急 *jū jí*] and inhibited turning of the waist. Pain is worse during the night and in yīn-type weather. The tongue has a white, slimy coating [苔白腻 *tāi bái nì*]. Deep slow pulse [脉沉迟 *mài chén chí*] or moderate pulse [脉缓 *mài huǎn*].

19.3 TREATMENT OF CHRONIC LUMBAR STRAIN USING CHINESE MEDICINALS

19.3.1 Accumulation of Taxation Injury, Qì-Blood Stagnation [积劳损伤，气血郁滞 *jī láo sǔn shāng, qì xuè yù zhì*]

Treatment Method for Accumulation of Taxation Injury, Qì-Blood Stagnation

Move qì and quicken blood, free the channels and check pain [行气活血，通经止痛 *xíng qì huó xuè, tōng jīng zhǐ tòng*].

Luxuriance-Regulating and Network-Quickening Beverage [调荣活络饮 *tiáo róng huó luò yǐn*]	
Chinese angelica [当归 *dāng guī*, Angelicae Sinensis Radix]	15g
red peony [赤芍 *chì sháo*, Paeoniae Radix Rubra]	12g
peach kernel [桃仁 *táo rén*, Persicae Semen]	9g
carthamus [红花 *hóng huā*, Carthami Flos]	9g
rhubarb [大黄 *dà huáng*, Rhei Rhizoma et Radix]	6g
pubescent angelica [独活 *dú huó*, Angelicae Pubescentis Radix]	9g
large gentian [秦艽 *qín jiāo*, Gentianae Macrophyllae Radix]	9g
achyranthes [牛膝 *niú xī*, Achyranthis Bidentatae Radix]	15g
cinnamon twig [桂枝 *guì zhī*, Cinnamomi Ramulus]	6g
bitter orange [枳壳 *zhǐ ké*, Aurantii Fructus]	10g
unripe tangerine peel [青皮 *qīng pí*, Citri Reticulatae Pericarpium Viride]	10g
Directions: Take decocted with water [水煎服 *shuǐ jiān fú*].	

Prescription Analysis

Chief Medicinals

Chinese angelica supplements and quickens blood. Peach kernel quickens blood and transforms stasis, thus treating the accumulation of taxation injury.

Support Medicinals

Red peony and carthamus quicken blood and transform stasis, thereby helping the chief medicinals to treat accumulation of taxation injury.

Assistant Medicinals

Rhubarb quickens blood, transforms stasis, and drains turbidity [泻浊 *xiè zhuó*]. Pubescent angelica and large gentian dispel wind, overcome dampness, and check pain [祛风，胜湿，止痛 *qū fēng, shèng shī, zhǐ tòng*]. Achyranthes dispels wind-damp, strengthens sinews and bones, supplements the kidneys, and quickens blood and transforms stasis. Cinnamon twig warms and frees the channels. Bitter orange and unripe tangerine peel move qì to help move blood.

This combination of medicinals is used to move qì and quicken blood and to free the channels and check pain.

Variation According to Signs

For severe blood stasis, add frankincense [乳香 *rǔ xiāng*] and myrrh [没药 *mò yào*]. For hypertonicity [拘急 *jū jí*] of the sinews, add ground pine [*shēn jīn cǎo*] and clematis [*wēi líng xiān*].

19.3.2   Wind-Cold-Damp Evil Obstructing the Channels and Network Vessels [风寒湿邪，痹阻经络 *fēng hán shī xié, bì zǔ jīng luò*]

Method of Treatment for Wind-Cold-Damp Evil Obstructing the Channels and Network Vessels

Warm the channels and dissipate cold, dispel wind and eliminate dampness [温经散寒，祛风除湿 *wēn jīng sàn hán, qū fēng chú shī*].

Pubescent Angelica and Mistletoe Decoction [独活寄生汤 *dú huó jì shēng tāng*]	
pubescent angelica [独活 *dú huó*, Angelicae Pubescentis Radix]	9g
mistletoe [桑寄生 *sāng jì shēng*, Taxilli Herba]	18g
eucommia [杜仲 *dù zhòng*, Eucommiae Cortex]	9g
achyranthes [牛膝 *niú xī*, Achyranthis Bidentatae Radix]	9g
asarum [细辛 *xì xīn*, Asari Herba]	3g
large gentian [秦艽 *qín jiāo*, Gentianae Macrophyllae Radix]	9g
poria [茯苓 *fú líng*, Poria]	12g
cinnamon bark [肉桂 *ròu guì*, Cinnamomi Cortex]	1.5g
saposhnikovia [防风 *fáng fēng*, Saposhnikoviae Radix]	9g
chuanxiong [川芎 *chuān xiōng*, Chuanxiong Rhizoma]	6g
ginseng [人参 *rén shēn*, Ginseng Radix]	12g
Chinese angelica [当归 *dāng guī*, Angelicae Sinensis Radix]	12g
white peony [白芍 *bái sháo*, Paeoniae Radix Alba]	9g
dried rehmannia [干地黄 *gān dì huáng*, Rehmanniae Radix Exsiccata]	15g
licorice [甘草 *gān cǎo*, Glycyrrhizae Radix]	6g
Directions: Take decocted with water [水煎服 *shuǐ jiān fú*].	

Prescription Analysis

Chief Medicinals

Pubescent angelica and mistletoe dispel wind and dissipate cold, overcome dampness and check pain [祛风散寒，胜湿止痛 *qū fēng sàn hán, shèng shī zhǐ tòng*].

Support Medicinals

Large gentian, saposhnikovia, asarum, eucommia, and achyranthes help the chief medicinals to dispel wind and overcome dampness and to dissipate cold and check pain. Eucommia and achyranthes supplement the kidneys and strengthen the sinews and bones.

Assistant Medicinals

Poria and ginseng supplement qì. Chinese angelica, dried rehmannia, chuanxiong, and white peony comprise Four Agents Decoction [四物汤 *sì wù tāng*], which supplements blood. Cinnamon bark warms yáng and frees the channels.

Licorice harmonizes the properties of all the medicinals [调和药性 *tiáo hé yào xìng*] and, together with white peony, relaxes tension [缓急 *huǎn jí*] and checks pain.

This combination of medicinals dispels wind and overcomes dampness, dissipates cold and checks pain, and supplements qì-blood and boosts the kidney.

Variation According to Signs

Pubescent Angelica and Mistletoe Decoction is a warming and supplementing prescription that dissipates with acridity. It also dispels wind and overcomes dampness, warms the channels and dissipates cold, supplements qì-blood and boosts the liver and kidney.

If cold evil is pronounced and the pain is severe, add aconite main tuber [*chuān wū tóu*] to emphasize warming the channels, dissipating cold, and checking pain.

If damp evil is pronounced, add atractylodes [*cāng zhú*], coix [*yì yǐ rén*], and fangji [*fáng jǐ*] to eliminate damp evil.

For enduring wind-damp, add scorpion [*quán xiē*], earthworm [*dì lóng*], centipede [*wú gōng*], and pangolin scales [*chuān shān jiǎ*] to track wind and free the network vessels [搜风通络 *sōu fēng tōng luò*].

19.4 ACUPUNCTURE TREATMENT FOR CHRONIC LUMBAR PAIN

19.4.1 Base Acupuncture Prescription for Chronic Lumbar Pain

This base prescription should be modified according to the identified patterns that are discussed below and according to the condition of the individual patient.

Method of Treatment for Chronic Lumbar Pain

Fortify the spleen and supplement the kidney, invigorate the lumbus and check pain [健脾补肾，壮腰止痛 *jiàn pí bǔ shèn, zhuàng yāo zhǐ tòng*].

Base Acupuncture Prescription for Chronic Lumbar Pain
BL-20 Spleen Transport [脾俞 *pí shū*]
BL-23 Kidney Transport [肾俞 *shèn shū*]
GV-4 Life Gate [命门 *mìng mén*]
BL-25 Large Intestine Transport [大肠俞 *dà cháng shū*]

Prescription Analysis

The lumbus is the house of the kidney [腰为肾之府 *yāo wéi shèn zhī fǔ*]; the spleen governs the flesh [脾主肌肉 *pí zhǔ jī ròu*]. Damage to the kidney and spleen constitutes the main cause for chronic lumbar strain, hence the points above are selected to fortify the spleen and kidney and invigorate the lumbus. Moxibustion may be added.

19.4.2 Points to Add to the Base Prescription

Points for Accumulation of Taxation Injury, Qì-Blood Stagnation   **[积劳损伤，气血郁滞 *jī láo sǔn shāng, qì xuè yù zhì*]**
BL-40 Bend Center [委中 *wěi zhōng*]
SP-6 Three Yīn Intersection [三阴交 *sān yīn jiāo*]
LR-3 Supreme Surge [太冲 *tài chōng*]

These points are added to the base prescription to course the liver and rectify qì and to quicken blood and check pain [疏肝理气，活血止痛 *shū gān lǐ qì, huó xuè zhǐ tòng*].

Wind-Cold-Damp Evil Obstructing the Channels and Network Vessels [风寒   **湿邪，痹阻经络 *fēng hán shī xié, bì zǔ jīng luò*]**
TB-5 Outer Pass [外关 *wài guān*]
BL-40 Bend Center [委中 *wěi zhōng*]

This pair of points dissipates wind and quickens blood [散风活血 *sàn fēng huó xuè*].

CHAPTER 20

Prolapse of Lumbar Intervertebral Disc

Prolapse of a lumbar intervertebral disc occurs when the fibrous outer coat of the intervertebral disc ruptures and the pulpiform nucleus protrudes, pressing on the adjacent nerve roots. This manifests as lumbar pain or as other symptoms attributable to impaired nerve function.

There are four main forms:

- liver and kidney depletion [肝肾亏损 *gān shèn kuī sǔn*]
- wind-cold obstruction [风寒闭阻 *fēng hán bì zǔ*]
- damp-heat congestion [湿热壅滞 *shī rè yōng zhì*]
- blood stasis collecting internally [瘀血内停 *yū xuè nèi tíng*]

20.1 POINTS OF ATTENTION FOR PROLAPSE OF LUMBAR INTERVERTEBRAL DISC

20.1.1 Physiology

The lumbus is the house of the kidney [腰为肾之府 *yāo wéi shèn zhī fǔ*]. If kidney essence is vacuous, the lumbus is not warmed and nourished properly, and the result is lumbar pain. Kidney vacuity is the root of this disease [本 *běn*] and wind-cold-damp evil is the tip [标 *biāo*] because it exploits [乘 *chéng*] vacuity and enters the body.

20.1.2 Pathomechanism

This disease tends to start with wind-cold-damp evil entering the sinews and bones, and dampness obstructing the network vessels, causing acute pain. If the disease endures and wind-cold-damp remains lodged in the lumbar area, kidney essence becomes increasingly vacuous and causes continuous aching pain [酸痛 *suān tòng*].

Another cause for lumbar strain is accumulation of taxation injury that repeatedly damages the sinew vessels and blocks the channels and network vessels.

20.1.3 Considerations for Diagnosis

Patients with long-standing vacuity patterns easily contract external evils (such as wind, cold, and/or damp evils) that result in a vacuity-repletion complex [虚实错杂 *xū shí cuò zá*]. In these circumstances one has to distinguish between the primary and secondary cause, the tip and the root [标本 *biāo běn*].

20.1.4   Treatment

In addition to treatment using Chinese medicinals and acupuncture, certain traditional exercises, e.g., Huá Tuó's "five animal exercises" [五禽戏 *wǔ qín xì*], are excellent for helping treat or prevent this disease.

20.2 CAUSES AND PATHOMECHANISM OF PROLAPSED LUMBAR INTERVERTEBRAL DISC; IDENTIFYING PATTERNS

20.2.1   Liver and Kidney Depletion [肝肾亏损 *gān shèn kuī sǔn*]

Causes and Pathomechanism of Liver and Kidney Depletion

This pattern results from overexertion by a patient with a weak constitution [素体虚弱 *sù tǐ xū ruò*] or from weakness in old age that leads to liver-kidney depletion. The liver stores blood and governs the sinews [肝藏血主筋 *gān cáng xuè zhǔ jīn*]; the kidney stores essence and governs the bones [肾藏精主骨 *shèn cáng jīng zhǔ gǔ*]. When both sinews and bones lose their source of nourishment and moisture, pain arises.

Important Signs of Liver and Kidney Depletion

Aching pain in the lumbus and back, which comes and goes and is relieved by rubbing and pressing. Pain is exacerbated by exertion and relieved by rest. Fatigue. There may be aching shins and painful heels, dizziness, and tinnitus.

When there is a tendency towards liver and kidney yīn vacuity [肝肾阴虚 *gān shèn yīn xū*], other symptoms will include vexation [心烦 *xīn fán*], sleeplessness, dry mouth and throat, flushed face, and vexing heat in the five hearts [五心烦热 *wǔ xīn fán rè*], as well as red tongue with scant fur [舌红少苔 *shé hóng shǎo tāi*] and a fine rapid pulse [脉细数 *mài xì shuò*].

When there is a tendency towards kidney yáng insufficiency [肾阳不足 *shèn yáng bù zú*], other symptoms will include lesser abdominal pain, swollen legs, aversion to cold, and cold limbs, as well as pale tongue with moist coating [舌淡苔润 *shé dàn tāi rùn*] and a deep weak pulse [脉沉弱 *mài chén ruò*].

20.2.2   Wind-Cold Obstruction [风寒闭阻 *fēng hán bì zǔ*]

Causes and Pathomechanism of Wind-Cold Obstruction

Wind-cold evil assails [侵袭 *qīn xí*] the body and blocks the channels and network vessels. This inhibits the free flow of qì-blood, causing pain.

Important Signs of Wind-Cold Obstruction

Pain in the lumbus and legs that is exacerbated by cold and relieved by warmth. The lumbus and legs feel heavy. The leg on the affected side is cold and numb. Pain is exacerbated by yīn-type weather. Aversion to cold and liking for warmth. The tongue with white slimy coating [苔白腻 *tāi bái nì*]. Deep slow pulse [脉沉迟 *mài chén chí*].

20.2.3   Damp-Heat Congestion [湿热壅滞 *shī rè yōng zhì*]

Causes and Pathomechanism of Damp-Heat Congestion

If damp-heat congests in the lumbar area, the sinews slacken [筋脉弛缓 *jīn mài chí huǎn*] and the channel qì stops. When there is stoppage, there is pain [不通则痛 *bù tōng zé tòng*].

Important Signs of Damp-Heat Congestion

Heavy, cumbersome, and painful lumbar area and leg(s). The pain feels hot and is exacerbated by hot and humid weather. The affected leg feels numb. Red tongue, yellow slimy coating [舌红, 苔黄腻 *shé hóng, tāi huáng nì*]. Soggy rapid pulse [脉濡数 *mài rú shuò*].

20.2.4   Blood Stasis Collecting Internally [瘀血内停 *yū xuè nèi tíng*]

Causes and Pathomechanism of Blood Stasis Collecting Internally

Knocks and falls cause sprains and bruises [闪挫 *shǎn cuò*] and give rise to qì stagnation and blood stasis [气滞血瘀 *qì zhì xuè yū*]. When there is stoppage, there is pain [不通则痛 *bù tōng zé tòng*].

Important Signs of Blood Stasis Collecting Internally

Stabbing pain [刺痛 *cì tòng*] in the lumbar region. The pain is in a fixed location. Inhibited bending, stretching, and turning of the waist. Purple tongue, or tongue with stasis macules [舌紫或有瘀斑 *shé zǐ huò yǒu yū bān*]. Rough pulse [涩脉 *sè mài*].

20.3   TREATMENT OF PROLAPSED LUMBAR INTERVERTEBRAL DISC USING CHINESE MEDICINALS

20.3.1   Liver and Kidney Depletion [肝肾亏损 *gān shèn kuī sǔn*]

Method of Treatment for Liver and Kidney Depletion

Enrich and supplement liver and kidney, strengthen the sinews and bones [滋补肝肾，强筋壮骨 *zī bǔ gān shèn, qiáng jīn zhuàng gǔ*].

Kidney-Supplementing Bone-Strengthening Decoction [补肾壮骨汤 *bǔ shèn zhuàng gǔ tāng*]	
cooked rehmannia [熟地黄 *shú dì huáng*, Rehmanniae Radix Conquita]	12g
Chinese angelica [当归 *dāng guī*, Angelicae Sinensis Radix]	12g
achyranthes [牛膝 *niú xī*, Achyranthis Bidentatae Radix]	9g
cornus [山茱萸 *shān zhū yú*, Corni Fructus]	12g
poria [茯苓 *fú líng*, Poria]	12g
dipsacus [续断 *xù duàn*, Dipsaci Radix]	12g
eucommia [杜仲 *dù zhòng*, Eucommiae Cortex]	12g
white peony [白芍 *bái sháo*, Paeoniae Radix Alba]	9g
unripe tangerine peel [青皮 *qīng pí*, Citri Reticulatae Pericarpium Viride]	9g
acanthopanax [五加皮 *wǔ jiā pí*, Acanthopanacis Cortex]	9g
Directions: Take decocted with water [水煎服 *shuǐ jiān fú*].	

Prescription Analysis

Chief Medicinals

Cooked rehmannia and cornus enrich and supplement the liver and kidney and strengthen the sinews and bones.

Support Medicinals

Chinese angelica, achyranthes, eucommia, white peony, and dipsacus help the chief medicinals supplement the liver and kidney and strengthen sinews and bones, thus treating the root [治本 *zhì běn*].

Assistant Medicinals

Acanthopanax supplements the liver and kidney; it also dispels wind-damp. Poria disinhibits dampness by bland percolation [淡渗利湿 *dàn shèn lì shī*] to fortify the spleen. Unripe tangerine peel courses depression-stagnation of liver qì [疏肝气之郁滞 *shū gān qì zhī yù zhì*].

This combination of medicinals is used to enrich and supplement the liver and kidney and to strengthen the sinews and bones.

Variation According to Signs

If there is a tendency towards kidney yīn vacuity, combine the prescription given above with Six-Ingredient Rehmannia Pill [六味地黄丸 *liù wèi dì huáng wán*]. If there is a tendency towards kidney yáng vacuity, combine the prescription given above with Golden Coffer Kidney Qì Pill [金匮肾气丸 *jīn guì shèn qì wán*]. If there is strong kidney vacuity, add velvet deerhorn [*lù róng*] to reinforce the prescription's function of enriching and supplementing. If there are signs of wind-damp, add eucommia [*dù zhòng*] and mistletoe [*sāng jì shēng*] to eliminate wind-damp.

20.3.2 Wind-Cold Obstruction [风寒闭阻 *fēng hán bì zǔ*]

Method of Treatment for Wind-Cold Obstruction

Dispel wind and eliminate dampness, dissipate cold and check pain [祛风除湿，散寒止痛 *qū fēng chú shī, sàn hán zhǐ tòng*].

Pubescent Angelica and Mistletoe Decoction [独活寄生汤 *dú huó jì shēng tāng*]	
pubescent angelica [独活 *dú huó*, Angelicae Pubescentis Radix]	10g
mistletoe [桑寄生 *sāng jì shēng*, Taxilli Herba]	15g
large gentian [秦艽 *qín jiāo*, Gentianae Macrophyllae Radix]	10g
saposhnikovia [防风 *fáng fēng*, Saposhnikoviae Radix]	10g
asarum [细辛 *xì xīn*, Asari Herba]	3g
chuanxiong [川芎 *chuān xiōng*, Chuanxiong Rhizoma]	9g
Chinese angelica [当归 *dāng guī*, Angelicae Sinensis Radix]	10g
cooked rehmannia [熟地黄 *shú dì huáng*, Rehmanniae Radix Conquita]	15g
white peony [白芍 *bái sháo*, Paeoniae Radix Alba]	10g
cinnamon twig [桂枝 *guì zhī*, Cinnamomi Ramulus]	10g
poria [茯苓 *fú líng*, Poria]	10g
eucommia [杜仲 *dù zhòng*, Eucommiae Cortex]	10g
achyranthes [牛膝 *niú xī*, Achyranthis Bidentatae Radix]	10g
codonopsis [党参 *dǎng shēn*, Codonopsis Radix]	10g
licorice [甘草 *gān cǎo*, Glycyrrhizae Radix]	6g
Directions: Take decocted with water [水煎服 *shuǐ jiān fú*].	

Prescription Analysis

Chief Medicinals

Pubescent angelica, large gentian, and saposhnikovia dispel wind-damp and check impediment pain [止痹痛 *zhǐ bì tòng*], thus treating the root [治本 *zhì běn*].

Support Medicinals

Asarum dissipates [散 *sàn*] wind-cold and checks pain. Eucommia, achyranthes, and mistletoe supplement liver and kidney and dispel wind-damp. Chinese angelica, cooked rehmannia, and white peony supplement blood. Codonopsis and poria supplement qì.

Assistant Medicinals

Chuanxiong and cinnamon twig quicken blood and free the channels to check pain.

Licorice not only harmonizes the properties of all the other medicinals [调和药性 *tiáo hé yào xìng*] in this formula, but also combines with white peony to comprise Peony and Licorice Decoction [芍药甘草汤 *sháo yào gān cǎo tāng*], which relaxes tension and checks pain [缓急止痛 *huǎn jí zhǐ tòng*].

This combination of medicinals is used to dispel wind and eliminate dampness and to dissipate cold and check pain. By dispelling wind-damp, supplementing qì-blood, dispelling evil, and supporting right [祛邪扶正 *qū xié fú zhèng*], the root and tip are treated simultaneously [标本同治 *biāo běn tóng zhì*].

Variation According to Signs

For cold pain [冷痛 *lěng tòng*] in both the lumbus and the legs, add aconite main tuber [*chuān wū tóu*] and wild aconite [*cǎo wū tóu*] to dissipate cold and check pain. For numbness in the lower limbs, add clematis [*wēi líng xiān*], chaenomeles [*mù guā*], and loofah [*sī guā luò*] to quicken blood and free the network vessels.

20.3.3   Damp-Heat Congestion [湿热壅滞 *shī rè yōng zhì*]

Method of Treatment for Damp-Heat Congestion

Clear heat, disinhibit dampness, check pain [清热, 利湿, 止痛 *qīng rè, lì shī, zhǐ tòng*].

Mysterious Three Pill [三妙丸 *sān miào wán*]	
atractylodes [苍术 *cāng zhú*, Atractylodis Rhizoma]	10g
phellodendron [黄柏 *huáng bǎi*, Phellodendri Cortex]	10g
achyranthes [牛膝 *niú xī*, Achyranthis Bidentatae Radix]	10g

Directions: The original prescription was taken as pills, 6g at a time, three times a day. The prescription can also be taken as a decoction [水煎服 *shuǐ jiān fú*] using the quantities given above.

Prescription Analysis

Chief Medicinals

Atractylodes is an acrid warm-drying medicinal [辛温而燥 *xīn wēn ér zào*] that dispels dampness. Phellodendron is a bitter cold-drying medicinal [苦寒而燥 *kǔ hán ér zào*] that dispels dampness and clears heat. The two medicinals together clear heat and dry dampness, thus treating the root [治本 *zhì běn*].

Support Medicinal

Achyranthes strengthens the sinews and bones, supplements and boosts the liver and kidney, and disinhibits dampness and quickens blood.

All three medicinals together clear heat and dry dampness, free the network vessels and check pain. There are only a few medicinals in this prescription, yet its function and power are focused and strong.

Variation According to Signs

If heat evil dominates (marked by signs such as a red tongue, thirst, and short voidings of reddish urine [小便短赤 *xiǎo biàn duǎn chì*]), add gardenia [*zhī zǐ*], alisma [*zé xiè*], and trifoliate akebia [*mù tōng*] to clear heat and disinhibit dampness. If dampness evil dominates (cumbersome and heavy lumbus and legs [腰腿困重 *yāo tuǐ kùn zhòng*]), add alisma [*zé xiè*], plantago seed [*chē qián zǐ*], and fangji [*fáng jǐ*]. For red, swollen, and painful joints, add large gentian [*qín jiāo*] and siegesbeckia [*xī xiān cǎo*].

20.3.4 Blood Stasis Collecting Internally [瘀血内停 *yū xuè nèi tíng*]

Method of Treatment for Blood Stasis Collecting Internally

Quicken blood and transform stasis, free the network vessels and check pain [活血祛瘀，通络止痛 *huó xuè qū yū, tōng luò zhǐ tòng*].

Peach Kernel and Carthamus Four Agents Decoction [桃红四物汤 *táo hóng sì wù tāng*]	
peach kernel [桃仁 *táo rén*, Persicae Semen]	10g
carthamus [红花 *hóng huā*, Carthami Flos]	10g
Chinese angelica [当归 *dāng guī*, Angelicae Sinensis Radix]	10g
chuanxiong [川芎 *chuān xiōng*, Chuanxiong Rhizoma]	10g
cooked rehmannia [熟地黄 *shú dì huáng*, Rehmanniae Radix Conquita]	15g
red peony [赤芍 *chì sháo*, Paeoniae Radix Rubra]	10g
Directions: Take decocted with water [水煎服 *shuǐ jiān fú*].	

Prescription Analysis

Chief Medicinal

Peach kernel and carthamus quicken blood, transform stasis, and check pain.

Support Medicinals

Chuanxiong and red peony help the chief medicinals quicken blood and transform stasis.

Assistant Medicinals

Chinese angelica and cooked rehmannia supplement blood.

This combination of medicinals quickens blood, dispels stasis, and checks pain. When blood stasis is dispelled, the pain will stop.

Variation According to Signs

For severe blood stasis, add frankincense [*rǔ xiāng*], myrrh [*mò yào*], and ground beetle [*zhè chóng*] to emphasize quickening blood and transforming stasis. For signs of wind-damp, add medicinals such as notopterygium [*qiāng huó*], pubescent angelica [*dú huó*], mistletoe [*sāng jì shēng*], and eucommia [*dù zhòng*] to dispel wind and check pain. For kidney vacuity, add eucommia [*dù zhòng*], cornus [*shān zhū yú*], and velvet deerhorn [*lù róng*] to supplement and boost the liver and kidney and to check pain.

20.4 ACUPUNCTURE TREATMENTS FOR PROLAPSED INTERVERTEBRAL LUMBAR DISC

20.4.1 Base Acupuncture Prescription for Prolapsed Intervertebral Lumbar Disc

This base prescription should be modified according to the identified patterns that are discussed below and according to the condition of the individual patient.

Treatment Method for Prolapsed Intervertebral Lumbar Disc

Quicken the blood and free the vessels [活血通脉 *huó xuè tōng mài*].

Base Acupuncture Prescription for Prolapsed Intervertebral Lumbar Disc
Stimulate Huá Tuó's paravertebral points [华佗夹脊穴 *huá tuó jiā jǐ xué*] in the lumbar region

Prescription Analysis

This selection of local points [局部取穴 *jú bù qǔ xué*] directly quickens blood and frees the vessels, and strengthens the muscles alongside the lumbar vertebrae. Although this treatment is simple, it is sufficient for minor cases of prolapsed discs.

20.4.2 Points to Add to the Base Prescription

Points for Liver and Kidney Depletion [肝肾亏损 *gān shèn kuī sǔn*]
BL-23 Kidney Transport [肾俞 *shèn shū*]
KI-3 Great Ravine [太溪 *tài xī*]
LR-8 Spring at the Bend [曲泉 *qū quán*]

These points supplement the liver and boost the kidneys [补肝益肾 *bǔ gān yì shèn*].

BL-23 is a back transport point, and back transport points are particularly indicated for yīn patterns, e.g., interior patterns, cold patterns, chronic diseases, and vacuity patterns.

KI-3, the source point [原穴 *yuán xué*] of the foot lesser yīn kidney channel, supplements both kidney yīn and kidney yáng [阴阳双补 *yīn yáng shuāng bǔ*].

LR-8 is the uniting point [合穴 *hé xué*] of the liver and corresponds to water. LR-8 can be used in relation to the five-phase correspondences, which is also called the "supplement the mother, drain the child" method [补母泻子法]. The liver corresponds to wood and LR-8 corresponds to water. Wood is engendered by water, as water is the mother of wood [水为木之母]. LR-8 therefore supplements the liver.

Points for Wind-Cold Obstruction [风寒闭阻 *fēng hán bì zǔ*]
TB-5 Outer Pass [外关 *wài guān*]
GV-3 Lumbar Yáng Pass [腰阳关 *yāo yáng guān*]
BL-60 Kunlun Mountains [昆仑 *kūn lún*]

These points dispel wind and dissipate cold, warm yáng and free the channels [祛风散寒，温阳通脉 *qū fēng sàn hán, wēn yáng tōng mài*].

TB-5 is an important point for releasing the exterior and treating pain induced by wind. GV-3 invigorates the lumbus and legs, supplements yáng, and dissipates cold [温阳散寒 *wēn yáng sàn hán*]. It is indicated in lumbar and leg pain. BL-60 warms the foot greater yáng bladder channel [足太阳膀胱经 *zú tài yáng páng guāng jīng*].

Points for Damp-Heat Congestion [湿热壅滞 *shī rè yōng zhì*]
GB-34 Yáng Mound Spring [阳陵泉 *yáng líng quán*]
KI-7 Recover Flow [复溜 *fù liū*]

This pair of points clears heat and disinhibits dampness [清热利湿 *qīng rè lì shī*]. GB-34 clears and disinhibits damp-heat, while KI-7 disinhibits dampness in the lower burner.

Points for Blood Stasis Collecting Internally [瘀血内停 *yū xuè nèi tíng*]
BL-40 Bend Center [委中 *wěi zhōng*]
SP-10 Sea of Blood [血海 *xuè hǎi*]
SP-6 Three Yīn Intersection [三阴交 *sān yīn jiāo*]

These points quicken blood and transform stasis [活血化瘀 *huó xuè huà yū*].

BL-40, which is discussed in Section 4.4.9, and SP-6, which is discussed in Section 5.4.2, are used here to quicken blood.

SP-10, an important point for all blood patterns [血证 *xuè zhèng*], is used in this combination to quicken blood and transform blood stasis.

CHAPTER 21

Sciatica

Sciatica is a form of impediment pattern [痹证 *bì zhèng*]; it specifically refers to pain felt along the back and/or outer side of the leg, along the area of distribution of the sciatic nerve.

There are six main forms of sciatica:

- wind evil obstructing the network vessels [风邪阻络 *fēng xié zǔ luò*]
- cold evil obstructing the network vessels [寒邪阻络 *hán xié zǔ luò*]
- damp evil obstructing the network vessels [湿邪阻络 *shī xié zǔ luò*]
- damp-heat obstructing the network vessels [湿热阻络 *shī rè zǔ luò*]
- static blood obstructing the network vessels [瘀血阻络 *yū xuè zǔ luò*]
- kidney vacuity improper nourishment[18] [肾虚失养 *shèn xū shī yǎng*]

21.1 POINTS OF ATTENTION FOR SCIATICA

21.1.1 Physiology

The area of distribution of the sciatic nerve, the back and outer side of the leg, overlaps with the area of distribution of the three yáng channels of the foot [足三阳经 *zú sān yáng jīng*]: the foot greater yáng bladder channel [足太阳膀胱经 *zú tài yáng páng guāng jīng*], the foot yáng brightness stomach channel [足阳明胃经 *zú yáng míng wèi jīng*], and the foot lesser yáng gallbladder channel [足少阳胆经 *zú shào yáng dǎn jīng*].

Both external evils [外邪 *wài xié*] and internal damage [内伤 *nèi shāng*] can cause channel qì obstruction of the three yáng channels of the foot, which impedes the smooth flow of qì-blood [气血运行不畅 *qì xuè yùn xíng bú chàng*] and gives rise to pain.

---

[18] In this pattern, kidney vacuity is responsible for improper nourishment of the sinews. (Ed.)

**21.2   CAUSES AND PATHOMECHANISM OF SCIATICA; IDENTIFYING
          PATTERNS**

**21.2.1   Wind, Cold and/or Damp Evil Obstructing the Network
            Vessels [风寒湿邪阻络 *fēng hán shī xié zǔ luò*]**

*Causes and Pathomechanism of Wind, Cold and/or Damp Evil Obstructing the
Network Vessels*

Wind, cold, and damp evils can individually or collectively exploit vacuity
[乘虚 *chéng xū*] to assail the body and block the channels and network vessels.
This inhibits the free flow of qì-blood and causes pain.

*Important Signs of Wind, Cold and/or Damp Evil Obstructing the Network
Vessels*

Wind Evil Obstructing the Network Vessels [风邪阻络 *fēng xié zǔ luò*]

Wandering pain [疼痛游走不定 *téng tòng yóu zǒu bú dìng*] that is
sometimes light and sometimes severe; aversion to wind and heat effusion [恶风
发热 *wù fēng fā rè*]. The tongue has a thin white coating [苔薄白 *tāi bó bái*].
Floating pulse [脉浮 *mài fú*].

Cold Evil Obstructing the Network Vessels [寒邪阻络 *hán xié zǔ luò*]

Acute cold pain in a fixed location that is exacerbated by cold and relieved by
warmth. Inhibited bending, stretching and turning of the waist. Physical cold and
cold limbs [形寒肢冷 *xíng hán zhī lěng*]. The tongue has a white coating [苔白 *tāi
bái*]. Stringlike tight pulse [脉弦紧 *mài xián jǐn*].

Dampness Evil Obstructing the Network Vessels [湿邪阻络 *shī xié zǔ luò*]

Pain in a fixed location that feels heavy. Disinclination to move. Heaviness
of the legs. Insensitivity of the skin [肌肤不仁 *jī fū bù rén*]. The pain tends to be
set off by yīn-type weather [阴雨天 *yīn yǔ tiān*]. The tongue has a white slimy
coating [苔白腻 *tāi bái nì*]. Soggy moderate pulse [脉濡缓 *mài rú huǎn*].

21.2.2   Damp-Heat Obstructing the Network Vessels [湿热阻络 *shī rè zǔ luò*]

Causes and Pathomechanism of Damp-Heat Obstructing the Network Vessels

There are three possible causes of this pattern:

- contraction of wind-damp-heat evil, e.g., during long summer [长夏 *cháng
  xià*] (the last half of the sixth month in the Chinese calendar, i.e., six months
  after Chinese New Year).

- wind, cold and/or dampness evil remain in the body for a long time, and the evil that lodges in the channels and network vessels undergoes depression and transformation into heat [郁而化热 *yù ér huà rè*].

- the patient has a constitutional tendency to yīn vacuity with heat brewing internally [内有蕴热 *nèi yǒu yùn rè*], which easily transforms contracted external evils into heat.

In all three of the above scenarios, the damp-heat that forms then blocks the channels, obstructs qì-blood, and causes pain.

Important Signs of Damp-Heat Obstructing the Network Vessels

Scorching pain [灼痛 *zhuó tòng*] that is worse on hot, humid days. Pain is relieved by moving the affected body parts. Generalized sensation of heaviness. Heat effusion [发热 *fā rè*]. Thirst, but no desire to drink [口渴不喜饮 *kǒu kě bù xǐ yǐn*]. Red tongue, yellow slimy tongue fur [舌红苔黄腻 *shé hóng tāi huáng nì*]. Slippery rapid pulse [脉滑数 *mài huá shuò*].

21.2.3 Static Blood Obstructing the Network Vessels [瘀血阻络 *yū xuè zǔ luò*]

Causes and Pathomechanism of Static Blood Obstructing the Network Vessels

Knocks and falls [跌打 *dié dǎ*] and trauma [外伤 *wài shāng*], incorrect posture, overstraining or incorrect use of force in the lumbar region, or enduring illness that impedes the smooth flow of qì-blood can all cause blood stasis collecting internally [瘀血内停 *yū xuè nèi tíng*] and qì-blood stagnating in the channels and network vessels, which result in stoppage and pain.

Important Signs of Static Blood Obstructing the Network Vessels

Severe stabbing pain that refuses pressure [拒按 *jù àn*]. Pain stays in a fixed location. Inhibited bending, stretching, and turning of the waist. Pain gets worse with movement. As blood stasis is an evil that has a physical form and is thus considered yīn [属阴 *shǔ yīn*], the pain caused by blood stasis is lighter during daytime and worse during nighttime. Dark purple tongue, or tongue with stasis macules [舌暗紫或有瘀斑 *shé àn zǐ huò yǒu yū bān*]. Rough pulse [涩脉 *sè mài*].

21.2.4 Kidney Vacuity Improper Nourishment [肾虚失养 *shèn xū shī yǎng*]

Causes and Pathomechanism of Kidney Vacuity Improper Nourishment

This pattern is often the result of a weak constitution, taxation fatigue, vacuity after enduring illness, old age bodily weakness, or sexual taxation [房室

劳伤 *fáng shì láo shāng*] that leads to kidney qì depletion. A depleted kidney improperly nourishes the sinews. This leads to loss of luxuriance, causing pain [不荣而痛 *bù róng ér tòng*].

Important Signs of of Kidney Vacuity Improper Nourishment

Continuous pain [疼痛绵绵 *téng tòng mián mián*] that is relieved by rest and exacerbated by fatigue. Aching lumbus and limp knees [腰酸膝软 *yāo suān xī ruǎn*]. Dizziness, tinnitus. Aversion to cold, cold limbs. Or hair loss, loosening of the teeth, seminal emission and impotence [遗精阳痿 *yí jīng yáng wěi*], menstrual irregularities [月经不调 *yuè jīng bù tiáo*]. Pale tongue or enlarged and tender tongue [舌质淡或胖嫩 *shé zhì dàn huò pàng nèn*]. Deep fine pulse [脉沉细 *mài chén xì*].

21.3   TREATMENT OF SCIATICA USING CHINESE MEDICINALS

21.3.1   Wind Evil Obstructing the Network Vessels [风邪阻络 *fēng xié zǔ luò*]

Method of Treatment for Wind Evil Obstructing the Network Vessels

Course wind and free the network vessels [疏风通络 *shū fēng tōng luò*].

Saposhnikovia Decoction [防风汤 *fáng fēng tāng*]	
saposhnikovia [防风 *fáng fēng*, Saposhnikoviae Radix]	30g
licorice [甘草 *gān cǎo*, Glycyrrhizae Radix]	30g
Chinese angelica [当归 *dāng guī*, Angelicae Sinensis Radix]	30g
poria [茯苓 *fú líng*, Poria]	30g
apricot kernel [杏仁 *xìng rén*, Armeniacae Semen]	30g
cinnamon bark [肉桂 *ròu guì*, Cinnamomi Cortex]	30g
scutellaria [黄芩 *huáng qín*, Scutellariae Radix]	10g
large gentian [秦艽 *qín jiāo*, Gentianae Macrophyllae Radix]	10g
pueraria [葛根 *gé gēn*, Puerariae Radix]	10g
ephedra [麻黄 *má huáng*, Ephedrae Herba]	15g

Directions: Grind all medicinals into a powder; mix 15g of the powder with 3 slices of fresh ginger [生姜 *shēng jiāng*, Zingiberis Rhizoma Recens] and 3 pieces of jujube [大枣 *dà zǎo*, Jujubae Fructus]; and cook with water and medicinal wine.

In modern times, the prescription is taken as a decoction [水煎服 *shuǐ jiān fú*] with the quantities of the medicinals proportionally reduced according to the ratio in the original prescription.

Prescription Analysis

Chief Medicinals

Both saposhnikovia and ephedra are warm-acrid [辛温 *xīn wēn*] medicinals that effuse and dissipate [发散 *fā sàn*] and dispel wind evil to treat the root [治本 *zhì běn*].

Support Medicinals

Large gentian dispels wind and overcomes dampness. Pueraria resolves the flesh and effuses and dissipates [解肌发散 *jiě jī fā sàn*]. Chinese angelica supplements and quickens blood. Poria disinhibits water and percolates dampness [利水渗湿 *lì shuǐ shèn shī*]. Cinnamon bark warms and frees the channels.

Assistant Medicinals

Apricot kernel diffuses and downbears lung qì [宣降肺气 *xuān jiàng fèi qì*] to dispel wind evil. Scutellaria clears heat and dries dampness. Adding a bitter-cold [苦寒 *kǔ hán*] medicinal to the otherwise warm and hot medicinals prevents excessive warming and drying.

Licorice harmonizes the actions of all the other medicinals.

This combination of medicinals dispels wind, overcomes dampness, and checks pain.

Variation According to Signs

Saposhnikovia Decoction is indicated for moving impediment [行痹 *xíng bì*], which is characterized by wandering pain [疼痛游走不定 *téng tòng yóu zǒu bú dìng*]. If the pain is pronounced, add notopterygium [*qiāng huó*], pubescent angelica [*dú huó*], asarum [*xì xīn*], aconite main tuber [*chuān wū tóu*], and wild aconite [*cǎo wū tóu*] to dissipate wind and check pain. If there is severe lumbus pain, add eucommia [*dù zhòng*] and achyranthes [*niú xī*] to dispel wind-damp, supplement liver and kidney, and strengthen the lumbus and knees. If there is numbness and tingling [麻木 *má mù*], add clematis [*wēi líng xiān*], chaenomeles [*mù guā*], and ground pine [*shēn jīn cǎo*] to quicken blood and free the network vessels.

21.3.2 Cold Evil Obstructing the Network Vessels [寒邪阻络 *hán xié zǔ luò*]

Method of Treatment for Cold Evil Obstructing the Network Vessels

Dissipate cold and eliminate dampness, free the network vessels and check pain [散寒除湿，通络止痛 *sàn hán chú shī, tōng luò zhǐ tòng*].

> **Aconite Main Tuber Variant Decoction [乌头汤加减 *wū tóu tāng jiā jiǎn*]**
>
> wild aconite [草乌头 *cǎo wū tóu*, Aconiti Tsao-Wu-Tou Tuber]   6g
> ephedra [麻黄 *má huáng*, Ephedrae Herba]   6g
> astragalus [黄芪 *huáng qí*, Astragali Radix]   12g
> white peony [白芍 *bái sháo*, Paeoniae Radix Alba]   9g
> asarum [细辛 *xì xīn*, Asari Herba]   3g
>
> ***Directions:*** Take decocted with water [水煎服 *shuǐ jiān fú*].

Prescription Analysis

Chief Medicinal

Wild aconite, which is very acrid and very hot [大辛大热 *dà xīn dà rè*], dissipates cold and checks pain.

Support Medicinals

Ephedra dissipates wind-cold. Asarum dissipates cold and checks pain.

Assistant Medicinals

Astragalus supplements the center and boosts qì [补中益气 *bǔ zhōng yì qì*]. White peony nourishes blood and supplements yīn.

This combination of medicinals warms the channels and dissipates cold. When cold evil is dispelled, the channels and collaterals are freed and pain stops.

Variation According to Signs

Aconite Main Tuber Variant Decoction is an excellent prescription for warming the channels and dissipating cold. In clinical practice, its main indication is for cold impediment and cold pain [寒痹冷痛 *hán bì lěng tòng*]. If the lumbus and legs feel heavy (an indication that damp evil predominates), add pubescent angelica [*dú huó*] and notopterygium [*qiāng huó*] to overcome dampness and check pain.

21.3.3   Dampness Evil Obstructing the Network Vessels [湿邪阻络 *shī xié zǔ luò*]

Method of Treatment

Dispel dampness and free the network vessels [祛湿通络 *qū shī tōng luò*].

Coix Decoction [薏苡仁汤 *yì yǐ rén tāng*]	
coix [薏苡仁 *yì yǐ rén*, Semen Coicis]	15g
atractylodes [苍术 *cāng zhú*, Atractylodis Rhizoma]	9g
notopterygium [羌活 *qiāng huó*, Notopterygii Rhizoma et Radix]	9g
pubescent angelica [独活 *dú huó*, Angelicae Pubescentis Radix]	9g
saposhnikovia [防风 *fáng fēng*, Saposhnikoviae Radix]	9g
aconite main tuber [川乌头 *chuān wū tóu*, Aconiti Tuber]	6g
ephedra [麻黄 *má huáng*, Ephedrae Herba]	6g
cinnamon twig [桂枝 *guì zhī*, Cinnamomi Ramulus]	6g
chuanxiong [川芎 *chuān xiōng*, Chuanxiong Rhizoma]	6g
licorice [甘草 *gān cǎo*, Glycyrrhizae Radix]	3g
Directions: Take decocted with water [水煎服 *shuǐ jiān fú*].	

Prescription Analysis

Chief Medicinal

Coix disinhibits water and percolates dampness [渗湿 *shèn shī*], treating the root [治本 *zhì běn*].

Support Medicinals

Notopterygium, pubescent angelica, atractylodes, and saposhnikovia dispel wind and overcome dampness. They help the chief medicinal overcome dampness and check pain.

Assistant Medicinals

Aconite main tuber warms the channels, dissipates cold, and checks pain. Acrid-warm ephedra dissipates wind-cold. Cinnamon twig warms and frees the channels. Chuanxiong quickens blood and frees the channels to check pain.

Licorice harmonizes the actions of all the other medicinals.

This combination of medicinals dispels dampness, frees the network vessels, and checks pain.

Variation According to Signs

The indication for Coix Decoction is damp impediment, which is marked by heaviness of the limbs that are painful. For numbness and tingling, add clematis [*wēi líng xiān*], chaenomeles [*mù guā*], and loofah [*sī guā luò*] to free the channels and quicken the network vessels. For inhibited urination [小便不利 *xiǎo biàn bú lì*], add trifoliate akebia [*mù tōng*], plantago seed [*chē qián zǐ*], alisma [*zé xiè*], and poria [*fú líng*] to disinhibit water and percolate dampness.

21.3.4   Damp-Heat Obstructing the Network Vessels [湿热阻络 *shī rè zǔ luò*]

Method of Treatment for Damp-Heat Obstructing the Network Vessels

Clear heat and eliminate dampness, free the network vessels and check pain [清热除湿，通络止痛 *qīng rè chú shī, tōng luò zhǐ tòng*].

Mysterious Three Pill [三妙丸 *sān miào wán*]	
atractylodes [苍术 *cāng zhú*, Atractylodis Rhizoma]	10g
phellodendron [黄柏 *huáng bǎi*, Phellodendri Cortex]	10g
achyranthes [牛膝 *niú xī*, Achyranthis Bidentatae Radix]	10g
Directions: The original prescription was taken in pill form. In modern times, it is often taken decocted with water [水煎服 *shuǐ jiān fú*].	

Prescription Analysis

Chief Medicinals

Atractylodes and phellodendron clear heat and dry dampness to treat the root [治本 *zhì běn*].

Support Medicinal

Achyranthes supplements the liver and kidney and strengthens sinews and bones.

All three medicinals together clear heat, eliminate dampness, free the network vessels, and check pain.

Variation According to Signs

For severe pain that is worse at night, add moutan [*mǔ dān pí*] and red peony [*chì sháo*] to cool blood and check pain. For dry mouth, thirst, and short voidings of reddish urine [小便短赤 *xiǎo biàn duǎn chì*], add trifoliate akebia [*mù tōng*], alisma [*zé xiè*], and gardenia [*zhī zǐ*] to clear and disinhibit damp-heat. For vexing heat in the five hearts [五心烦热 *wǔ xīn fán rè*] and for tidal heat and night sweating [潮热盗汗 *cháo rè dào hàn*], add ligustrum [*nǚ zhēn zǐ*], lycium berry [*gǒu qǐ zǐ*], and eclipta [*hàn lián cǎo*] to enrich yīn and clear heat [滋阴清热 *zī yīn qīng rè*].

21.3.5   Static Blood Obstructing the Network Vessels [瘀血阻络 *yū xuè zǔ luò*]

Method of Treatment for Static Blood Obstructing the Network Vessels

Quicken blood and move qì, free the network vessels and check pain [活血行气，通络止痛 *huó xuè xíng qì, tōng luò zhǐ tòng*].

Generalized Pain Stasis-Expelling Variant Decoction **[身痛逐瘀汤加减 *shēn tòng zhú yū tāng jiā jiǎn*]**	
large gentian [秦艽 *qín jiāo*, Gentianae Macrophyllae Radix]	3g
chuanxiong [川芎 *chuān xiōng*, Chuanxiong Rhizoma]	6g
peach kernel [桃仁 *táo rén*, Persicae Semen]	9g
carthamus [红花 *hóng huā*, Carthami Flos]	9g
licorice [甘草 *gān cǎo*, Glycyrrhizae Radix]	6g
notopterygium [羌活 *qiāng huó*, Notopterygii Rhizoma et Radix]	3g
myrrh [没药 *mò yào*, Myrrha]	6g
Chinese angelica [当归 *dāng guī*, Angelicae Sinensis Radix]	9g
flying squirrel's droppings [五灵脂 *wǔ líng zhī*, Trogopteri Faeces]	6g
cyperus [香附 *xiāng fù*, Cyperi Rhizoma]	3g
achyranthes [牛膝 *niú xī*, Achyranthis Bidentatae Radix]	9g
earthworm [地龙 *dì lóng*, Pheretima]	6g
Directions: Take decocted with water [水煎服 *shuǐ jiān fú*].	

Prescription Analysis

Chief Medicinals

Peach kernel and carthamus quicken blood, transform stasis, and check pain.

Support Medicinals

Chuanxiong, myrrh, flying squirrel's droppings, and earthworm help the chief medicinals quicken blood and transform stasis.

Assistant Medicinals

Notopterygium and large gentian dispel wind-damp and relieve impediment pain [止痹痛 *zhǐ bì tòng*]. Chinese angelica supplements and quickens blood. Cyperus quickens blood and moves qì. Achyranthes quickens blood and strengthens the sinews and bones.

Licorice harmonizes the actions of all the other medicinals.

This combination of medicinals is used to quicken blood and transform stasis and to free the network vessels and check pain.

Variation According to Signs

Generalized Pain Stasis-Expelling Variant Decoction is a potent prescription for quickening blood and dispelling stasis. It is indicated in cases of static blood obstructing the network vessels that causes pain in the lumbus and the legs. If there are signs of liver and kidney insufficiency and limp aching lumbus and knees [腰膝酸软 *yāo xī suān ruǎn*], add eucommia [*dù zhòng*], acanthopanax [*wǔ jiā pí*], and dipsacus [*xù duàn*] to supplement the liver and kidney and strengthen the lumbus and knees.

21.3.6   Kidney Vacuity Improper Nourishment [肾虚失养 *shèn xū shī yǎng*]

Method of Treatment for Kidney Vacuity Improper Nourishment

Supplement the kidney and strengthen the lumbus [补肾强腰 *bǔ shèn qiáng yāo*].

Golden Coffer Kidney Qì Pill [金匮肾气丸 *jīn guì shèn qì wán*]	
cooked rehmannia [熟地黄 *shú dì huáng*, Rehmanniae Radix Conquita]	20g
dioscorea [山药 *shān yào*, Dioscoreae Rhizoma]	15g
cornus [山茱萸 *shān zhū yú*, Corni Fructus]	15g
alisma [泽泻 *zé xiè*, Alismatis Rhizoma]	10g
poria [茯苓 *fú líng*, Poria]	10g
moutan [牡丹皮 *mǔ dān pí*, Moutan Cortex]	10g
cinnamon twig [桂枝 *guì zhī*, Cinnamomi Ramulus]	10g
(or cinnamon bark [肉桂 *ròu guì*, Cinnamomi Cortex]	6g)
aconite [附子 *fù zǐ*, Aconiti Tuber Laterale]	6g

Directions: The original prescription was taken as a pill, 6g at a time, three times a day. In modern times the prescription is often taken decocted in water [水煎服 *shuǐ jiān fú*]; in this case, aconite has to be pre-decocted [先煎 *xiān jiān*] for 30 minutes in order to dispel its toxins.

Prescription Analysis

Chief Medicinals

Cooked rehmannia enriches and supplements kidney yīn. Aconite warms and supplements kidney yáng. Supplementing both yīn and yáng treats the root [治本 *zhì běn*].

Support Medicinals

Dioscorea, cornus, and cinnamon twig assist the chief medicinals in using yīn to help yáng [以阴助阳 *yǐ yīn zhù yáng*].

Assistant Medicinals

Alisma, poria, and moutan drain kidney turbidity [泻肾浊 *xiè shèn zhuó*] and thereby make it easier to supplement the kidney.

This combination of medicinals can supplement fire within water [水中补火 *shuǐ zhōng bǔ huǒ*]; it supplements both yīn and yáng and fortifies the sinews and bones, thus stopping pain.

Variation According to Signs

Golden Coffer Kidney Qì Pill is Zhāng Zhòng-Jǐng's [张仲景] representative prescription for warming and supplementing kidney yáng. If there are signs of wind-damp, add mistletoe [*sāng jì shēng*] and acanthopanax [*wǔ jiā pí*]. For severe aching in the lumbus, add eucommia [*dù zhòng*] and gastrodia [*tiān má*].

21.4 ACUPUNCTURE TREATMENTS FOR SCIATICA

21.4.1 Base Acupuncture Prescription for Sciatica

This base prescription should be modified according to the identified patterns that are discussed below and according to the condition of the individual patient.

Treatment Method for Sciatica

Free the network vessels and check pain [通络止痛 *tōng luò zhǐ tòng*].

Base Acupuncture Prescription for Sciatica
GB-30 Jumping Round [环跳 *huán tiào*]
BL-54 Sequential Limit [秩边 *zhì biān*]
BL-63 Metal Gate [金门 *jīn mén*]
BL-58 Taking Flight [飞扬 *fēi yáng*]
BL-67 Reaching Yīn [至阴 *zhì yīn*]

Prescription Analysis

BL-67 is the well point [井穴 *jǐng xué*] of the foot greater yáng bladder channel, and its functions are freeing, coursing, and discharging [宣通疏泄 *xuān tōng shū xiè*]. Well points are located at the meeting point of channels that stand in interior-exterior relationship, the point where yīn changes into yáng or vice versa. They effectively resolve qì, free the channels, and promote interaction between yīn and yáng [解气通经, 交通阴阳 *jiě qì tōng jīng, jiāo tōng yīn yáng*]. Thus, well points are often used to treat repletion channel qì stagnation patterns of both the channel that the point is located on and the channel that stands in interior-exterior relation.

BL-58 is the network point [络穴 *luò xué*] and BL-63 is the cleft point [郄穴 *xī xué*] of the foot greater yáng bladder channel. This pair of points quickens the network vessels and checks pain [活络止痛 *huó luò zhǐ tòng*].

GB-30 and BL-54 are both located along the distribution of the sciatic nerve. Needling GB-30 and BL-54 courses and frees the channels and dissipates external evil [疏通经脉， 祛散外邪 *shū tōng jīng mài, qū sàn wài xié*].

21.4.2   Points to Add to the Base Prescription

Points for Wind Evil Obstructing the Network Vessels [风邪阻络 *fēng xié zǔ luò*]
TB-5 Outer Pass [外关 *wài guān*] BL-40 Bend Center [委中 *wěi zhōng*]

Adding this pair of points to the base prescription above dissipates wind and quickens the network vessels [散风活络 *sàn fēng huó luò*].

TB-5 Outer Pass [外关 *wài guān*] connects to the yáng linking vessel [阳维脉 *yáng wéi mài*]. The yáng linking vessel runs along the sides of the body, including the lateral aspect of the leg, and can be used to treat pain symptoms in that area, e.g., sciatica. It links all yáng channels together and governs the exterior of the body [主一身之表 *zhǔ yì shēn zhī biǎo*]. Thus, TB-5 is an important point for resolving the exterior [解表 *jiě biǎo*].

Points for Cold Evil Obstructing the Network Vessels [寒邪阻络 *hán xié zǔ luò*]
GV-3 Lumbar Yáng Pass [腰阳关 *yāo yáng guān*]

Use GV-3 to warm yáng and dissipate cold [温阳散寒 *wēn yáng sàn hán*]; it invigorates the lumbus and legs and supplements yáng, and it is indicated for lumbar and leg pain.

Points for Dampness Evil Obstructing the Network Vessels [湿邪阻络 *shī xié zǔ luò*]
SP-9 Yīn Mound Spring [阴陵泉 *yīn líng quán*]

SP-9 is the uniting water point [合水穴 *hé shuǐ xué*] of the foot greater yīn channel and a very important point for disinhibiting dampness [利湿 *lì shī*] in the lower burner.

Points for Damp-Heat Obstructing the Network Vessels [湿热阻络 *shī rè zǔ luò*]
GB-34 Yáng Mound Spring [阳陵泉 *yáng líng quán*]

GB-34 clears heat and disinhibits dampness [清热利湿 *qīng rè lì shī*].

Points for Static Blood Obstructing the Network Vessels
[瘀血阻络 *yū xuè zǔ luò*]

BL-40 Bend Center [委中 *wěi zhōng*]
SP-10 Sea of Blood [血海 *xuè hǎi*]

These points quicken blood and transform stasis [活血化瘀 *huó xuè huà yū*].

BL-40 frees the channels and quickens the network vessels, moves blood and dispels stasis [通经活络，行血祛瘀 *tōng jīng huó luò, xíng xuè qū yū*].

SP-10, called "Sea of Blood," is an important point for treating all blood patterns; it is frequently used to move blood.

Points for Kidney Vacuity Improper Nourishment
[肾虚失养 *shèn xū shī yǎng*]

BL-23 Kidney Transport [肾俞 *shèn shū*]
GV-4 Life Gate [命门 *mìng mén*]
KI-3 Great Ravine [太溪 *tài xī*]

These three points supplement and nourish kidney qì [补养肾气 *bǔ yǎng shèn qì*].

BL-23 is a back transport point [背俞 *bèi shū*]. Because back transport points predominantly treat the bowels and viscera they are connected with, BL-23 treats the kidney. Back transport points are particularly indicated in yīn patterns, i.e., interior patterns, cold patterns, vacuity patterns, and chronic diseases.

GV-4 is an important point for supplementing kidney yáng and invigorating the life gate fire [补肾阳壮命门火 *bǔ shèn yáng zhuàng mìng mén huǒ*].

KI-3 is the source point [原穴 *yuán xué*] of the foot lesser yīn kidney channel, the point where source qì of the kidney collects. Source points are mostly used to treat the five viscera. KI-3 supplements the kidneys and invigorates original yáng [元阳 *yuán yáng*] as well as kidney yīn.

CHAPTER 22
Knee Pain

Knee pain is the result of wind, cold, and/or damp assailing the knee, blocking the channels and network vessels, impeding the smooth flow of qì-blood, and causing the knee joint, sinews, and muscles to hurt. The main signs are aching pain [酸痛 *suān tòng*] and inhibited movement.

There are three main forms of knee pain:

- prevalence of wind [风重型 *fēng zhòng xíng*]
- prevalence of cold [寒重型 *hán zhòng xíng*]
- prevalence of dampness [湿重型 *shī zhòng xíng*]

22.1 POINTS OF ATTENTION FOR KNEE PAIN

22.1.1 Physiology

The liver governs the sinews [肝主筋 *gān zhǔ jīn*]; the kidney governs the bones [肾主骨 *shèn zhǔ gǔ*]. Knee pain easily occurs when, owing to liver-kidney yīn and essence insufficiency, wind-cold-damp evils exploit vacuity [乘虚 *chéng xū*] and assail the knee.

22.1.2 Pain Characteristics

***Prevalence of Wind* [风重型 *fēng zhòng xíng*]**

Wind is swift and changeable [风善行数变 *fēng shàn xíng shuò biàn*]; it is marked by a rapid onset of disease and swift changes in the disease manifestations. Thus, wind causes wandering pain that has no fixed location.

***Prevalence of Cold* [寒重型 *hán zhòng xíng*]**

Cold governs congealing [凝滞 *níng zhì*] and contracture and tautness [收引 *shōu yǐn*]; it inhibits the normal flow of qì and blood, blocks the channels, and/or causes tension of the sinews, thus causing pain.

Pain caused by cold is characterized by acuteness (intensity) and fixed location. It is relieved by the application of warmth and exacerbated by exposure to cold.

Prevalence of Dampness [湿重型 *shī zhòng xíng*]

Dampness has a downward tendency and is heavy [重浊 *zhòng zhuó*], viscous [黏滞 *nián zhì*], and lingering, meaning that dampness patterns are especially tenacious and hard to cure. This sort of pain feels heavy and remains in a fixed location.

22.2 CAUSES AND PATHOMECHANISM OF KNEE PAIN; IDENTIFYING PATTERNS

22.2.1 All Forms

Causes and Pathomechanism of Knee Pain

Wind-cold-damp assails the knee, blocks the channels and network vessels, impedes the smooth flow of qì-blood, and causes the joint, sinews, and muscles of the knee to hurt.

22.2.2 Prevalence of Wind [风重型 *fēng zhòng xíng*]

Important Signs of Prevalence of Wind

A prevalence of wind is characterized by wandering pain in the knee. Aversion to wind [恶风 *wù fēng*]. Pain gets worse when exposed to wind. Inhibited movement in the knee joint. The tongue has a white coating [苔白 *tāi bái*]. Floating pulse [脉浮 *mài fú*].

22.2.3 Prevalence of Cold [寒重型 *hán zhòng xíng*]

Important Signs of *Prevalence* of Cold

Cold pain in the knee. Cold limbs. Aversion to cold. Pain is relieved by the application of warmth and exacerbated by exposure to cold. The tongue has a white coating [苔白 *tāi bái*]. Deep slow pulse [脉沉迟 *mài chén chí*].

22.2.4 Prevalence of Dampness [湿重型 *shī zhòng xíng*]

Important Signs of Prevalence of Dampness

Swollen knee with distending pain [胀痛 *zhàng tòng*]. Heaviness in the knee joint. Pain gets worse in yīn-type weather [阴雨天 *yīn yǔ tiān*]. Tongue with white, slimy coating [苔白腻 *tāi bái nì*]. Soggy moderate pulse [脉濡缓 *mài rú huǎn*].

22.3   TREATMENT OF KNEE PAIN USING CHINESE MEDICINALS

22.3.1   Prevalence of Wind [风重型 *fēng zhòng xíng*]

Method of Treatment for Prevalence of Wind

Dispel wind, overcome dampness, check pain [祛风，胜湿，止痛 *qū fēng, shèng shī, zhǐ tòng*].

Saposhnikovia Decoction [防风汤 *fáng fēng tāng*]	
saposhnikovia [防风 *fáng fēng*, Saposhnikoviae Radix]	9g
Chinese angelica [当归 *dāng guī*, Angelicae Sinensis Radix]	9g
poria [茯苓 *fú líng*, Poria]	12g
stir-fried apricot kernel [炒杏仁 *chǎo xìng rén*, Armeniacae Semen Frictum]	9g
notopterygium [羌活 *qiāng huó*, Notopterygii Rhizoma et Radix]	9g
large gentian [秦艽 *qín jiāo*, Gentianae Macrophyllae Radix]	9g
cinnamon twig [桂枝 *guì zhī*, Cinnamomi Ramulus]	6g
fresh ginger [生姜 *shēng jiāng*, Zingiberis Rhizoma Recens]	5g
licorice [甘草 *gān cǎo*, Glycyrrhizae Radix]	3g
Directions: Take decocted with water [水煎服 *shuǐ jiān fú*].	

Prescription Analysis

  Chief Medicinal

Acrid-warm [辛温 *xīn wēn*] saposhnikovia effuses and dissipates [发散 *fā sàn*]; it dispels wind, overcomes dampness, and checks pain.

  Support Medicinals

Acrid-warm [辛温 *xīn wēn*] notopterygium effuses and dissipates [发散 *fā sàn*]. Cinnamon twig warms and frees the channels [温通经脉 *wēn tōng jīng mài*]. Both support medicinals help the chief medicinal effuse and dissipate wind evil, overcome dampness, and check pain.

  Assistant Medicinals

Poria disinhibits dampness by bland percolation [淡渗利湿 *dàn shèn lì shī*]. Apricot kernel diffuses and downbears lung qì [宣降肺气 *xuān jiàng fèi qì*] to dispel wind evil. Acrid-warm [辛温 *xīn wēn*] fresh ginger dissipates wind-cold. Chinese angelica quickens and supplements blood.

Licorice harmonizes the characteristics of all the medicinals [调和药性 *tiáo hé yào xìng*].

This combination of medicinals dispels wind, overcomes dampness, and checks pain.

Variation According to Signs

Saposhnikovia Decoction dispels wind while simultaneously warming yáng and dispeling cold. For inhibited bending and stretching of the joints [关节屈伸 不利 *guān jié qū shēn bú lì*], add ground pine [*shēn jīn cǎo*] and star jasmine stem [*luò shí téng*] to soothe the sinews and quicken the network vessels [舒筋活 络 *shū jīn huó luò*]. If knee pain is severe, add asarum [*xì xīn*], corydalis [*yán hú suǒ*], aconite main tuber [*chuān wū tóu*], and wild aconite [*cǎo wū tóu*] to dissipate cold, quicken blood, move qì, and check pain.

22.3.2 Prevalence of Cold [寒重型 *hán zhòng xíng*]

Method of Treatment for Prevalence of Cold

Warm the channels, dissipate cold, check pain [温经, 散寒, 止痛 *wēn jīng, sàn hán, zhǐ tòng*].

Aconite Main Tuber Decoction [乌头汤 *wū tóu tāng*]	
processed aconite tuber [制川乌头 *zhì chuān wū tóu*, Aconiti Tuber Praeparata]	6g
ephedra [麻黄 *má huáng*, Ephedrae Herba]	9g
white peony [白芍 *bái sháo*, Paeoniae Radix Alba]	12g
astragalus [黄芪 *huáng qí*, Astragali Radix]	18g
licorice [甘草 *gān cǎo*, Glycyrrhizae Radix]	6g

Directions: Predecoct [先煎 *xiān jiān*] the processed aconite tuber for 30 minutes. Decoct with remaining ingredients in water [水煎服 *shuǐ jiān fú*].

Prescription Analysis

Chief Medicinals

Processed aconite tuber, which is very acrid and very hot [大辛大热 *dà xīn dà rè*], warms the channels, dissipates cold, and checks pain.

Support Medicinal

Acrid-warm [辛温 *xīn wēn*] ephedra effuses and dissipates [发散 *fā sàn*] and helps the chief medicinal to effuse and dissipate wind-cold evil.

Assistant Medicinals

Astragalus supplements qì and upbears yáng [补气升阳 *bǔ qì shēng yáng*]. White peony nourishes yīn and supplements blood; it also prevents acrid-hot/warm [辛热/温 *xīn rè/ wēn*] processed aconite tuber and ephedra from excessively effusing and dissipating [发散 *fā sàn*].

Licorice harmonizes the characteristics of all the medicinals [调和药性 *tiáo hé yào xìng*]. Used together with white peony, it relaxes tension and checks pain [缓急止痛 *huǎn jí zhǐ tòng*].

This combination of medicinals warms the channels, dissipates cold, and checks pain.

Variation According to Signs

Aconite Main Tuber Decoction warms the channels, dissipates cold, and checks pain. If there are strong signs of wind-damp, add notopterygium [*qiāng huó*], pubescent angelica [*dú huó*], and asarum [*xì xīn*] to dissipate cold, overcome dampness, and check pain. For inhibited bending and straightening of the joints, add ground pine [*shēn jīn cǎo*], chaenomeles [*mù guā*], and clematis [*wēi líng xiān*] to soothe the sinews and quicken the network vessels [舒筋活络 *shū jīn huó luò*].

22.3.3   Prevalence of Dampness [湿重型 *shī zhòng xíng*]

Method of Treatment for Prevalence of Dampness

Dispel dampness, free the network vessels, and check pain [祛湿, 通络, 止痛 *qū shī, tōng luò, zhǐ tòng*].

Coix Decoction [薏苡仁汤 *yì yǐ rén tāng*]	
coix [薏苡仁 *yì yǐ rén*, Semen Coicis]	30g
atractylodes [苍术 *cāng zhú*, Atractylodis Rhizoma]	15g
white atractylodes [白术 *bái zhú*, Atractylodis Macrocephalae Rhizoma]	15g
cinnamon twig [桂枝 *guì zhī*, Cinnamomi Ramulus]	9g
ephedra [麻黄 *má huáng*, Ephedrae Herba]	6g
Chinese angelica [当归 *dāng guī*, Angelicae Sinensis Radix]	12g
astragalus [黄芪 *huáng qí*, Astragali Radix]	15g
lindera [乌药 *wū yào*, Linderae Radix]	12g
fresh ginger [生姜 *shēng jiāng*, Zingiberis Rhizoma Recens]	9g
licorice [甘草 *gān cǎo*, Glycyrrhizae Radix]	6g
Directions: Take decocted with water [水煎服 *shuǐ jiān fú*].	

Prescription Analysis

Chief Medicinals

Coix disinhibits water and percolates dampness [利水渗湿 *lì shuǐ shèn shī*], frees impediment and checks pain [通痹止痛 *tōng bì zhǐ tòng*].

Support Medicinals

Atractylodes dries dampness. White atractylodes disinhibits dampness. Ephedra diffuses the lung [宣肺 *xuān fèi*] and frees and disinhibits the urinary bladder to dispel dampness. Astragalus fortifies the spleen and disinhibits dampness. These support medicinals all help the chief medicinal disinhibit water and percolate dampness.

Assistant Medicinals

Cinnamon twig assists yáng and promotes qì transformation [助阳化气 *zhù yáng huà qì*], disinhibits the urinary bladder and dispels water. It also warms and frees the channels. Chinese angelica supplements and quickens blood to free the channels. Lindera warms the lower burner, moves qì, and disinhibits water. Fresh ginger effuses and dissipates [发散 *fā sàn*] wind-cold.

Licorice harmonizes the characteristics of all medicinals [调和药性 *tiáo hé yào xìng*].

This combination of medicinals disinhibits dampness.

Variation According to Signs

For inhibited bending and stretching of the knee joints [膝关节屈伸不利 *guān jié qū shēn bú lì*], add ground pine [*shēn jīn cǎo*], star jasmine stem [*luò shí téng*], and clematis [*wēi líng xiān*] to soothe and free the channels. If pain is severe, add corydalis [*yán hú suǒ*], asarum [*xì xīn*], and aconite main tuber [*chuān wū tóu*] to check pain.

22.4 ACUPUNCTURE TREATMENT FOR KNEE PAIN

22.4.1 Base Acupuncture Prescription for Knee Pain

This base prescription should be modified according to the identified patterns discussed below and according to the individual patient's condition.

Treatment Method for Knee Pain

Quicken blood, free the network vessels, and check pain [活血, 通络, 止痛 *huó xuè, tōng luò, zhǐ tòng*].

Base Acupuncture Prescription for Knee Pain
M-LE-16 (Extra Point) Inner Eye of Knee [内膝眼 *nèi xī yǎn*]
ST-34 Beam Hill [梁丘 *liáng qiū*]

Prescription Analysis

M-LE-16 is a local point [局部取穴 *jú bù qǔ xué*] that is selected to directly quicken blood and free the network vessels.

ST-34, the cleft point [郄穴 *xī xué*] of the foot yáng brightness channel, has an exceptionally strong capacity to check pain. Cleft points are indicated for (1) acute patterns of the associated internal organs or along the distribution of the channel—especially acute pain, and (2) bleeding patterns [出血证 *chū xuè zhèng*]. The cleft points of the yáng channels are predominantly used for the former, and the cleft points of the yīn channels are predominantly used for the latter.

22.4.2 Points to Add to the Base Prescription

Points for Prevalence of Wind [风重型 *fēng zhòng xíng*]
ST-34 Beam Hill [梁丘 *liáng qiū*] Extra point Heding [鹤顶 *hè dǐng*]

Extra point Heding is located in the depression just above the middle of the upper rim of the patella; it dissipates wind evil [散风邪 *sàn fēng xié*] and is often used to treat the knee area.

Points for Prevalence of Cold [寒重型 *hán zhòng xíng*]
ST-36 Leg Three Lǐ [足三里 *zú sān lǐ*] ST-41 Ravine Divide [解溪 *jiě xī*]

These points warm yáng and free the network vessels [温阳通络 *wēn yáng tōng luò*].

Points for Prevalence of Dampness [湿重型 *shī zhòng xíng*]
SP-9 Yīn Mound Spring [阴陵泉 *yīn líng quán*]

SP-9 disinhibits dampness and dispels evil [利湿祛邪 *lì shī qū xié*]. SP-9 is used to fortify the spleen and percolate dampness [健脾渗湿 *jiàn pí shèn shī*] and to disinhibit the lower burner [通利下焦 *tōng lì xià jiāo*]. As the uniting water point [合水穴 *hé shuǐ xué*] of the foot greater yīn spleen channel, its special indication is dampness. SP-9 warms and moves the middle burner [温运中焦 *wēn yùn zhōng jiāo*], disinhibits water, and disperses swelling [利水消肿 *lì shuǐ xiāo zhǒng*]. Because of its location and its channel distribution, SP-9 is often used in treating knee problems.

CHAPTER 23

Heel Pain

Pain in the heel makes it difficult to put weight on the affected foot and thus impairs walking.

There are three main forms of heel pain:

- kidney yīn depletion [肾阴亏损 *shèn yīn kuī sǔn*]
- kidney yáng vacuity [肾阳虚亏 *shèn yáng xū kuī*]
- static blood internal obstruction [瘀血内阻 *yū xuè nèi zǔ*]

23.1 POINTS OF ATTENTION FOR HEEL PAIN

23.1.1 Physiology

The foot lesser yīn kidney channel [足少阴肾经 *zú shào yīn shèn jīng*] passes through, and thus affects, the heel. Heel pain is often due to kidney vacuity and is often seen in elderly people.

23.2 CAUSES AND PATHOMECHANISM OF HEEL PAIN; IDENTIFYING PATTERNS

23.2.1 Kidney Yīn Depletion [肾阴亏损 *shèn yīn kuī sǔn*] and Kidney Yáng Vacuity [肾阳虚亏 *shèn yáng xū kuī*]

Causes and Pathomechanism of Kidney Yīn Depletion and Kidney Yáng Vacuity

Conditions such as a weak constitution, taxation fatigue [劳倦 *láo juàn*], sexual taxation [房室劳伤 *fáng shì láo shāng*], and long standing illness damage the kidney. The kidney governs the bones [肾主骨 *shèn zhǔ gǔ*], and the health of the bones depends on the nourishment provided by the kidney.

Important Signs of Kidney Yīn Depletion and Kidney Yáng Vacuity

Kidney Yīn Depletion [肾阴亏损 *shèn yīn kuī sǔn*]

Aching pain in the heel, difficulty standing on the affected heel, fatigue, and lack of strength [倦怠乏力 *juàn dài fá lì*]. Kidney yīn depletion signs include intermittent heat in the foot and shin [足胫时热 *zú jìng shí rè*]; dizziness and dizzy vision [头晕目眩 *tóu yūn mù xuàn*]; dry mouth and throat; and short voidings of reddish urine [小便短赤 *xiǎo biàn duǎn chì*]. Pale red tongue with scant fur [舌淡红少苔 *shé dàn hóng shǎo tāi*]. Sunken fine forceless pulse [脉沉细无力 *mài chén xì wú lì*] or fine and rapid [细数 *xì shuò*].

Kidney Yáng Vacuity [肾阳虚亏 *shèn yáng xū kuī*]

Painful heel, difficulty standing on the affected heel. Kidney yáng vacuity signs include: Inability to stand for long periods; cold heel, sole, and toes; aching pain and lack of strength in lumbus and legs; aversion to cold; long voidings of clear urine [小便清长 *xiǎo biàn qīng cháng*]; pale tongue, pale with thin white coating [舌质淡苔薄白 *shé zhì dàn tāi bó bái*]. Sunken fine forceless pulse [脉沉细无力 *mài chén xì wú lì*].

23.2.2   Static Blood Internal Obstruction [瘀血内阻 *yū xuè nèi zǔ*]

Causes and Pathomechanism of Static Blood Internal Obstruction

Excessive walking damages the sinews, or else external trauma [外伤 *wài shāng*] or persistent depressed cold-damp obstruction gives rise to blood stasis. Blood stasis blocks the channels in the heel and causes stoppage [不通 *bù tōng*] and pain.

Important Signs of Static Blood Internal Obstruction

Stabbing pain [刺痛 *cì tòng*] in the heel and sole of the foot. Severe pain like a knife cutting into the foot when trying to stand on the affected heel. Local sensation of scorching heat [灼热 *zhuó rè*]. Purple tongue, possibly with stasis macules [舌质紫或有瘀斑 *shé zhì zǐ huò yǒu yū bān*]. Rough pulse [涩脉 *sè mài*].

23.3   TREATMENT OF HEEL PAIN USING CHINESE MEDICINALS

23.3.1   Kidney Yīn Depletion [肾阴亏损 *shèn yīn kuī sǔn*]

Method of Treatment for Kidney Yīn Depletion

Invigorate water and enrich yīn [壮水滋阴 *zhuàng shuǐ zī yīn*].

Left-Restoring (Kidney Yīn) Pill [左归丸 *zuǒ guī wán*]	
cooked rehmannia [熟地黄 *shú dì huáng*, Rehmanniae Radix Conquita]	240g
dioscorea [山药 *shān yào*, Dioscoreae Rhizoma]	120g
cornus [山茱萸 *shān zhū yú*, Corni Fructus]	120g
lycium berry [枸杞子 *gǒu qǐ zǐ*, Lycii Fructus]	120g
cuscuta [菟丝子 *tù sī zǐ*, Cuscutae Semen]	120g
deerhorn glue [鹿角胶 *lù jiǎo jiāo*, Cervi Cornus Gelatinum]	120g
tortoise plastron glue [龟版胶 *guī bǎn jiāo*, Testudinis Plastri Gelatinum]	120g
cyathula [川牛膝 *chuān niú xī*, Cyathulae Radix]	90g

Directions: Grind the above medicinals into powder, mix with honey, and form into pills. Take 6g at a time, twice a day.

Prescription Analysis

Chief Medicinal

Cooked rehmannia strongly supplements liver-kidney yīn [大补肝肾之阴 *dà bǔ gān shèn zhī yīn*], treating the root [治本 *zhì běn*].

Support Medicinals

Cornus, lycium berry, cuscuta, deerhorn glue, and tortoise plastron glue help the chief medicinal enrich and supplement liver-kidney yīn.

Assistant Medicinals

Dioscorea fortifies the spleen and promotes the source of engendering transformation of later heaven [资后天生化之源 *zī hòu tiān shēng huà zhī yuán*]. Cyathula supplements the liver and kidney, strengthens sinews and bones, and quickens blood and checks pain.

This combination of medicinals invigorates water and enriches yīn. The kidney governs the bones [肾主骨 *shèn zhǔ gǔ*].

Variation According to Signs

Left-Restoring (Kidney Yīn) Pill enriches yīn. For effulgent yīn-vacuity fire [阴虚火旺 *yīn xū huǒ wàng*], vexing heat in the five hearts [五心烦热 *wǔ xīn fán rè*], and tidal heat effusion and night sweating [潮热盗汗 *cháo rè dào hàn*], add anemarrhena [*zhī mǔ*] and phellodendron [*huáng bǎi*]. For dizziness, add dragon bone [*lóng gǔ*], oyster shell [*mǔ lì*], and loadstone [*cí shí*] to settle and subdue floating yáng [镇潜浮阳 *zhèn qián fú yáng*]. For disturbed sleep, sleeplessness, and profuse dreaming, add spiny jujube kernel [*suān zǎo rén*], biota seed [*bǎi zǐ rén*], and polygala [*yuǎn zhì*] to nourish the heart and quiet the spirit [养心安神 *yǎng xīn ān shén*].

23.3.2   Kidney Yáng Vacuity [肾阳虚亏 *shèn yáng xū kuī*]

Method of Treatment

Warm the kidney and invigorate yáng [温肾壮阳 *wēn shèn zhuàng yáng*].

Right-Restoring (Life Gate) Pill [右归丸 *yòu guī wán*]	
cooked rehmannia [熟地黄 *shú dì huáng*, Rehmanniae Radix Conquita]	240g
dioscorea [山药 *shān yào*, Dioscoreae Rhizoma]	120g
cornus [山茱萸 *shān zhū yú*, Corni Fructus]	90g
lycium berry [枸杞子 *gǒu qǐ zǐ*, Lycii Fructus]	120g
cuscuta [菟丝子 *tù sī zǐ*, Cuscutae Semen]	120g
deerhorn glue [鹿角胶 *lù jiǎo jiāo*, Cervi Cornus Gelatinum]	120g
eucommia [杜仲 *dù zhòng*, Eucommiae Cortex]	120g
Chinese angelica [当归 *dāng guī*, Angelicae Sinensis Radix]	90g
cinnamon bark [肉桂 *ròu guì*, Cinnamomi Cortex]	90g
aconite [附子 *fù zǐ*, Aconiti Tuber Laterale]	60g

Directions: Grind the above medicinals into powder, mix with honey, and form into pills. Take 6g at a time, three times a day. Can also be taken as a decoction [水煎服 *shuǐ jiān fú*] with the quantity of the medicinals decreased according to the original ratio.

Prescription Analysis

Chief Medicinals

Cooked rehmannia and cinnamon bark supplement fire within water [水中补火 *shuǐ zhōng bǔ huǒ*], and warm and supplement kidney yáng.

Support Medicinals

Cornus, lycium berry, and deerhorn glue enrich and supplement kidney yīn [滋补肾阴 *zī bǔ shèn yīn*]. Cuscuta, eucommia, and aconite warm and supplement kidney yáng.

Assistant Medicinals

Dioscorea supplements the spleen and promotes later heaven [资后天 *zī hòu tiān*]. Chinese angelica supplements blood and boosts yīn.

This combination of medicinals warms the kidney and invigorates yáng.

Variation According to Signs

Right-Restoring (Life Gate) Pill warms and supplements kidney yáng. For severe lumbar pain, add mistletoe [*sāng jì shēng*], acanthopanax [*wǔ jiā pí*], pubescent angelica [*dú huó*], and asarum [*xì xīn*] to dispel wind-damp, dissipate cold, and check pain. If there is sloppy diarrhea [大便溏泻 *dà biàn táng xiè*] due to spleen-kidney yáng vacuity, or fifth-watch diarrhea [五更泄 *wǔ gēng xiè*], add evodia [*wú zhū yú*], nutmeg [*ròu dòu kòu*], and psoralea [*bǔ gǔ zhī*] to warm and supplement spleen and kidney yáng and to astringe the intestines and check diarrhea [涩肠止泻 *sè cháng zhǐ xiè*].

23.3.3   Static Blood Internal Obstruction [瘀血内阻 *yū xuè nèi zǔ*]

Method of Treatment for Static Blood Internal Obstruction

Quicken blood, transform stasis, and check pain [活血化瘀止痛 *huó xuè huà yū zhǐ tòng*].

Peach Kernel and Carthamus Four Agents Decoction [桃红四物汤 *táo hóng sì wù tāng*]	
peach kernel [桃仁 *táo rén*, Persicae Semen]	10g
carthamus [红花 *hóng huā*, Carthami Flos]	10g
Chinese angelica [当归 *dāng guī*, Angelicae Sinensis Radix]	10g
chuanxiong [川芎 *chuān xiōng*, Chuanxiong Rhizoma]	10g
white peony [白芍 *bái sháo*, Paeoniae Radix Alba]	10g
cooked rehmannia [熟地黄 *shú dì huáng*, Rehmanniae Radix Conquita]	20g
Directions: Take decocted with water [水煎服 *shuǐ jiān fú*].	

Prescription Analysis

Chief Medicinals

Peach kernel and carthamus quicken blood, transform stasis, and check pain.

Support Medicinals

Chuanxiong, white peony and Chinese angelica help the chief medicinals quicken and regulate blood [活血调血 *huó xuè tiáo xuè*].

Assistant Medicinal

Cooked rehmannia nourishes blood and supplements yīn.

This combination of medicinals quickens blood, transforms stasis, and checks pain.

Variation According to Signs

Peach Kernel and Carthamus Four Agents Decoction quickens blood and transforms stasis. For severe blood stasis and pain, add corydalis [*yán hú suǒ*], sparganium [*sān léng*], and curcuma rhizome [*é zhú*] to emphasize quickening blood and transforming stasis.

23.4 Acupuncture Treatments for Heel Pain

23.4.1 Kidney Yīn Depletion [肾阴亏损 *shèn yīn kuī sǔn*] and Kidney Yáng Vacuity [肾阳虚亏 *shèn yáng xū kuī*]

Treatment Method for Kidney Yīn Depletion and Kidney Yáng Vacuity

Supplement the kidneys, free the network vessels, and check pain [补肾通络止痛 *bǔ shèn tōng luò zhǐ tòng*].

> **Points for Kidney Yīn Depletion and Kidney Yáng Vacuity Heel Pain**
>
> BL-60 Kunlun Mountains [昆仑 *kūn lún*]
> **joining** [透 *tòu*] KI-3 Great Ravine [太溪 *tài xī*]
> BL-23 Kidney Transport [肾俞 *shèn shū*]

Prescription Analysis

BL-60, the river fire point [经火穴 *jīng huǒ xué*] of the foot greater yáng channel, warms and nourishes the channel [温养经脉 *wēn yǎng jīng mài*].

The heel is governed by the kidney [足跟为肾所主 *zú gēn wéi shèn suǒ zhǔ*], the kidney governs the bones [肾主骨 *shèn zhǔ gǔ*], and the kidney channel passes posterior to the medial malleolus and into the heel. KI-3 is the source point [原穴 *yuán xué*] of the foot lesser yīn kidney channel, the point where source qì of the kidney collects. Thus, KI-3 supplements the kidneys and invigorates original yáng [元阳 *yuán yáng*].

The foot lesser yīn channel passes the inner aspect and the foot greater yáng channel passes the outer aspect of the heel. Joining [相透 *xiāng tòu*] KI-3 and BL-60 connects the interior-exterior related channels and frees qì-blood, checking pain.

23.4.2 Static Blood Internal Obstruction [瘀血内阻 *yū xuè nèi zǔ*]

Treatment Method

Quicken the blood and transform stasis, free the network vessels and check pain [活血化瘀，通络止痛 *huó xuè huà yū, tōng luò zhǐ tòng*].

Perform bloodletting [放血 *fàng xuè*] at BL-57 Mountain Support [承山 *chéng shān*] and bloodletting [放血 *fàng xuè*] at the heel.

Prescription Analysis

The foot greater yáng channel passes through the gastrocnemius muscle down to the posterior aspect of the lateral malleolus. Because BL-57 is an acupuncture point on that channel, bloodletting at BL-57 improves the flow of qì-blood at the heel and thereby frees the channel and network vessels and checks pain.

CHAPTER 24
Arthritis (Impediment Pattern)

Impediment pattern is caused by the external evils wind, cold, dampness, and/or heat invading the fleshy exterior and joints, blocking the channels and network vessels, and affecting sinews, bones, and muscles. Impediment pattern manifests in signs such as aching pain [酸痛 *suān tòng*] or inhibited movement [屈伸不利 *qū shēn bú lì*] of the joints, sinews, and bones as well as in and numbness and tingling [麻木 *má mù*] or heaviness of the limbs.

There are two main impediment patterns.

- wind-cold-damp impediment [风寒湿痹 *fēng hán shī bì*], which can be further divided into:
    1) moving impediment [行痹 *xíng bì*]
    2) painful impediment [痛痹 *tòng bì*]
    3) fixed impediment [着痹 *zhuó bì*]
- wind-damp-heat impediment [风湿热痹 *fēng shī rè bì*]

24.1   POINTS OF ATTENTION FOR IMPEDIMENT

24.1.1   Considerations for Diagnosis

When treating impediment pattern, first differentiate the main two forms. This is quite easy due to the clear differences in signs. Wind-damp-heat impediment [风湿热痹 *fēng shī rè bì*] signs include: hot, red, swollen, painful joints [关节红肿灼热痛 *guān jié hóng zhǒng zhuó rè tòng*]; heat effusion [发热 *fā rè*]; thirst; red tongue, yellow tongue fur, and rapid pulse; and usually a rapid onset. Wind-cold-damp impediment [风寒湿痹 *fēng hán shī bì*] also manifests in painful limbs and joints, but there is no sign of heat or swelling, the tongue fur is white, the pulse is moderate [缓脉 *huǎn mài*], onset is relatively slow, and the pain is aggravated by yīn-type weather [阴雨天 *yīn yǔ tiān*].

Next, if necessary, differentiate within wind-cold-damp impediment [风寒湿痹 *fēng hán shī bì*] patterns. Establish which of the three evils is most prevalent. Wind, cold, and damp tend to cause impediment in combination. However, the signs and symptoms will differ according to which one is prevailing.

A prevalence of wind gives rise to moving impediment [行痹 *xíng bì*] and is characterized by wandering pain in the joints [关节疼痛游走不定 *guān jié téng tòng yóu zǒu bú dìng*]. Wind, which is swift and changeable [风善行数变 *fēng shàn xíng shuò biàn*], has a rapid onset of disease and swift changes in manifestations. Thus, wind causes wandering pain that has no fixed location.

A prevalence of cold gives rise to painful impediment [痛痹 *tòng bì*] and is characterized by acute pain in a fixed location; it is aggravated by cold and relieved by warmth. Cold governs congealing [凝滞 *níng zhì*] and contracture and tautness [收引 *shōu yǐn*]. Pain caused by cold is characterized by acuteness (intenseness) and fixed location; it is relieved by the application of warmth and exacerbated by exposure to cold.

A prevalence of damp gives rise to fixed impediment [着痹 *zhuó bì*] and is characterized by pain in the joints of fixed location, heaviness of the limbs, and numbness of the skin [肌肤不仁 *jī fū bù rén*]. The pain tends to be set off by yīn-type weather [阴雨天 *yīn yǔ tiān*]. Dampness has a downward tendency and is heavy [重浊 *zhòng zhuó*], viscous [黏滞 *nián zhì*], and lingering.

Complications

- Impediment is easily complicated if the illness persists and causes qì and blood vacuity, phlegm obstructing the network vessels [痰阻络脉 *tán zǔ luò mài*], or damage to the internal organs.

- Enduring impediment that obstructs the blood vessels and congeals the fluids [津液凝聚 *jīn yè níng jù*] brings about blood stasis and phlegm turbidity [痰浊 *tán zhuó*] obstruction in the channels and network vessels. Signs of this development include stasis macules [瘀斑 *yū bān*] on the skin and swollen knotty joints.

- Enduring impediment damages and wears [伤耗 *shāng hào*] qì-blood, which leads to qì-blood depletion or liver-kidney depletion [肝肾亏损 *gān shèn kuī sǔn*].

- If impediment pattern is not cured, the enduring illness can affect the internal organs, e.g., heart impediment [心痹 *xīn bì*].

24.2 CAUSES AND PATHOMECHANISM OF IMPEDIMENT; IDENTIFYING PATTERNS

24.2.1 Wind-Cold-Damp Impediment [风寒湿痹 *fēng hán shī bì*]

Causes and Pathomechanism of Wind-Cold-Damp Impediment

Wind-cold-damp impediment is caused by wind, cold, and/or dampness evil exploiting vacuity [风寒湿邪乘虚 *fēng hán shī xié chéng xū*], assailing [侵袭 *qīn xí*] the body, and blocking the channels and network vessels. This inhibits the free flow of qì-blood and causes pain, numbness, heaviness, and impeded movement in joints and flesh. Furthermore, vacuity of right qì [正气亏虚 *zhèng qì kuī xū*] allows external evil to assail the body.

Important Signs of Wind-Cold-Damp Impediment

Moving Impediment [行痹 *xíng bì*] *(Prevalence of Wind)*

Wandering pain in the joints. Inhibited bending and stretching of the joints, aversion to wind and heat effusion [恶风发热 *wù fēng fā rè*]. The tongue has a white coating [苔白 *tāi bái*]. Floating pulse [脉浮 *mài fú*].

Painful Impediment [痛痹 *tòng bì*] *(Prevalence of Cold)*

Acute pain in a fixed location; pain is aggravated by cold and relieved by warmth. Inhibited bending and stretching of the joints. The tongue has a white coating [苔白 *tāi bái*]. Stringlike and tight pulse [脉弦紧 *mài xián jǐn*].

Fixed Impediment [着痹 *zhuó bì*] *(Prevalence of Damp)*

Pain in the joints of fixed location, heaviness of the limbs, and numbness of the skin [肌肤不仁 *jī fū bù rén*]. Disinclination to move. The pain tends to be set off by yīn-type weather [阴雨天 *yīn yǔ tiān*]. The tongue has a white, slimy coating [苔白腻 *tāi bái nì*]. Soggy moderate pulse [脉濡缓 *mài rú huǎn*].

24.2.2 Wind-Damp-Heat Impediment [风湿热痹 *fēng shī rè bì*]

Causes and Pathomechanism of Wind-Damp-Heat Impediment

Wind-damp-heat impediment is caused by contraction of wind-damp-heat evil, e.g., during long summer [长夏 *cháng xià*].

Another possible cause is wind-cold-damp evil transforming into heat. This may be due to (1) a constitutional tendency to yīn vacuity, with heat brewing internally [内有蕴热 *nèi yǒu yùn rè*], that easily transforms contracted external evils into heat, or (2) enduring wind-cold-damp impediment [风寒湿痹 *fēng hán shī bì*], with the evil lodged in the channels and network vessels becoming depressed and transforming into heat [郁而化热 *yù ér huà rè*].

Important Signs of Wind-Damp-Heat Impediment

Scorching hot, red, swollen, painful joints; heat effusion [发热 *fā rè*]; thirst; aversion to wind [恶风 *wù fēng*]; and generally rapid onset. Red tongue, yellow tongue fur [舌红苔黄 *shé hóng tāi huáng*]. Slippery rapid pulse [脉滑数 *mài huá shuò*].

24.3 TREATMENT OF IMPEDIMENT USING CHINESE MEDICINALS

24.3.1 Wind-Cold-Damp Impediment [风寒湿痹 *fēng hán shī bì*]

Moving Impediment [行痹 *xíng bì*]

Method of Treatment

Dispel wind and dissipate cold, eliminate dampness and check pain [祛风散寒，除湿止痛 *qū fēng sàn hán, chú shī zhǐ tòng*].

Saposhnikovia Decoction [防风汤 *fáng fēng tāng*]	
saposhnikovia [防风 *fáng fēng*, Saposhnikoviae Radix]	9g
Chinese angelica [当归 *dāng guī*, Angelicae Sinensis Radix]	9g
poria [茯苓 *fú líng*, Poria]	12g
stir-fried apricot kernel [炒杏仁 *chǎo xìng rén*, Armeniacae Semen Frictum]	9g
notopterygium [羌活 *qiāng huó*, Notopterygii Rhizoma et Radix]	9g
cinnamon twig [桂枝 *guì zhī*, Cinnamomi Ramulus]	6g
fresh ginger [生姜 *shēng jiāng*, Zingiberis Rhizoma Recens]	5g
licorice [甘草 *gān cǎo*, Glycyrrhizae Radix]	3g
Directions: Take decocted with water [水煎服 *shuǐ jiān fú*].	

Prescription Analysis

Chief Medicinal

Saposhnikovia dispels wind and eliminates dampness to treat the root [治本 *zhì běn*].

Support Medicinals

Acrid-warm and dry [辛温而燥 *xīn wēn ér zào*] notopterygium dispels wind and dissipates cold, dries dampness and checks pain. Cinnamon twig warms and frees the channels [温通经脉 *wēn tōng jīng mài*]. Chinese angelica supplements and quickens blood.

Assistant Medicinals

Poria disinhibits dampness by bland percolation [淡渗利湿 *dàn shèn lì shī*]. Apricot kernel diffuses and effuses lung qì [宣发肺气 *xuān fā fèi qì*]. Fresh ginger dissipates cold. The assistant medicinals help the chief and support medicinals dispel wind, dissipate cold, and disinhibit dampness.

Licorice harmonizes the properties of all the medicinals [调和药性 *tiáo hé yào xìng*].

This combination of medicinals is used to dispel wind and dissipate cold and to eliminate dampness and check pain.

Variation According to Signs

Saposhnikovia Decoction treats. moving impediment [行痹 *xíng bì*]. For severe pain, add pubescent angelica [*dú huó*], aconite main tuber [*chuān wū tóu*], and wild aconite [*cǎo wū tóu*] to dissipate cold and check pain. For inhibited bending and stretching of the joints [关节屈伸不利 *guān jié qū shēn bú lì*], add ground pine [*shēn jīn cǎo*] and star jasmine stem [*luò shí téng*]. For numbness and tingling, add clematis [*wēi líng xiān*], loofah [*sī guā luò*], and vaccaria [*wáng bù liú xíng*] to quicken blood and free the network vessels.

Painful Impediment [痛痹 *tòng bì*]

Method of Treatment

Warm the channels, dissipate cold, check pain [温经散寒止痛 *wēn jīng sàn hán zhǐ tòng*].

Aconite Main Tuber Decoction [乌头汤 *wū tóu tāng*]	
processed aconite tuber [制川乌头 *zhì chuān wū tóu*, Aconiti Tuber Praeparata]	6g
ephedra [麻黄 *má huáng*, Ephedrae Herba]	9g
white peony [白芍 *bái sháo*, Paeoniae Radix Alba]	12g
astragalus [黄芪 *huáng qí*, Astragali Radix]	18g
licorice [甘草 *gān cǎo*, Glycyrrhizae Radix]	6g

Directions: Predecoct [先煎 *xiān jiān*] the processed aconite root for 30 minutes. Decoct with remaining ingredients in water [水煎服 *shuǐ jiān fú*].

Prescription Analysis

Chief Medicinal

Processed aconite tuber warms the channels, dissipates cold, and checks pain.

Support Medicinal

Acrid-warm [辛温 *xīn wēn*] ephedra effuses and dissipates [发散 *fā sàn*] and helps the chief medicinal dissipate wind-cold evil [散风寒之邪 *sàn fēng hán zhī xié*].

Assistant Medicinals

White peony nourishes blood and emolliates the liver [养血柔肝 *yǎng xuè róu gān*] and also relaxes tension and checks pain [缓急止痛 *huǎn jí zhǐ tòng*]. Astragalus supplements qì, upbears yáng, and secures the exterior [补气升阳固表 *bǔ qì shēng yáng gù biǎo*].

Licorice harmonizes the properties of all the medicinals [调和药性 *tiáo hé yào xìng*].

This combination of medicinals warms the channels, dissipates cold, and checks pain.

Variation According to Signs

For severe wind-cold, add notopterygium [*qiāng huó*], pubescent angelica [*dú huó*], and asarum [*xì xīn*] to dissipate wind-damp, dissipate cold, and check pain. For inhibited bending and stretching of the joints [关节屈伸不利 *guān jié qū shēn bú lì*], add large gentian [*qín jiāo*], fangji [*fáng jǐ*], and ground pine [*shēn jīn cǎo*]. For numbness and tingling, add clematis [*wēi líng xiān*], loofah [*sī guā luò*], and vaccaria [*wáng bù liú xíng*] to free the channels and quicken the network vessels. For physical cold and cold limbs [形寒肢冷 *xíng hán zhī lěng*], add cinnamon bark [*ròu guì*] to warm yáng.

Fixed impediment [着痹 *zhuó bì*]

Method of Treatment

Dispel dampness, free the network vessels, and check pain [祛湿，通络，止痛 *qū shī, tōng luò, zhǐ tòng*].

Coix Decoction [薏苡仁汤 *yì yǐ rén tāng*]	
coix [薏苡仁 *yì yǐ rén*, Semen Coicis]	30g
atractylodes [苍术 *cāng zhú*, Atractylodis Rhizoma]	15g
white atractylodes [白术 *bái zhú*, Atractylodis Macrocephalae Rhizoma]	15g
cinnamon twig [桂枝 *guì zhī*, Cinnamomi Ramulus]	9g
ephedra [麻黄 *má huáng*, Ephedrae Herba]	6g
Chinese angelica [当归 *dāng guī*, Angelicae Sinensis Radix]	12g

astragalus [黄芪 *huáng qí*, Astragali Radix]	15g
lindera [乌药 *wū yào*, Linderae Radix]	12g
fresh ginger [生姜 *shēng jiāng*, Zingiberis Rhizoma Recens]	9g
licorice [甘草 *gān cǎo*, Glycyrrhizae Radix]	6g

Directions: Take decocted with water [水煎服 *shuǐ jiān fú*].

Prescription Analysis

Chief Medicinal

Coix disinhibits water and percolates dampness [利水渗湿 *lì shuǐ shèn shī*] and also frees impediment and checks pain [通痹止痛 *tōng bì zhǐ tòng*].

Support Medicinals

Atractylodes dries dampness. White atractylodes disinhibits dampness. Astragalus disinhibits water. These support medicinals all help the chief medicinal dispel damp evil.

Assistant Medicinals

Cinnamon twig warms and frees the channels. Acrid-warm [辛温 *xīn wēn*] ephedra effuses and dissipates [发散 *fā sàn*], diffuses the lung [宣肺 *xuān fèi*], and disinhibits dampness. Chinese angelica supplements and quickens blood to free the channels. Lindera dissipates cold and moves qì. Fresh ginger effuses and dissipates [发散 *fā sàn*] wind-cold.

Licorice harmonizes the properties of all the medicinals [调和药性 *tiáo hé yào xìng*].

This combination of medicinals dispels dampness, frees the network vessels, and checks pain.

Variation According to Signs

The indication for Coix Decoction is fixed impediment [着痹 *zhuó bì*]. For severe pain, add notopterygium [*qiāng huó*], pubescent angelica [*dú huó*], asarum [*xì xīn*], aconite main tuber [*chuān wū tóu*], and wild aconite [草乌头 *cǎo wū tóu*] to warm the channels, dissipate cold, and check pain. For numbness and tingling of the limbs, add chaenomeles [*mù guā*], clematis [*wēi líng xiān*], and earthworm [*dì lóng*] to free the channels and quicken the network vessels [通经活络 *tōng jīng huó luò*]. For inhibited bending and stretching of the joints [关节屈伸不利 *guān jié qū shēn bú lì*], add ground pine [*shēn jīn cǎo*] and star jasmine stem [*luò shí téng*].

24.3.2   Wind-Damp-Heat Impediment [风湿热痹 *fēng shī rè bì*]

Method of Treatment for Wind-Damp-Heat Impediment

Dispel wind-damp, free the channels and network vessels, and resolve heat toxin [祛风湿，通经络，解热毒 *qū fēng shī, tōng jīng luò, jiě rè dú*].

Siegesbeckia and Clerodendron Pill [豨桐丸 *xī tóng wán*]

siegesbeckia [豨莶草 *xī xiān cǎo*, Siegesbeckiae Herba]
clerodendron [臭梧桐 *chòu wú tóng*, Clerodendri Folium]

Directions: Take equal amounts of the two above medicinals and grind into a fine powder. Form into pills, and take 6g at a time, three times a day.

Prescription Analysis

Chief Medicinals

Siegesbeckia and clerodendron are both cool/cold medicinals, and both have a strong capacity to dispel wind-damp, free the channels and network vessels, and resolve heat toxin [解热毒 *jiě rè dú*].

Variation According to Signs

The indication for Siegesbeckia and Clerodendron Pill is wind-damp-heat impediment [风湿热痹 *fēng shī rè bì*]. If the prescription is used as a decoction, one may enhance the prescription by adding large gentian [*qín jiāo*], fangji [*fáng jǐ*], erythrina [*hǎi tóng pí*], lonicera stem and leaf [*rěn dōng téng*], and star jasmine stem [*luò shí téng*]. For severe red swelling, add moutan [*mǔ dān pí*], red peony [*chì sháo*], atractylodes [*cāng zhú*], and phellodendron [*huáng bǎi*] to clear heat and dry dampness, cool blood and resolve toxins. For rigid joints [关节强直 *guān jié qiáng zhí*] and for inhibited bending and stretching of the joints [关节屈伸不利 *guān jié qū shēn bú lì*], add Solomon's seal [*yù zhú*], white peony [*bái sháo*], and dendrobium [*shí hú*] to nourish yīn and emolliate the sinews [养阴柔筋 *yǎng yīn róu jīn*].

24.4   ACUPUNCTURE TREATMENT FOR IMPEDIMENT

24.4.1   Base Acupuncture Prescription for Wind-Cold-Damp Impediment [风寒湿痹 *fēng hán shī bì*]

This base prescription should be modified according to the identified patterns discussed below and according to the patient's individual condition.

Treatment Method for Wind-Cold-Damp Impediment

Warm the channels and dissipate cold, dispel wind and free the channels, eliminate dampness and check pain [温经散寒，祛风通经，除湿止痛 *wēn jīng sàn hán, qū fēng tōng jīng, chú shī zhǐ tòng*].

Base Acupuncture Prescription for Wind-Cold-Damp Impediment

GB-20 Wind Pool [风池 *fēng chí*]
BL-17 Diaphragm Transport [膈俞 *gé shū*]
SP-10 Sea of Blood [血海 *xuè hǎi*]
CV-4 Pass Head [关元 *guān yuán*]
BL-23 Kidney Transport [肾俞 *shèn shū*]
SP-9 Yīn Mound Spring [阴陵泉 *yīn líng quán*]
KI-7 Recover Flow [复溜 *fù liū*]

Prescription Analysis

GB-20 dispels and dissipates wind evil [祛散风邪 *qū sàn fēng xié*].

BL-17 and SP-10 are chosen according to the principle: "To treat wind, first treat the blood; when the blood moves, wind naturally disappears" [治风先治血。血行风自灭 *zhì fēng xiān zhì xuè. xuè xíng fēng zì miè*]. BL-17 is the meeting point of the blood [血会 *xuè huì*] and SP-10 treats the blood.

CV-4 and BL-23 boost the source of fire [益火之原 *yì huǒ zhī yuán*], warm and supplement yáng qì, and dispel cold evil.

SP-9 and KI-7 disinhibit dampness and fortify the spleen [利湿健脾 *lì shī jiàn pí*].

24.4.2 Points to Add to the Base Prescription for Wind-Cold-Damp Impediment

Add points to the base prescription according to the predominance of signs and symptoms of any of the three types of wind-cold-damp impediment. Then, select local points [局部取穴 *jú bù qǔ xué*] according to the location of the impediment.

Points for Wind-Cold-Damp Impediment of the Shoulder

LI-15 Shoulder Bone [肩髃 *jiān yú*]
TB-14 Shoulder Bone Hole [肩髎 *jiān liáo*]
LI-16 Great Bone [巨骨 *jù gǔ*]

Points for Wind-Cold-Damp Impediment of the Elbow

LI-11 Pool at the Bend [曲池 *qū chí*]
TB-10 Celestial Well [天井 *tiān jǐng*]
LI-10 Arm Three Lǐ [手三里 *shǒu sān lǐ*]

Points for Wind-Cold-Damp Impediment of the Wrist
LI-4 Union Valley [合谷 *hé gǔ*]
TB-4 Yáng Pool [阳池 *yáng chí*]
LI-5 Yáng Ravine [阳溪 *yáng xī*]
SI-4 Wrist Bone [腕骨 *wàn gǔ*]

Points for Wind-Cold-Damp Impediment of the Knee
GB-33 Knee Yáng Joint [膝阳关 *xī yáng guān*]
joining [透 *tòu*] LR-8 Spring at the Bend [曲泉 *qū quán*]
ST-36 Leg Three Lǐ [足三里 *zú sān lǐ*]
ST-34 Beam Hill [梁丘 *liáng qiū*]
Extra Point Heding [鹤顶 *hè dǐng*]
ST-35 Calf's Nose [犊鼻 *dú bí*]

Points for Wind-Cold-Damp Impediment of the Ankle
GB-40 Hill Ruins [丘墟 *qiū xū*]
ST-41 Ravine Divide [解溪 *jiě xī*]
BL-62 Extending Vessel [申脉 *shēn mài*]

24.4.3 Wind-Damp-Heat Impediment [风湿热痹 *fēng shī rè bì*]

This prescription should be modified according to the condition of the individual patient.

Treatment Method for Wind-Damp-Heat Impediment

Clear heat, dispel wind, and eliminate dampness [清热祛风除湿 *qīng rè qū fēng chú shī*].

Acupuncture Prescription for Wind-Damp-Heat Impediment
GV-14 Great Hammer [大椎 *dà zhuī*]
LI-11 Pool at the Bend [曲池 *qū chí*]
LI-4 Union Valley [合谷 *hé gǔ*]
LR-2 Moving Between [行间 *xíng jiān*]

Prescription Analysis

LI-11, LI-4, and LR-2 all clear heat. GV-14 harmonizes construction and defense [调和营卫 *tiáo hé yíng wèi*] and diffuses yáng qì [宣通阳气 *xuān tōng yáng qì*]. When yáng qì is diffused, heat evil is dispelled.

Chinese-Latin Table of Medicinals Used in This Book

ài yè [艾叶]	Artemisiae Argyi Folium
bài jiàng cǎo [败酱草]	Patriniae Herba
bái jiè zǐ [白芥子]	Brassica Albae Semen
bái jí lí [白蒺藜]	Tribuli Fructus
bái máo gēn [白茅根]	Imperatae Rhizoma
bái sháo [白芍]	Paeoniae Radix Alba
bái tóu wēng [白头翁]	Pulsatillae Radix
bái wēi [白薇]	Cynanchi Baiwei Radix
bái zhǐ [白芷]	Angelicae Dahuricae Radix
bái zhú [白术]	Atractylodis Macrocephalae Rhizoma
bǎi zǐ rén [柏子仁]	Biota Semen
bǎn lán gēn [板蓝根]	Isatidis Radix
bàn xià [半夏]	Pinelliae Rhizoma
bèi mǔ [贝母]	Fritillariae Bulbus
běi shā shēn [北沙参]	Glehniae Radix
biǎn xù [萹蓄]	Polygoni Avicularis Herba
biē jiǎ [鳖甲]	Amydae Carapax
bīng láng [槟榔]	Arecae Semen
bīng táng [冰糖]	Rock sugar
bì xiè [萆薢]	Dioscoreae Hypoglaucae Rhizoma

bò hé [yè] [薄荷叶]	Menthae Herba
bǔ gǔ zhī [补骨脂]	Psoraleae Fructus
cāng zhú [苍术]	Atractylodis Rhizoma
cǎo wū tóu [草乌头]	Aconiti Tsao-Wu-Tou tuber
cè bǎi yè [侧柏叶]	Biotae Folium
chái hú [柴胡]	Bupleuri Radix
chǎo xìng rén [炒杏仁]	Armeniacae Semen Frictum
chén pí [陈皮]	Citri Reticulatae Pericarpium
chén xiāng [沉香]	Aquilariae Lignum Resinatum
chē qián zǐ [车前子]	Plantaginis Semen
chì sháo [赤芍]	Paeoniae Radix Rubra
chòu wú tóng [臭梧桐]	Clerodendri Folium
chuān huáng lián [川黄连]	Coptidis Rhizoma Sichuanense
chuān liàn zǐ [川楝子]	Toosendan Fructus
chuān niú xī [川牛膝]	Cyathulae Radix
chuān shān jiǎ [穿山甲]	Manitis Squama
chuān wū tóu [川乌头]	Aconiti Tuber
chuān xiōng [川芎]	Chuanxiong Rhizoma
cí shí [磁石]	Magnetitum
dà huáng [大黄]	Rhei Rhizoma et Radix
dàn dòu chǐ [淡豆豉]	Sojae Semen Praeparatum
dàn zhú yè [竹叶]	Lophatheri Folium
dāng guī [当归]	Angelicae Sinensis Radix
dǎng shēn [党参]	Codonopsis Radix
dǎn nán xīng [胆南星]	see *Dǎn Xīng*
dǎn xīng [胆星]	Arisaematis cum Felle Bovis
dān shēn [丹参]	Salviae Miltiorrhizae Radix
dà zǎo [大枣]	Jujubae Fructus
dà fù pí [大腹皮]	Arecae Pericarpium
dà qīng yè [大青叶]	Isatidis Folium
dēng xīn cǎo [灯心草]	Junci Medulla

dì gǔ pí [地骨皮]	Lycii Radicus Cortex
dì lóng [地龙]	Pheretima
dì yú [地榆]	Sanguisorbae Radix
dōng kuí zǐ [冬葵子]	Malvae Semen
dú huó [独活]	Angelicae Pubescentis Radix
dù zhòng [杜仲]	Eucommiae Cortex
é zhú [莪术]	Curcumae Rhizoma
fáng fēng [防风]	Saposhnikoviae Radix
fáng jǐ [防己]	Fang Ji Radix
fēng huà xiāo [风化硝]	Mirabilitum Efflorescentia
fó shǒu [佛手]	Citri Sarcodactylidis Fructus
fú líng [茯苓]	Poria
fù pén zǐ [覆盆子]	Rubi Fructus
fú shén [茯神]	Poria cum Pini Radice
fù zǐ [附子]	Aconiti Tuber Laterale
gān cǎo [甘草]	Glycyrrhizae Radix
gān dì huáng [干地黄]	Rehmanniae Radix Exsiccata
gān jiāng [干姜]	Zingiberis Rhizoma
gǎo běn [藁本]	Ligustici Rhizoma
gé gēn [葛根]	Puerariae Radix
gǒu qǐ zǐ [枸杞子]	Lycii Fructus
gōu téng [钩藤]	Uncariae Ramulus cum Uncis
guā lóu [瓜蒌]	Trichosanthis Fructus
guā lóu rén [瓜蒌仁]	Trichosanthis Seminis
guī bǎn [龟版]	Testudinis Plastrum
guī bǎn jiāo [龟版胶]	Testudinis Plastri Gelatinum
guì zhī [桂枝]	Cinnamomi Ramulus
hǎi jīn shā [海金沙]	Lygodii Spora
hàn lián cǎo [旱莲草]	Ecliptae Herba
hé shǒu wū [何首乌]	Polygoni Multiflori Radix
hóng huā [红花]	Carthami Flos

hòu pò [厚朴]	Magnoliae Officinalis Cortex
huáng bǎi [黄柏]	Phellodendri Cortex
huáng lián [黄连]	Coptidis Rhizoma
huáng qí [黄芪]	Astragali Radix
huáng qín [黄芩]	Scutellariae Radix
huá shí [滑石]	Talcum
huò xiāng [藿香]	Agastaches Seu Pogostemi Herba
bái jiāng cán [白僵蚕]	Bombyx Batryticatus
jiāng huáng [姜黄]	Curcumae Longae Rhizoma
jié gěng [桔梗]	Platycodonis Radix
jīng jiè [荆芥]	Schizonepetae Herba
jīn qián cǎo [金钱草]	Lysimachiae Herba
jīn yín huā [金银花]	Lonicerae Flos
jī xuè téng [鸡血藤]	Spatholobi Caulis
jú huā [菊花]	Chrysanthemi Flos
jú pí [橘皮]	Citri Reticulatae Pericarpium (see *chén pí*)
lái fú zǐ [莱菔子]	Raphani Semen
lián qiào [连翘]	Forsythiae Fructus
liú jì nú [刘寄奴]	Artemisiae Anomalae Herba
lóng dǎn cǎo [龙胆草]	Gentianae Radix
lóng gǔ [龙骨]	Mastodi Ossis Fossilia
lú gēn [芦根]	Phragmitis Rhizoma
lú huì [芦荟]	Aloe
lù jiǎo jiāo [鹿角胶]	Cervi Cornus Gelatinum
luò shí téng [络石藤]	Trachelospermi Caulis
lù róng [鹿茸]	Cervi Cornu Paravum
mǎ bó [马勃]	Lasiosphaera seu Calvatia
má huáng [麻黄]	Ephedrae Herba
mài dōng [麦冬]	Ophiopogonis Radix
mài yá [麦芽]	Hordei Fructus Germinatus
màn jīng zǐ [蔓荆子]	Viticis Fructus

máng xiāo [芒硝]	Mirabilitum
má zǐ rén [麻子仁]	Cannabis Fructus
mò yào [没药]	Myrrha
mǔ dān pí [牡丹皮]	Moutan Cortex
mù guā [木瓜]	Chaenomelis Fructus
mǔ lì [牡蛎]	Ostreae Concha
mù tōng [木通]	Akebiae Trifoliatae Caulis
mù xiāng [木香]	Aucklandiae Radix
niú bàng zǐ [牛蒡子]	Arctii Fructus
niú xī [牛膝]	Achyranthis Bidentatae Radix
nǚ zhēn zǐ [女贞子]	Ligustri Lucidi Fructus
pèi lán [佩兰]	Eupatorii Herba
pú gōng yīng [蒲公英]	Taraxaci Herba cum Radice
pú huáng [蒲黄]	Typhae Pollen
qiāng huó [羌活]	Notopterygii Rhizoma et Radix
qīng hāo [青蒿]	Artemisiae Apiaceae seu Annuae Herba
qīng pí [青皮]	Citri Reticulatae Pericarpium Viride
qín pí [秦皮]	Fraxini Cortex
qín jiāo [秦艽]	Gentianae Macrophyllae Radix
quán xiē [全蝎]	Buthus
ǒu jié [藕节]	Nelumbinis Rhizomatis Nodus
qū mài [瞿麦]	Dianthi Herba
rěn dōng téng [忍冬藤]	Lonicerae Caulis et Folium
rén shēn [人参]	Ginseng Radix
ròu dòu kòu [肉豆蔻]	Myristicae Semen
ròu guì [肉桂]	Cinnamomi Cortex
rǔ xiāng [乳香]	Olibanum
sān léng [三棱]	Rhizoma Sparganii
sāng jì shēng [桑寄生]	Taxilli Herba
sāng piāo xiāo [桑螵蛸]	Mantidis Oötheca
sān qī [三七]	Notoginseng Radix

shān yào [山药]	Dioscoreae Rhizoma
shān zhū yú [山萸肉]	Corni Fructus
shān zhā [山楂]	Crataegi Fructus
shān zhī zǐ [山栀子]	Gardeniae Fructus
shān zhū yú [山茱萸]	Corni Fructus
shā rén [砂仁]	Amomi Fructus
shā shēn [沙参]	Adenophorae Radix
shēng dì huáng [生地黄]	Rehmanniae Radix Exsiccata seu Recens
shēng jiāng [生姜]	Zingiberis Rhizoma Recens
shēng lóng gǔ [生龙骨]	Mastodi Ossis Fossilia Cruda
shēng má [升麻]	Cimicifugae Rhizoma
shēng mǔ lì] [生牡蛎	Ostreae Concha Cruda
shēng pú huáng [生蒲黄]	Typhae Pollen Crudum
shēng shí gāo [生石膏]	Gypsum Crudum
shēng zhě shí [生赭石]	Haematitum
shēn jīn cǎo [伸筋草]	Lycopodii Clavati Herba
shén qū [神曲]	Massa Medicata Fermentata
shè xiāng [麝香]	Moschus
shí hú [石斛]	Dendrobii Herba
shí chāng pú [石菖蒲]	Acori Tatarinowii Rhizoma
shí gāo [石膏]	Gypsum
shí jué míng [石决明]	Haliotidis Concha
shí wéi [石韦]	Pyrrosiae Folium
shú dì huáng [熟地黄]	Rehmanniae Radix Conquita
sī guā luò [丝瓜络]	Luffae Fasciculus Vascularis
suān zǎo rén [酸枣仁]	Ziziphi Spinosi Semen
táo rén [桃仁]	Persicae Semen
tiān dōng [天冬]	Asparagi Tuber
tiān má [天麻]	Gastrodiae Rhizoma
tiān nán xīng [天南星]	Arisaematis Rhizoma
tiān huā fěn [天花粉]	Trichosanthis Radix

tǔ bèi mǔ [土贝母]	Bolbostemmatis Rhizoma
tǔ fú ling [土茯苓]	Smilacis Glabrae Rhizoma
tù sī zǐ [菟丝子]	Cuscutae Semen
wǎ léng zǐ [瓦楞子]	Arcae Concha
wáng bù liú xíng [王不留行]	Vaccariae Semen
wēi líng xiān [威灵仙]	Clematidis Radix
wú gōng [蜈蚣]	Scolopendra
wǔ jiā pí [五加皮]	Acanthopanacis Cortex
wǔ líng zhī [五灵脂]	Trogopteri Faeces
wū tóu [乌头]	Aconiti Tuber
wǔ wèi zǐ [五味子]	Schisandrae Fructus
wū yào [乌药]	Linderae Radix
wú zhū yú [吴茱萸]	Evodiae Fructus
xià kū cǎo [夏枯草]	Prunellae Spica
xiāng fù [香附]	Cyperi Rhizoma
xiǎo huí xiāng [小茴香]	Foeniculi Fructus
xìng rén [杏仁]	Armeniacae Semen
xī xiān cǎo [豨莶草]	Siegesbeckiae Herba
xì xīn [细辛]	Asari Herba
xiè bái [薤白]	Allii Bulbus
xuán shēn [玄参]	Scrophulariae Radix
xù duàn [续断]	Dipsaci Radix
yè jiāo téng [夜交藤]	Polygoni Multiflori Caulis
yě jú huā [野菊花]	Chrysanthemi Indicae Flos
yì mǔ cǎo [益母草]	Leonuri Herba
yīn chén hāo [茵陈蒿]	Artemisiae Capillaris Herba
yí táng [饴糖]	Maltosum
yì yǐ rén [薏苡仁]	Semen Coicis
yì zhì rén [益智仁]	Alpiniae Oxyphyllae Fructus
yuán hú/yán hú suǒ [元胡/延胡索]	Corydalis Rhizoma
yuǎn zhì [远志]	Polygalae Radix

yù jīn [郁金]	Curcumae Radix
yù lǐ rén [郁李仁]	Pruni Japonicae Semen
yù zhú [玉竹]	Polygonati Odorati Rhizoma
zé xiè [泽泻]	Alismatis Rhizoma
zhè chóng [虫]	Eupolyphaga seu Steleophaga
zhì chuān wū tóu [制川乌头]	Aconiti Tuber Praeparata
zhì fù zǐ [制附子]	Aconiti Tuber Laterale Praeparata
zhì gān cǎo [炙甘草]	Glycyrrhizae Radix Preparata
zhī mǔ [知母]	Anemarrhenae Rhizoma
zhǐ ké [枳壳]	Aurantii Fructus
zhǐ shí [枳实]	Aurantii Fructus Immaturus
zhī zǐ [栀子]	Gardeniae Fructus
zhū líng [猪苓]	Polyporus
zǐ cǎo [紫草]	Lithospermi, Macrotomiae, seu Onosmatis Radix
zǐ huā dì dīng [紫花地丁]	Violae Herba

Pinyin-English Table of
Points and Channels Used in this Book

ā shì xué	Ouch point [阿是穴]
bǎi huì	GV-20 Hundred Convergences [百会]
chéng shān	BL-57 Mountain Support [承山]
cì liáo	BL-32 Second Bone Hole [次髎]
dà cháng shū	BL-25 Large Intestine Transport [大肠俞]
dà dū	SP-2 Great Metropolis [大都]
dà líng	PC-7 Great Mound [大陵]
dà zhuī	GV-14 Great Hammer [大椎]
èr jiān	LI-2 Second Space [二间]
fàng xuè	Bloodletting [放血]
fàng xuè(jú bù cì luò)	Local bloodletting (network vessel pricking) [局部刺络放血]
fēi yáng	BL-58 Taking Flight [飞扬]
fēng chí	GB-20 Wind Pool [风池]
fēng fǔ	GV-16 Wind Mansion [风府]
fēng lóng	ST-40 Bountiful Bulge [丰隆]
fù liū	KI-7 Recover Flow [复溜]
gé shū	BL-17 Diaphragm Transport [膈俞]
guān chōng	TB-1 Passage Hub [关冲]
guāng míng	GB-37 Bright Light [光明]
guān yuán	CV-4 Pass Head [关元]
hè dǐng	Extra Point Heding [鹤顶]
hé gǔ	LI-4 Union Valley [合谷]
hé xué	uniting point [合穴]
hòu xī	SI-3 Back Ravine [后溪]

huán tiào	GB-30 Jumping Round [环跳]
huá tuó jiā jǐ xué	M-BW-35 Huá Tuó's Paravertebral Points [华佗夹脊穴]
huì xué	meeting point [会穴]
jiā jǐ	Paravertebrals *Jiaji* (at the neck) [夹脊]
jiàn lǐ]	CV-11 Interior Strengthening [建里
jiān liáo	TB-14 Shoulder Bone Hole [肩髎]
jiān yú	LI-15 Shoulder Bone [肩髃]
jiāo huì xué	intersection point [交会穴]
jiě xī	ST-41 Ravine Divide [解溪]
jǐng xué	well point [井穴]
jīn mén	BL-63 Metal Gate [金门]
jù gǔ	LI-16 Great Bone [巨骨]
kūn lún	BL-60 Kunlun Mountains [昆仑]
liáng mén	ST-21 Beam Gate [梁门]
liáng qiū	ST-34 Beam Hill [梁丘]
lì duì	ST-45 Severe Mouth [厉兑]
liè quē	LU-7 Broken Sequence [列缺]
lǐ gōu	LR-5 Woodworm Canal [蠡沟]
luò xué	network point [络穴]
mìng mén	GV-4 Life Gate [命门]
mù xué	alarm point [募穴]
nèi guān	PC-6 Inner Pass [内关]
nèi tíng	ST-44 Inner Court [内庭]
pí shū	BL-20 Spleen Transport [脾俞]
qì hǎi	CV-6 Sea of Qì [气海]
qī mén	LR-14 Cycle Gate [期门]
qiū xū	GB-40 Hill Ruins [丘墟]
qū chí	LI-11 Pool at the Bend [曲池]
qū quán	LR-8 Spring at the Bend [曲泉]
rì yuè	GB-24 Sun and Moon [日月]
sān jiān	LI-3 Third Space [三间]
sān yīn jiāo	SP-6 Three Yīn Intersections [三阴交]
shàng jù xū	ST-37 Upper Great Hollow [上巨虚]
shāng yáng	LI-1 Shang yáng [商阳]
shào hǎi	HT-3 Lesser Sea [少海]
shào zé	SI-1 Lesser Marsh [少泽]
shēn mài	BL-62 Extending Vessel [申脉]

shén què	CV-8 Spirit Gate Tower [神阙]
shèn shū	BL-23 Kidney Transport [肾俞]
shí qī zhuī xué	M-BW-25 (Extra Point) Seventeenth Vertebra Point [十七椎穴]
shǒu jué yīn xīn bāo jīng	hand reverting yīn pericardium channel [手厥阴心包经]
shǒu sān lǐ	LI-10 Arm Three Lǐ [手三里]
shǒu shào yáng sān jiāo jīng	hand lesser yáng triple burner channel [手少阳三焦经]
shǒu shào yīn xīn jīng	hand lesser yīn heart channel [手少阴心经]
shǒu tài yáng xiǎo cháng jīng	hand greater yáng small intestine channel [手太阳小肠经]
shǒu tài yīn fèi jīng	hand greater yīn lung channel [手太阴肺经]
shǒu yáng míng dà cháng jīng	hand yáng brightness large intestine channel [手阳明大肠经]
sì shén cōng	M-HN-1 (Extra Point) Alert Spirit Quartet [四神聪]
tài bái	SP-3 Supreme White [太白]
tài chōng	LR-3 Supreme Surge [太冲]
tài xī	KI-3 Great Ravine [太溪]
tài yáng	M-HN-9 (Extra Point) Greater Yáng [太阳]
tài yuān	LU-9 Great Abyss [太渊]
tiān jǐng	TB-10 Celestial Well [天井]
tiān shū	ST-25 Celestial Pivot [天枢]
tiáo kǒu	ST-38 Ribbon Opening [条口]
tōng lǐ	HT-5 Connecting Lǐ [通里]
tòu	joining [透]
wài guān	TB-5 Outer Pass [外关]
wàn gǔ	SI-4 Wrist Bone [腕骨]
wèi shū	BL-21 Stomach Transport [胃俞]
wěi zhōng	BL-40 Bend Center [委中]
xià hé xué	lower uniting point [下合穴]
xià jù xū	ST-39 Lower Great Hollow [下巨虚]
xiá xī	GB-43 Pinched Ravine [侠溪]
xíng jiān	LR-2 Moving Between [行间]
xī xué	cleft point [郄穴 *xī xué*]
nèi xī yǎn	M-LE-16 (Extra Point) Inner Eye of Knee [内膝眼]

xī yáng guān	GB-33 Knee yáng Joint [膝阳关]
xuán zhōng	GB-39 Suspended Bell [悬钟]
xuè hǎi	SP-10 Sea of Blood [血海]
yáng chí	TB-4 Yáng Pool [阳池]
yǎng lǎo	SI-6 Nursing the Aged [养老]
yáng líng quán	GB-34 Yáng Mound Spring [阳陵泉]
yáng wéi mài	yang linking vessel [阳维脉]
yáng xī	LI-5 yáng Ravine [阳溪]
yāo yáng guān	GV-3 Lumbar yáng Pass [腰阳关]
yīn gǔ	KI-10 yīn Valley [阴谷]
yíng xué	spring point [荥穴]
yīn líng quán	SP-9 yīn Mound Spring [阴陵泉]
yìn táng	EXTRA Hall of Impression [印堂]
yǒng quán	KI-1 Gushing Spring [涌泉]
yuán xué	source point [原穴]
zhāng mén	LR-13 Camphorwood Gate [章门]
zhào hǎi	KI-6 Shining Sea [照海]
zhì biān	BL-54 Sequential Limit [秩边]
zhī gōu	TB-6 Branch Ditch [支沟]
zhì yīn	BL-67 Reaching Yīn [至阴]
zhī zhèng	SI-7 Branch to the Correct [支正]
zhōng jí	CV-3 Central Pole [中极]
zhōng wǎn	CV-12 Center Stomach Duct [中脘]
zú jué yīn gān jīng	foot reverting yīn liver channel [足厥阴肝经]
zú qiào yīn	GB-44 Foot Orifice Yīn [足窍阴]
zú sān lǐ	ST-36 Leg Three Lǐ [足三里]
zú shào yáng dǎn jīng	foot lesser yáng gallbladder channel [足少阳胆经]
zú shào yīn shèn jīng	foot lesser yīn kidney channel [足少阴肾经 *zú shào yīn shèn jīng*]
zú tài yáng páng guāng jīng	foot greater yáng bladder channel [足太阳膀胱经]
zú tài yīn pí jīng	foot greater yīn spleen channel [足太阴脾经]
zú yáng míng wèi jīng	foot yáng brightness stomach channel [足阳明胃经]

Bibliography

Chinese Works

三画

1. 广州中医学院，中国中医研究院主编。《中医大辞典》。北京：人民卫生出版社，1995。

四画

2. 中国中医研究院主编单位。《中医证候鉴别诊断学》。北京：人民卫生出版社，1987。

3. 王彦晖著。《中医湿病学》。北京：人民卫生出版社，1997。

4. 王云凯主编。《临床常用百穴精解》。天津：天津科学技术出版社，2000。

5. 邓铁涛主编。《中医诊断学》。北京：人民卫生出版社，1987。

6. 韦绪性主编。《疼痛学》。北京：中国中医药出版社，1996。

五画

7. 北京中医学院中医系中医基础理论教研室编。《濒湖脉学白话解》。北京：人民卫生出版社，1961。

8. 冯兴化等主编。《中医内科临床手册》。北京：人民卫生出版社，1996。

六画

9. 刘冠军编著。《脉诊》。上海：上海科学技术出版社，1979。

10. 金*李东垣著，贾成文主编。《脾胃论白话解》。西安：三秦出版社，2000。

11. 向宗暄主编。《中医辨脉症治》。北京：中国中医药出版社，1998。

12. 刘兰芳等编著。《新编中医痛证临床备要》。北京：科学技术文献出版社，1998。

13. 伊智雄，刘春英主编。《实用颈背腰痛中医治疗学》。北京：人民卫生出版社，1997。

七画

14. 肖永俭等主编。《骨关节病的针灸治疗》。北京：中国中医药出版社，1997。

15. 辛瑛主编。《中医舌诊知识》。北京：人民卫生出版社，1996。

16. 苏诚炼等主编。《中医痛证大成》。福州：福建科学技术出版社，1996。

17. 宋一同等主编。《骨伤痛证诊疗法》。北京：人民卫生出版社，1998。

八画

18. 罗元恺主编。《中医妇科学》。上海：上海科学技术出版社，1986。

19. 杨俏田等主编。《中医疼痛治疗学》。太原：山西科学技术出版社，1999。

20. 周超凡主编。《历代中医治则精华》。北京：中国中医药出版社，1991。

21. 张安桢主编。《中医骨伤科学》。北京：人民卫生出版社，1988。

22. 张宝生等主编。《颈肩腰腿痛的针灸推拿治疗》。北京：中医古籍出版社，1997。

十画

23. 秦伯未著。《中医入门》。北京：人民卫生出版社，1959。

24. 徐宜厚等编著。《皮肤病中医诊疗学》。北京：人民卫生出版社，1997。

25. 黄泰康主编。《中医疑难病方药手册》。北京：中国医药科技出版社，1994。

Non-Chinese Works

26. *Concise English-Chinese Medical Dictionary,* Laurence Urdang Associates Limited and People's Medical Publishing House, 1990.

27. Maciocia, Giovanni, *Foundations of Chinese Medicine,* Churchill Livingstone 1989.

28. Urban & Fischer, *Das MSD Manual,* CD-Rom Version 6.0, Haar: MSD Sharp & Dohme GmbH, 2000.

29. Wiseman, Nigel and Feng, Ye, *A Practical Dictionary of Chinese Medicine*, Brookline, Massachusetts: Paradigm Publications, 1998.

30. Yang, Shou-Zhong and Li, Jian-Yong, *Li Dong-yuan's Treatise on the Spleen & Stomach, A Translation of the Pi Wei Lun,* Boulder: Blue Poppy Press, 1993.

31. Zenz, Michael, *Taschenbuch der Schmerztherapie,* Stuttgart: Wiss. Verl.-Ges.,1995

Index

About the Authors

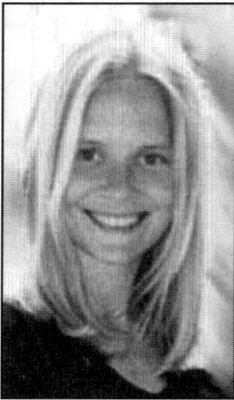

Dagmar Riley studied and practiced TCM in Běijīng, China for over 10 years. She studied Chinese medicine in the form of a traditional master-disciple relationship under Dr. Zhū Shēng-Ān, the former director of the Confucius Temple Traditional Chinese Medicine Clinic. She also studied under several other teachers, including Prof. Zhāng Chūn-Róng of the Běijīng University of Chinese Medicine [北京中医药大学], vice chief doctor Liú Dé-Quán of the Xuānwǔ TCM Hospital [北京宣武中医医院], Wáng Hán-Wén (master of *Shāng Hán Lùn*) and other professors in the China Academy of Traditional Chinese Medicine [中国中医研究院], and Běijīng Massage Hospital [北京按摩医院].

She was granted a scholarship to read 5 years of Chinese Sports Medicine and Rehabilitation Studies at the Běijīng University of Physical Education [北京体育大学], studying acupuncture and herbal medicine as they are used today on China's national athletes. Another focus of her studies was the role of qì-gōng in treatment and rehabilitation.

Upon completion of her studies, Mrs. Riley founded the Sino-European Traditional Chinese Medicine Practice in Běijīng. She currently heads a busy practice in Sydney, Australia.

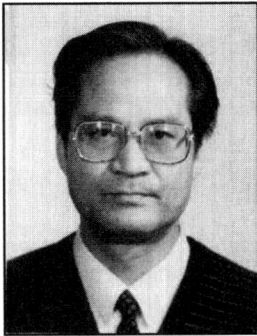

Zhāng Chūn-Róng [张春荣] is professor at the Běijīng University of Chinese Medicine [北京中医药大学]. Upon receiving his degree he Chinese Medicine in 1976 accepted a teaching position at the University. Since then, he has been teaching and conducting research in the fields of Chinese Medicine and Chinese Medicinals, next to his duties in the affiliated hospital.

Zhāng Chūn-Róng is the author of numerous books on Chinese Medicine, including 《中药学概论》，《家庭饮食保健法》，《常见病的饮食保健》，《趣味中药学》. He co-authored 《大百科全书*传统医学卷》，《老年百科全书》，《临床中药学》，《实用中成药学》，《中药学较学参考资料》，《中药学》, and 《本草纲目诠释》.

In the field of clinical practice, Zhāng Chūn-Róng successfully developed patent medicines that gained the approval of the authorities. His area of expertise includes chronic gastritis, chronic cholecystitis, duodenal ulcer, facial paralysis, diabetes, and trachitis.

The Chinese medicinal formulas in this book have been written by Professor Zhāng Chūn-Róng, who divides his time between researching, authoring, teaching and seeing patients at the Běijīng University of Chinese Medicine. Professor Zhāng's academic achievements are outstanding. Thus, his choices of formulas and variations are based on an extremely well-founded academic base. They can be apppreciated by anyone who has completed studies of Chinese medicinals and formulas and are an excellent means for furthering skill in applying the principles of Chinese Medicine to the treatment of pain.

In his free time, he loves to fish and, whenever he can, he drives several hours into the countryside to pursue his hobby in solitude and tranquility.

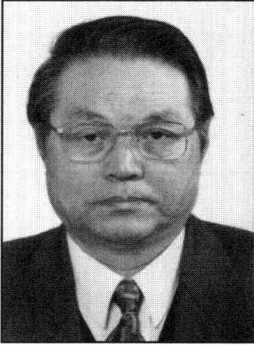

Liú Dé-Quán [刘德全] is vice chief doctor of the Běijīng Xuānwǔ TCM Hospital [北京宣武中医医院], on the board of directors of the China Association of Acupuncture and Moxibustion, Secretary of the Běijīng Association of Acupuncture and Moxibustion, and on the board of directors of the Běijīng Association of Physicians.

He developed a strong interest in Chinese Medicine when he was a child, following a family tradition, and graduated from Běijīng Union University Chinese Medicine College [北京联和大学中医药学院]. Today, Liú Dé-Quán has more than 40 years of clinical experience.

His area of expertise are difficult and complicated cases [疑难杂病] in the field of internal medicine, gynecology, and pediatrics.

The acupuncture prescriptions were written by Dr. Liú, who has seen patients all day, six days a week, for over 40 years, averaging more than 80 patients on a normal day. Because of this wealth of experience, and because he comes from a family tradition of CM practitioners, his treatments are often anything but "by the book" and are perfectly adapted to the individual case of the patient. Nevertheless, he strictly applies the principles of Chinese medicine in his therapeutic decision. Therefore, his acupuncture prescriptions are both a clinical treasury and a chance to step away from textbook knowledge and learn the "way of thought" (*sī lù*) that Dr. Liú Dé-Quán has developed using the principles of Chinese medicine according to the nature of change.